Second Edition

DERMATOLOGY
Visual Recognition and Case Reviews

Christine J. Ko, MD

Professor of Dermatology and Pathology
Dermatology
Yale University
New Haven, Connecticut

ELSEVIER

Elsevier
1600 John F. Kennedy Blvd.
Ste 1600
Philadelphia, PA 19103-2899

VISUAL RECOGNITION AND CASE REVIEWS, SECOND EDITION   ISBN: 978-0-323-69725-5

Library of Congress Control Number: 2020943706

Content Strategist: Charlotta Kryhl
Content Development Specialist: Kevin Travers
Content Development Manager: Meghan Andress
Publishing Services Manager: Shereen Jameel
Senior Project Manager: Kamatchi Madhavan
Design Direction: Patrick Ferguson

Printed in the United States of America

Last digit is the print number: 9   8   7   6   5   4   3   2   1

Dedication

To Jean, a true north

Contents

Preface

This atlas would not have been possible without the preexisting body of work, published and unpublished, of numerous dermatologists. Extensive credit is due to all authors and editors whose excellent photographs and schematics have been reproduced in this text, particularly those who worked on the third edition of *Dermatology* edited by Jean Bolognia, Joseph Jorizzo, and Julie Schaffer (Saunders, 2013), and to those who worked on other textbooks and journal articles. Every effort has been made to appropriately credit all of the contributors, and any errors or omissions are unintentional. Special thanks are also due to the many patients who consented to photography of their presentations, allowing us to learn from them.

This atlas is meant to be used as an introduction to dermatology and dermatopathology and as a rich resource of images that can hone the visual recognition skills of both the novice and the expert in dermatology and/or pathology and other specialties that involve examination of the skin. The main purpose of this text is to present classic visual clues that point to the correct diagnosis because that is the important first step in proper management and care. Given the above goals, the minimal text and the absence of treatment algorithms were deliberate, indicating the need to supplement this atlas with comprehensive textbooks and original articles.

Dermatology: Visual Recognition and Case Reviews came to fruition with the aid of various dermatology resources to enhance the key concepts, correlations, and learning opportunities within the text. Numerous illustrations from the following leading titles, collections, and colleagues have been incorporated throughout the chapters, and we gratefully acknowledge this volume of content and principally credit the following:

- Jean L. Bolognia, MD
- Julie V. Schaffer, MD
- Kalman Watsky, MD
- Karynne O. Duncan, MD
- Bolognia JL, Jorizzo JL, Schaffer JV, et al. *Dermatology*. 3rd ed. Philadelphia, PA: Elsevier Saunders; 2012.
- Bolognia JL, Schaffer JV, Duncan KO, Ko CJ. *Dermatology Essentials*. Philadelphia, PA: Elsevier Saunders; 2014.
- Yale Dermatology Residents' Slide Collection
- Yale Department of Dermatology faculty and residents, including Jennifer M. McNiff, MD; Richard Antaya, MD; Irwin Braverman, MD; Brittany Craiglow, MD; Leonard Milstone, MD; Peter Heald, MD; Jonathan Leventhal, MD; Mary Tomayko, MD, PhD; Jeff Gehlhausen, MD, PhD; Jacob Siegel, MD; Julie Cantatore-Francis, MD; Christopher Stamey, MD; Swapna Reddy, MD; Robert Stavert, MD; and Jennifer N. Choi, MD, and Jaehyuk Choi, MD, PhD (currently at Northwestern University).

- Other leading titles
Callen JP, Jorizzo JL. *Dermatological Signs of Internal Disease*. 4th ed. Philadelphia, PA: Elsevier Saunders; 2009.
Eichenfield LF, Frieden IJ, Zaenglein AL, Mathes E. *Neonatal and Infant Dermatology*. 3rd ed. London: Saunders; 2014.
Elston D. Clinical image collection. *Dermatopathology*. 2nd ed. London: Elsevier Saunders; 2014.
James WD, Berger T, Elston D. *Andrews' Diseases of the Skin*. 11th ed. Edinburgh: Saunders; 2011.
Patterson JW. *Weedon's Skin Pathology*. 4th ed. London: Churchill Livingstone; 2015.
Patterson JW. *Practical Skin Pathology: A Diagnostic Approach*. Philadelphia: Saunders; 2013.
Schachner LA, Hansen RE, eds. *Pediatric Dermatology*. 4th ed. London: Elsevier Mosby; 2011.
Tyring SK, Lupi O, Hengge UR. *Tropical Dermatology*. London: Churchill Livingstone; 2005.
Weston WL, Lane AT, Morelli JG. *Color Textbook of Pediatric Dermatology*. 4th ed. St. Louis: Mosby; 2007.

Many thanks to the Elsevier team as well, particularly Russell Gabbedy, Fiona Conn, and Anne Collett, for all their work on the first edition. For this second edition, deep appreciation to Kevin Travers, Kamatchi Madhavan, and Charlotta Kryhl.

Recently, I created a mini-quiz on more common skin diseases, including the one in Fig. 1, with the question, "What do you think this is?" I gave the quiz to my children, my husband, my babysitter, a Mohs surgeon, and a dermatopathologist. Their answers are in Table 1. Surprisingly (I mean no disrespect), my babysitter, who is a smart cookie but is not in the health care field at all, got it right, even using the word "plaque"!

When I asked my babysitter how she knew, her answer was telling. She said she has a coworker who has plaque psoriasis and that she has seen television commercials on psoriasis a fair number of times.

Psoriasis is familiar to her.

This, then, is what this atlas is about. Skin disease and, to a greater degree, the microscopic correlate, is not something that most people encounter on a daily basis, *unless you know someone with a given skin disease.* If the latter is true, that particular skin disease can become as familiar and recognizable as an individual book, house, or apple. The aim of this atlas is to provide the reader with as many images as possible so that knowledge about the diseases becomes entrenched in the brain on a more organic level, leading to (even more) easy recognition

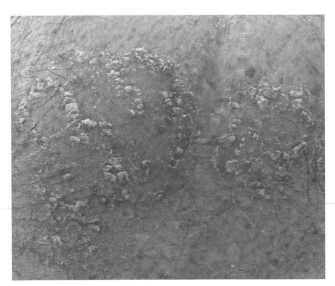

Fig. 1 Psoriasis, plaque type.

when encountered in daily life, for the first time or one of many.

Table 1 Answers to the question, "What is this?" when shown Fig. 1	
Child, age 7 years	A scab
Child, age 11 years	Something pink with white spots that is elevated
Babysitter, age 33 years	Plaque psoriasis
Orthopedic spine surgeon, age 45 years	A drug rash? Not sure
Dermatopathologist, age 57 years	Psoriasis
Mohs surgeon, age 59 years	Psoriasis

HOW TO READ THIS BOOK

This atlas is structured for a comfortable sit-down and front to back cover read. However, the book can be jumped into at will, in any desired order. The initial section is a general overview, an exploration of the gestalt concepts (see Table 1.1) that are used, often unconsciously, to formulate a dermatologic diagnosis, with emphasis on conscious recognition of key differences (Chapters 2 and 3). The second section is devoted to particular morphologies, and the case reviews apply these principles of visual recognition, focusing on the most important perceptual (and sometimes historical) features.

When we think about how we see the world around us on a daily basis, we usually do not spend much time dwelling on the fact that our eyes are always creating

two-dimensional images out of three-dimensional objects. Because of this, our brain learns, from a very early age, that the images supplied by our eyes need to be assigned depth and other properties that are lost in the transition from three dimensions to two dimensions. For most of us, this process occurs at the subconscious level and is something we barely think about. There are universal rules of vision that our brains tend to follow, without conscious direction, on the basis of what we come to learn is the most common thing a two-dimensional shape represents (Fig. 2).

Vision can be likened to speech. Thinking back to how we learned our first words in any language, most of us cannot consciously remember because we were just

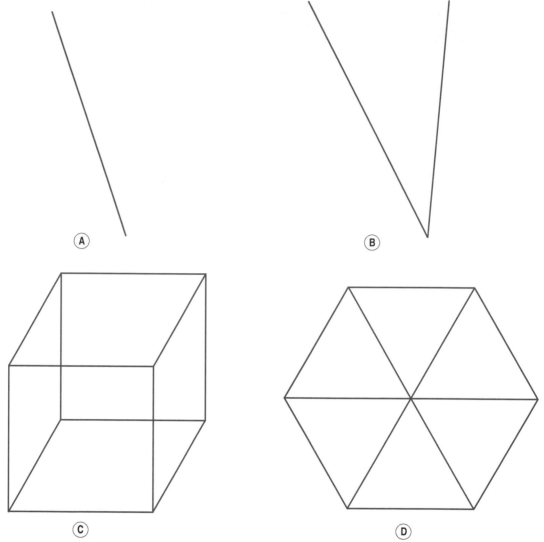

Fig. 2 Basic visual rules. **A** A line is generally interpreted as a line. **B** Two lines coming together to a point are generally interpreted as forming a corner, or vertex. Because of **A** and **B**, **C** is interpreted as a cube (Necker cube) more easily than the second image (Kopfermann figure). In **D**, most people's instinct is to interpret the image as a hexagonal boundary around three intersecting lines, rather than a cube.

babies. For most of us, it was not until formal schooling that we devoted time to learning how to speak. The initial rules of basic grammar for a given native language (e.g., subject–verb structure, verb conjugations, where to place an adjective) are acquired naturally over time. Although young children often need to be corrected in their phrasing early on, ultimately language ability develops in the correct manner because every day they hear others speak using the syntax of their primary language(s).

Key to the unconscious learning of the universal rules of vision and speech is seeing three-dimensional objects and hearing language, respectively, on a daily basis. In contrast, learning a different language at school can be challenging—a conscious process of parsing each unfamiliar word. The language will be learned more rapidly through immersion in an environment where that language is spoken primarily.

Eventually, one learns the language in school. More complex sentences and words that are not heard on a daily basis need to be consciously learned, for the same reason—lack of familiarity.

The rules of vision, however, are generally not formally taught, except perhaps in art classes. For our purposes, visual recognition in dermatology and dermatopathology is aided, in large part, by immersion—seeing the features of skin diseases on a daily basis in the clinic or under the microscope—and what we see more of becomes familiar. To aid in developing that familiarity and, ultimately, rapid recognition, this atlas presents visual details, including clinical (examples in Fig. 3), and histopathologic (examples in Fig. 4) features.

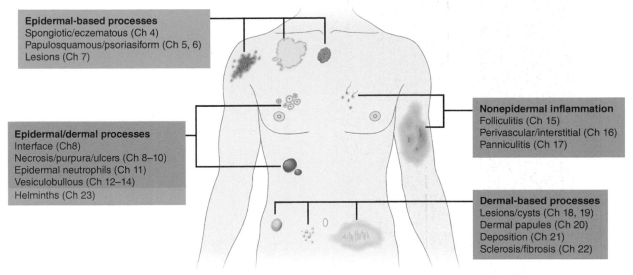

Epidermal-based processes
Spongiotic/eczematous (Ch 4)
Papulosquamous/psoriasiform (Ch 5, 6)
Lesions (Ch 7)

Epidermal/dermal processes
Interface (Ch8)
Necrosis/purpura/ulcers (Ch 8–10)
Epidermal neutrophils (Ch 11)
Vesiculobullous (Ch 12–14)
Helminths (Ch 23)

Nonepidermal inflammation
Folliculitis (Ch 15)
Perivascular/interstitial (Ch 16)
Panniculitis (Ch 17)

Dermal-based processes
Lesions/cysts (Ch 18, 19)
Dermal papules (Ch 20)
Deposition (Ch 21)
Sclerosis/fibrosis (Ch 22)

Fig. 3 Clinical examples of major categories of skin diseases. The features that cause the entities in these categories to look different make up the basic rules of clinical dermatology.

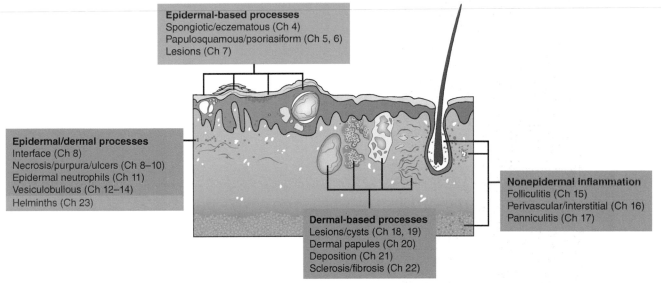

Epidermal-based processes
Spongiotic/eczematous (Ch 4)
Papulosquamous/psoriasiform (Ch 5, 6)
Lesions (Ch 7)

Epidermal/dermal processes
Interface (Ch 8)
Necrosis/purpura/ulcers (Ch 8–10)
Epidermal neutrophils (Ch 11)
Vesiculobullous (Ch 12–14)
Helminths (Ch 23)

Nonepidermal inflammation
Folliculitis (Ch 15)
Perivascular/interstitial (Ch 16)
Panniculitis (Ch 17)

Dermal-based processes
Lesions/cysts (Ch 18, 19)
Dermal papules (Ch 20)
Deposition (Ch 21)
Sclerosis/fibrosis (Ch 22)

Fig. 4 Histopathologic examples of major categories of skin diseases. The features that cause the entities in these categories to look different make up the basic rules of dermatopathology.

Key Concepts | 1

INTRODUCTION

The "how" of determining a diagnosis for visual specialties, such as dermatology and dermatopathology, is not transparent. Ultimately, the entire process is summed up with such phrases as "It just doesn't look like that" or "That's what it looks like to me" (Table 1.1). *You see it, and you know it.* This is akin to being told that an elephant is an elephant by a parent or a teacher, with the brain learning to recognize an elephant without explicitly being told that the elephant's key features include the trunk, the large ears, the large body, and the squat legs.

Breaking things down into key features can train the eye and brain to see and recognize things more readily (Table 1.2). This chapter goes over basic concepts that are involved in such gestalt recognition in dermatology. Such cognitive knowledge of why things are different (how to separate or categorize) is integral to visual recognition, especially for things that have overarching similarities. For example, a leopard, a cheetah, and a jaguar are all large cats of similar height, but each animal's spots are distinctive; knowing this is key to rapid gestalt recognition of these unique animals. This chapter will cover body site/region; age; distribution; patterns; linear lesions; epidermal vs dermal vs deeper; acute vs chronic eczematous, inflammatory cell types (epidermal and dermal); classic lesions; lesions with zones of color; lesional topography; types of scales; and color.

Table 1.1   Visual recognition in dermatology as related to cognitive psychology

Dermatologic concepts		Cognitive psychology concepts
Overview ("from the doorway")	**Close-up view (lesion itself)**	**Gestalt**
Age	Pattern (e.g. eczematous, psoriasiform, lichenoid, inflammatory)	Figure–ground separation
Body site		Similarity
Distribution	Morphology	Proximity
Pattern, including linearity	Color, including zonation	Continuity
Epidermal vs dermal vs deep soft tissue involvement	Topography (including scale)	Order
		Closure

Table 1.2   Visual recognition of three different big cats by their spots

Cheetah spots	Leopard spots	Jaguar spots
Round	Round to polygonal rosette	Polygonal rosette
Solid black	Solid color within rosette	Spots within rosette

BODY SITE/REGION

Key Differences

- **Scalp** – numerous anagen hair follicles with bulbs (arrows) in the fat (Fig. 1.1)
- **Ear** – vellus hair follicles (arrows) and central cartilage (*) (Fig. 1.2)
- **Face** – prominent hair follicles and sebaceous glands within the dermis (Fig. 1.3)
- **Eyelid** – vellus hair follicles (arrow) and underlying skeletal muscle (*) (Fig. 1.4)
- **Cutaneous lip** – epidermis with keratin and a granular layer (arrows); skeletal muscle (*) (Fig. 1.5)
- **Mucosal lip** – pale epithelium that lacks a granular layer and does not keratinize (Fig. 1.6)
- **Areola** – acanthotic, pigmented epidermis with dermal smooth muscle bundles (arrows) (Fig. 1.7)
- **Back** – thick dermis (Fig. 1.8)
- **Axilla** – undulating epidermis with deep apocrine glands (arrows) (Fig. 1.9)
- **Acral** – thick stratum corneum with stratum lucidum (arrow) (Fig. 1.10)
- **Nail** – nail plate (arrow), nail matrix (black bar), and nail bed (Fig. 1.11)

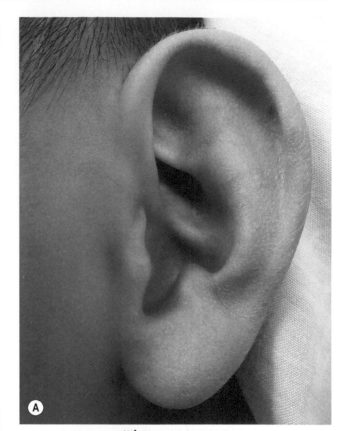

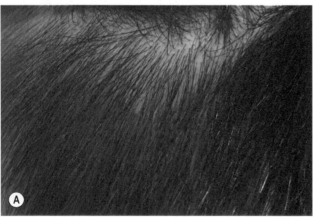

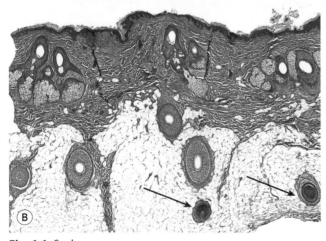

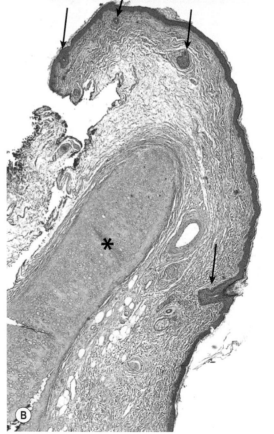

Fig. 1.1 Scalp.

Fig. 1.2 Ear.

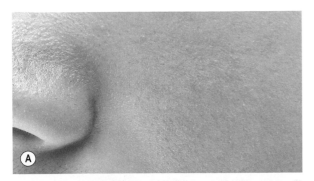

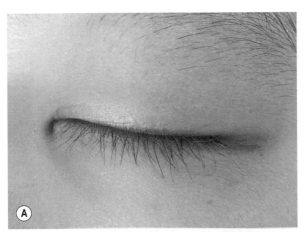

Fig. 1.3 Face.

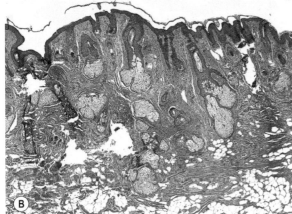

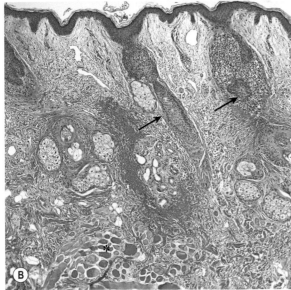

Fig. 1.4 Eyelid.

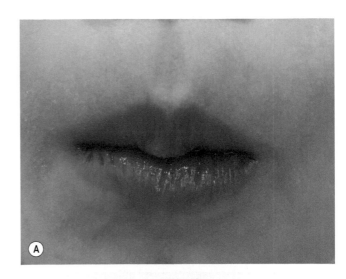

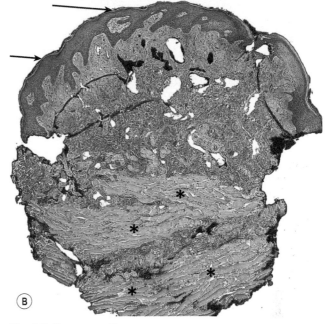

Fig. 1.5 Cutaneous lip.

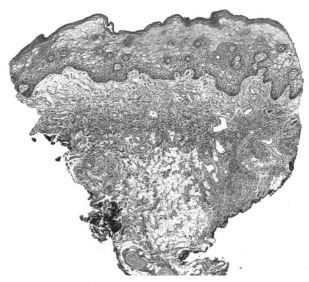

Fig. 1.6 Mucosal lip.

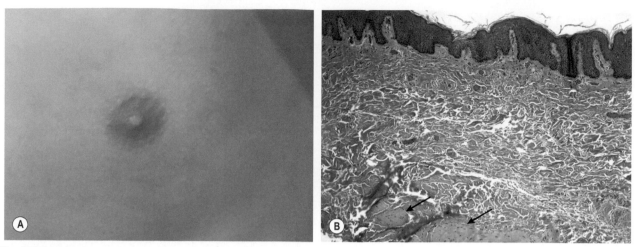

Fig. 1.7 Areola.

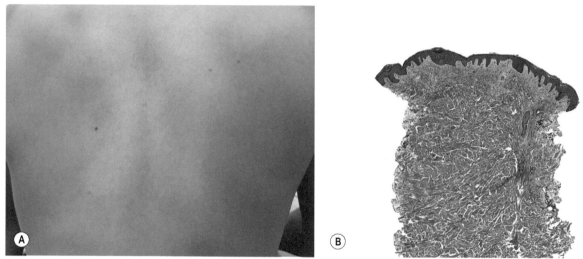

Fig. 1.8 Back.

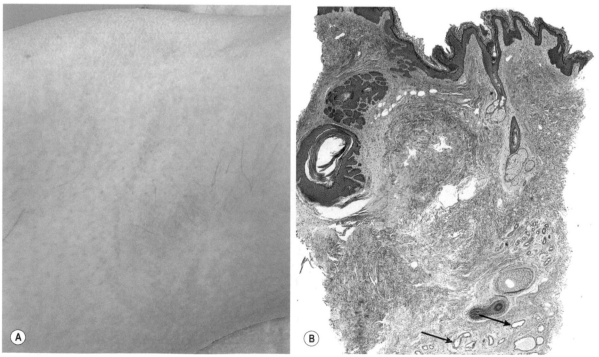

Fig. 1.9 Axilla.

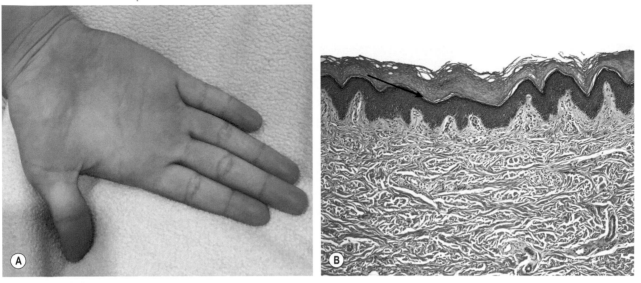

Fig. 1.10 Acral skin.

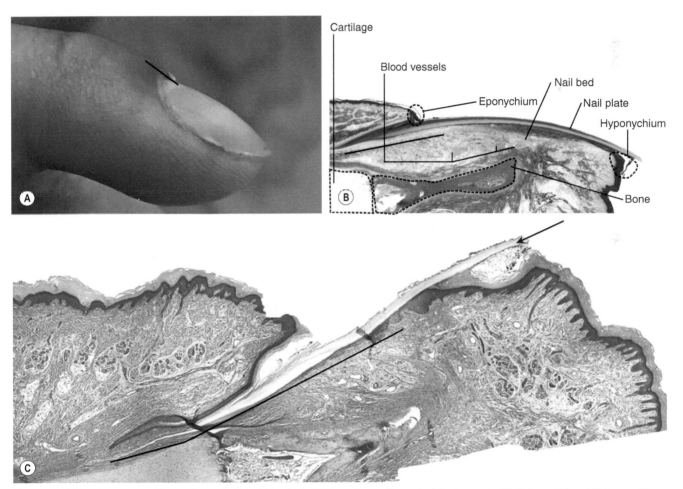

Fig. 1.11 Nail unit anatomy. The nail matrix (*black line* in A, B, C) produces the nail plate (*arrow* in B). *B, From Telser AG, Young JK, Baldwin KM. Integrated Histology, 1e. St Louis: Mosby, 2007, with permission.*

AGE

- **Young skin** – has small adnexal structures (arrows) and more compact dermis (Figs. 1.12, 1.13)
- **Older skin** – has characteristic solar elastosis (arrows) (Fig. 1.14)

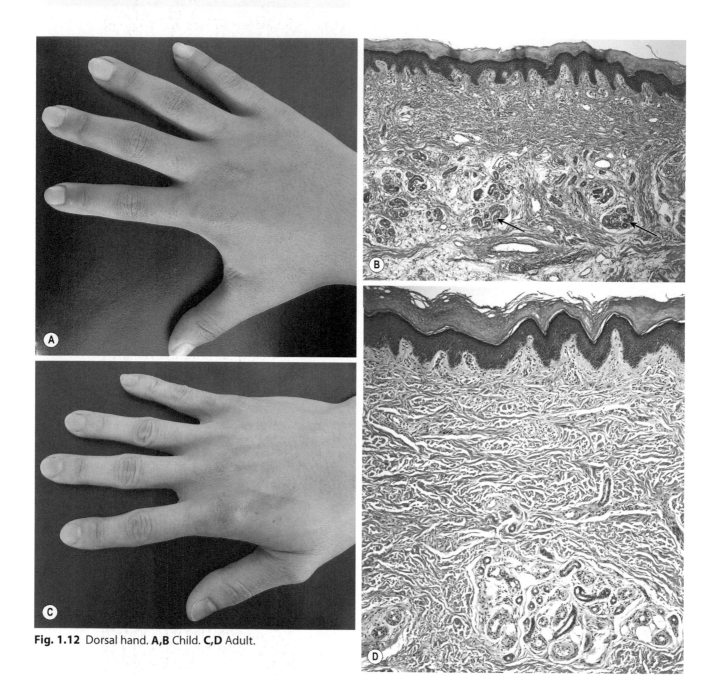

Fig. 1.12 Dorsal hand. **A,B** Child. **C,D** Adult.

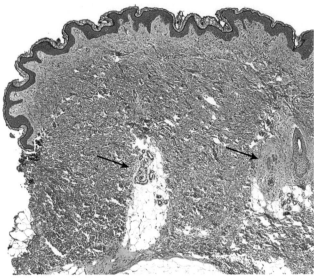

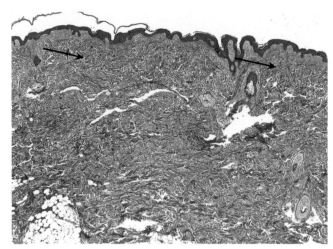

Fig. 1.14 Neck, 61-year-old.

Fig. 1.13 Groin, 2-year-old.

DISTRIBUTION

Extensive – more than one body part affected with multiple lesions; may preferentially affect extensor surfaces (e.g. elbows/knees) vs flexor surfaces (e.g. antecubital/popliteal fossae) or ventral vs dorsal surfaces (Fig. 1.15)

Photodistributed – can vary depending on the type of clothing worn; sun-protected sites of the face/neck generally include the central upper cutaneous lip and submental area (Fig. 1.16A; see Fig. 3.7)

Double-covered – generally includes sites covered by undergarments (Fig. 1.16B)

Acral – hands/feet but also the tips of the ears/nose (Fig. 1.16C)

Body folds – inframammary/intertriginous (Fig. 1.16D)

Generalized – involving the majority of the cutaneous surface (Fig. 1.17A)

Localized – limited to a discrete area (Fig. 1.17B)

Dermatomal – patterns of cutaneous innervation by spinal nerve roots (Fig. 1.18A)

Blaschkoid – follows patterns of embryonic cell migration; the linear pattern on the extremities is similar to the dermatomal pattern, whereas the V-shaped curves over the trunk and the S-shapes on the abdomen are characteristic (Fig. 1.18B)

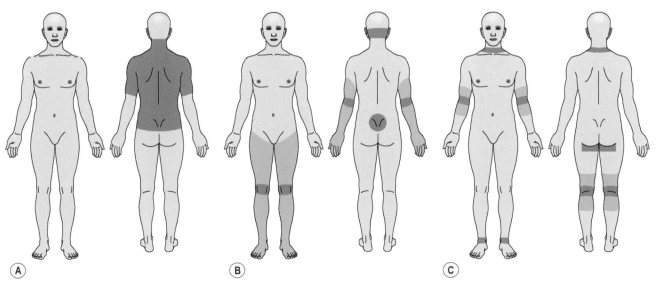

Fig. 1.15 Distribution. **A** Upper back and posterior arms. **B** Extensor surfaces. **C** Flexor surfaces. Areas shaded in red are classically involved; light pink areas may also be involved.

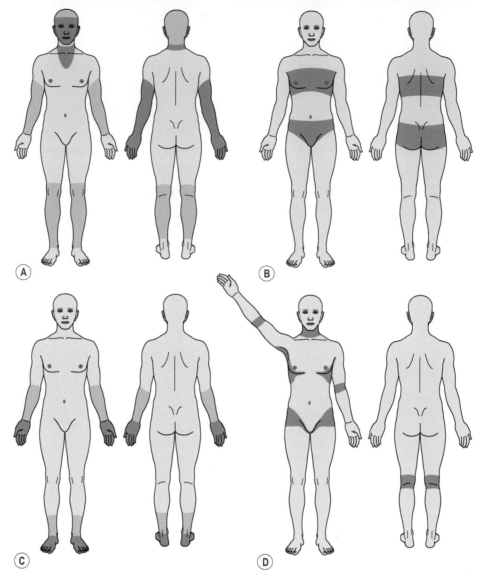

Fig. 1.16 Distribution. **A** Photodistribution. **B** Double-covered sites. **C** Acral. **D** Body folds. Areas shaded in red are classically involved; light pink areas may also be involved.

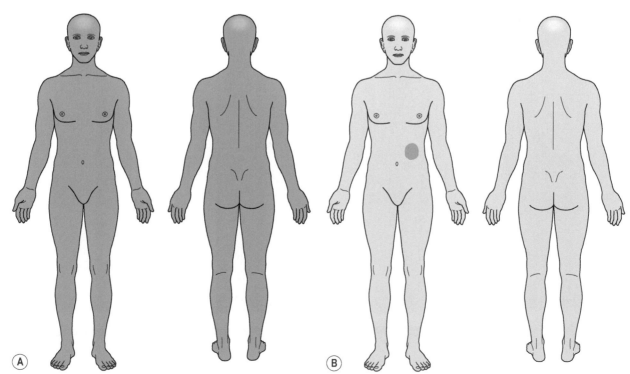

Fig. 1.17 Distribution – **A** Generalized. **B** Localized.

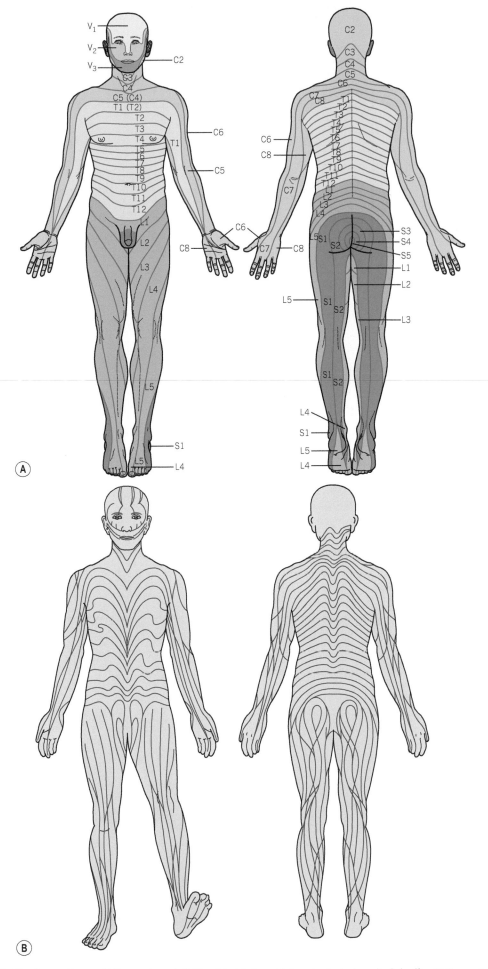

Fig. 1.18 Distribution patterns. **A** Dermatomal. **B** Blaschkoid. *From Bolognia JL, Jorizzo JL, Schaffer JV. Dermatology, 3e. London: Saunders, 2012, with permission.*

PATTERNS

Thin stripes – often corresponds to the Blaschko lines (see Fig. 1.18B; Fig. 1.19A); sometimes, when lesions are smaller, the blaschkoid/linear pattern is less obvious
Rarer patterns of mosaicism – include phylloid (Fig. 1.20) and checkerboard/segmental (Fig. 1.21)
Small net – regular with the "holes" of the net ≈1 cm in size (Fig. 1.22A,B)
Large net – irregular with the "holes" of an incomplete net usually >1 cm in size (Fig. 1.22C,D)

Serpiginous – (Fig. 1.23A)
Concentric rings – (Fig. 1.23B)
Circular (solid circle/oval) (Fig. 1.24)
Annular (ring with unaffected center) (Fig. 1.25)
Complex, connecting curves and lines, like Chinese letters (Fig. 1.26)
Exogenous – the shape corresponds to the contact area of the external inducer (Fig. 1.27)

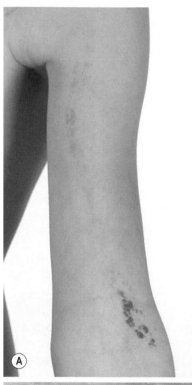

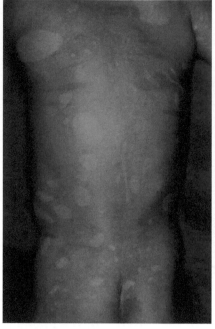

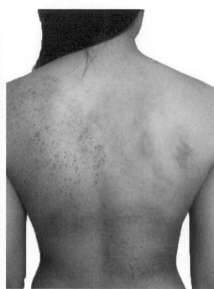

Fig. 1.21 Nevus spilus maculosa. *Courtesy, Jae hyuk Choi, MD PhD.*

Fig. 1.20 Phylloid hypomelanosis caused by mosaicism for trisomy 13. *Courtesy, Rudolf Happle, MD.*

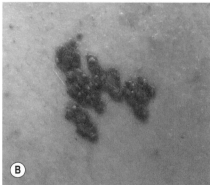

Fig. 1.19 Epidermal nevus. **A** A linear light tan to brown lesion along the upper arm extending down to the antecubital fossa. **B** When lesions are smaller, the linear distribution may be less obvious. *A, Courtesy, Celia Moss, MD. From Bolognia JL, Jorizzo JL, Schaffer JV. Dermatology, 3e. London: Saunders, 2012, with permission.*

Fig. 1.22 Small and large nets. **A,B** Livedo reticularis. **C,D** Livedo racemosa. Sneddon syndrome in D. *D, Courtesy, Christopher Baker and Robert Kelly, MD. B, Courtesy, Peter Heald, MD. A,C,D, From Bolognia JL, Jorizzo JL, Schaffer JV. Dermatology, 3e. London: Saunders, 2012, with permission.*

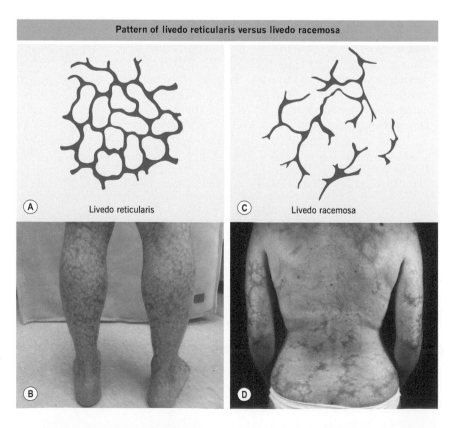

Pattern of livedo reticularis versus livedo racemosa

Livedo reticularis

Livedo racemosa

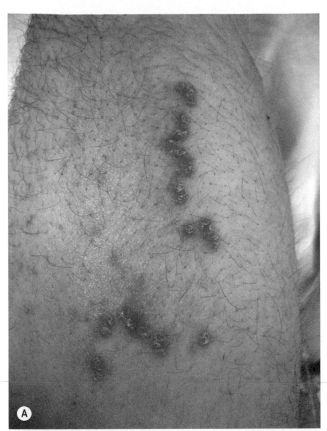

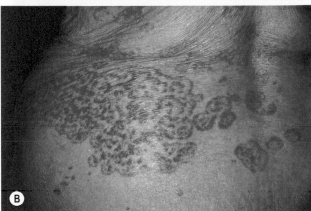

Fig. 1.23 **A** Elastosis perforans serpiginosa. **B** Erythema gyratum repens in a patient with breast carcinoma. *A, Courtesy, Yale Dermatology Residents' Slide Collection. B, Courtesy, Jeffrey Callen, MD. B, From Bolognia JL, Jorizzo JL, Schaffer JV. Dermatology, 3e. London: Saunders, 2012, with permission.*

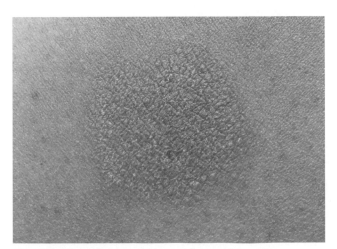

Fig. 1.24 Fixed drug eruption, resolving, with surface changes secondary to rubbing.

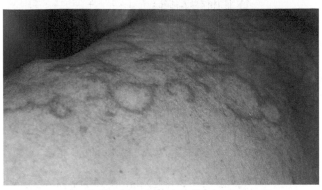

Fig. 1.25 Annular elastolytic giant cell granuloma. *Courtesy, Kalman Watsky, MD. From Bolognia JL, Jorizzo JL, Schaffer JV. Dermatology, 3e. London: Saunders, 2012, with permission.*

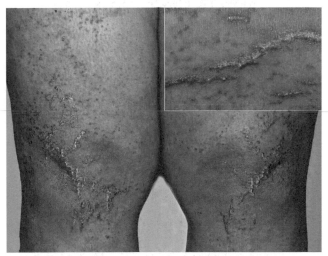

Fig. 1.26 Keratosis lichenoides chronica. *Courtesy, Kathryn Schwarzenberger, MD. From Bolognia JL, Jorizzo JL, Schaffer JV. Dermatology, 3e. London: Saunders, 2012, with permission.*

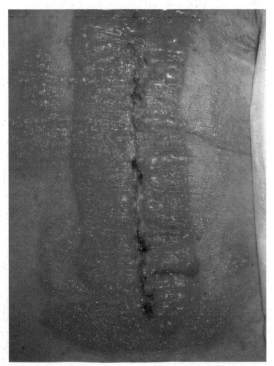

Fig. 1.27 Allergic contact dermatitis. *Courtesy, Yale Dermatology Residents' Slide Collection.*

LINEARITY

Inflammatory (Fig. 1.28), **mosaic** (Fig. 1.29), **vascular** (Fig. 1.30), **infectious**, and **externally induced** (Fig. 1.31) disorders – can present with linear lesions; lesions within a dermatome or embryonic lines (see Fig. 1.18) and koebnerized lesions can also be linear

Linear psoriasis – characteristic silvery scale is seen over red plaques; the presence of psoriatic lesions (see Fig. 1.28A; arrow) outside of the linear lesion distinguishes this clinically from inflammatory linear verrucous epidermal nevus

Linear lichen planus – typically composed of flat-topped purplish papules with Wickham striae

Lichen striatus – similar appearance to lichen planus, but lesions are usually small (1–2 mm) with minimal scale

Linear porokeratosis – subtle, discrete, raised rim of scale around thin, flat pink plaques

Incontinentia pigmenti – an initial vesicular stage becomes verrucous and hyperpigmented with late-stage hypopigmentation and absent adnexal structures (see Fig. 1.29)

Goltz syndrome (see Fig. 3.12E) – linear streaks are composed of yellowish papules (fat herniation), telangiectasias, hyperpigmented macules, atrophic foci, and hypopigmented splotches

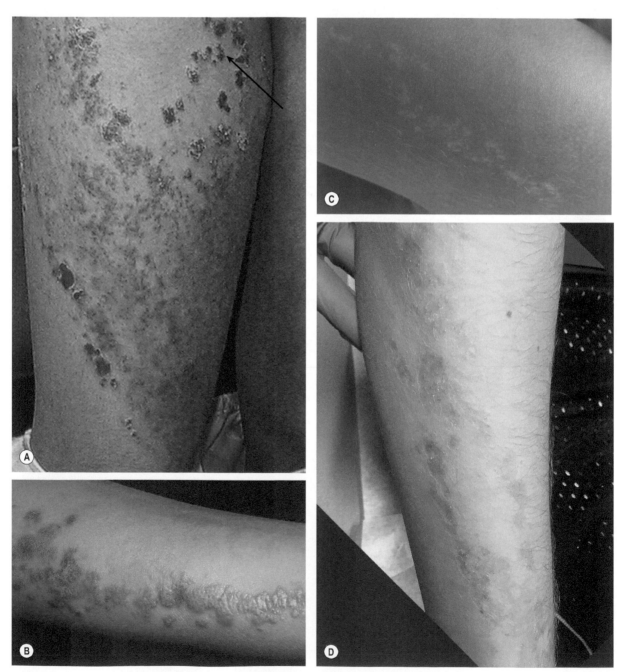

Fig. 1.28 Inflammatory. **A** Linear psoriasis. **B** Linear lichen planus. **C** Lichen striatus **D** Linear porokeratosis. *B, Courtesy, Joyce Rico, MD. From Bolognia JL, Jorizzo JL, Schaffer JV. Dermatology, 3e. London: Saunders, 2012, with permission. C, Courtesy, Brittany Craiglow, MD. D, Courtesy, Julie Cantatore-Francis, MD.*

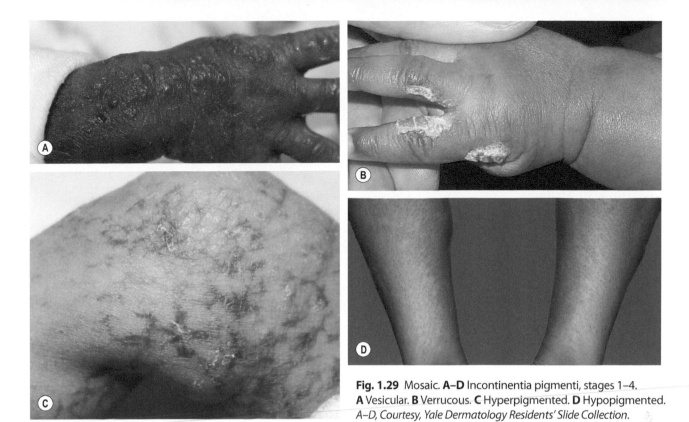

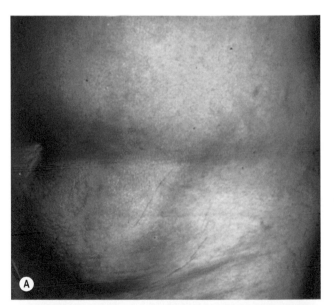

Fig. 1.29 Mosaic. **A–D** Incontinentia pigmenti, stages 1–4. **A** Vesicular. **B** Verrucous. **C** Hyperpigmented. **D** Hypopigmented. *A–D, Courtesy, Yale Dermatology Residents' Slide Collection.*

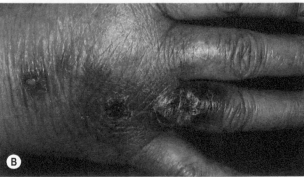

Fig. 1.30 Vascular. **A** Superficial thrombophlebitis in a patient with Behçet disease. **B** Sporotrichoid spread of an atypical mycobacterial infection. *A, Courtesy, Samuel Moschella, MD. B, Courtesy, Yale Dermatology Residents' Slide Collection. A, From Bolognia JB, Jorizzo JL, Rapini RP. Dermatology, 2e. London: Saunders, 2008, with permission.*

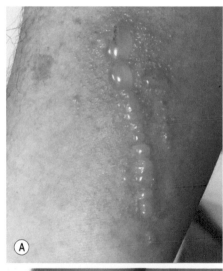

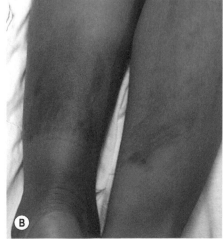

Fig. 1.31 Externally induced. **A** Poison ivy. **B** Phytophotodermatitis, postinflammatory pigmentary alteration. *A, Courtesy, Joyce Rico, MD. B, Courtesy, Yale Dermatology Residents' Slide Collection.*

EPIDERMAL VS DERMAL VS DEEP SOFT TISSUE INVOLVEMENT

Tumors, inflammation, edema, or other deposits can affect the epidermis, dermis, or deeper soft tissue (Fig. 1.32). Inflammation of the epidermis is addressed in the next section. Inflammation affecting the epidermis can be follicular (e.g. folliculitis) or nonfollicular (e.g. pustular psoriasis).

Basic Epidermal Patterns

Eczematous/Spongiotic*

Clinical:
Crust, "wet" appearance and/or vesicles (circles), erythema (arrow) (Fig. 1.33A)

Histopathologic:
Parakeratosis with serum, intercellular edema/vesicles (circles), perivascular inflammation, and slightly dilated vessels (arrow) (Fig. 1.33B)

Papulosquamous/psoriasiform*

Clinical:
Silvery to white scaly (arrow) plaque (bar), sharp demarcation from normal skin, bright red erythema underlying scale (Fig. 1.34A)

---

*Can have overlapping features, especially in chronic spongiotic conditions

Histopathologic:
Dry parakeratosis usually without serum (arrow), acanthosis; in psoriasis, the prototype disorder, acanthosis is regular (bar), often with neutrophils in the epidermis (Fig. 1.34B)

Lichenoid (Interface)†

Clinical:
Violaceous (arrow) to pink to gray, depending on skin tone, lesions often flat-topped (Fig. 1.35A)

Histopathologic:
Band-like lymphocytic infiltrate (arrow), pigment incontinence (more prominent in darker skin types) (Fig. 1.35B)

Vacuolar (Interface)†

Clinical:
Thin lesions, may be pink, red, gray or dusky in color, depending on acuity and skin tone (Fig. 1.36A)

Histopathologic:
Vacuoles in basal cells (arrows) (Fig. 1.36B)

---

†Interface disorders can have overlapping features; note that there is not a true clinical–pathologic correlate for the vacuolar pattern in the same way as there is for the other three basic patterns

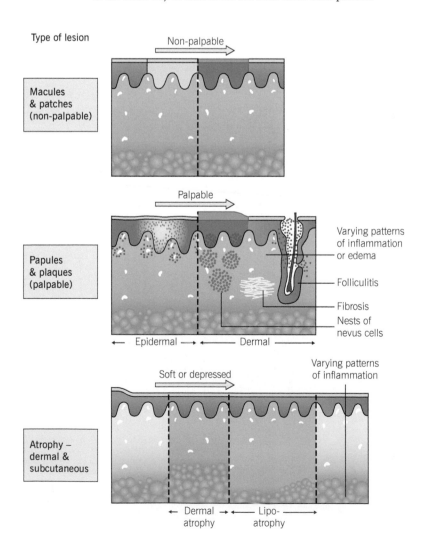

Fig. 1.32 Epidermal vs dermal vs deep soft tissue involvement. *Adapted from Bolognia JL, Jorizzo JL, Schaffer JV. Dermatology, 3e. London: Saunders, 2012, with permission.*

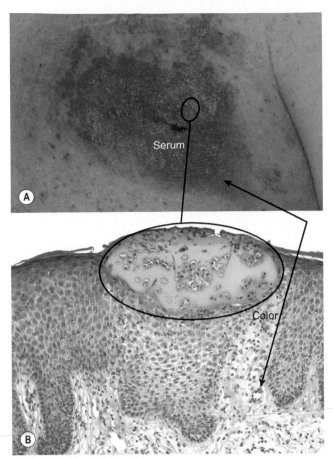

Fig. 1.33 Allergic contact dermatitis to adhesive. *A, Courtesy, Kalman Watsky, MD.*

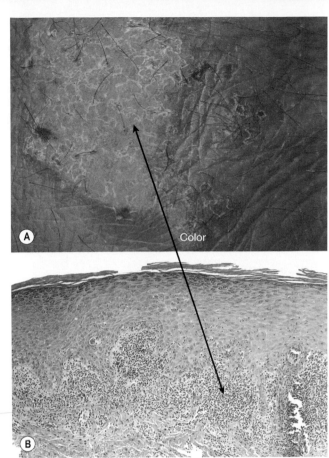

Fig. 1.35 Lichen planus. *A, Courtesy, Yale Dermatology Residents' Slide Collection.*

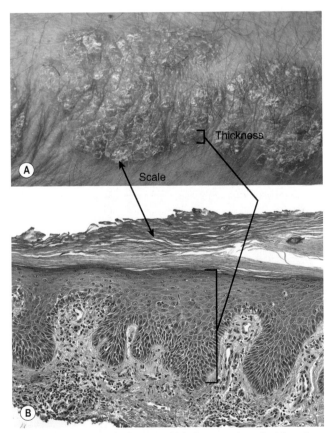

Fig. 1.34 Psoriasis. *A, Courtesy, Yale Dermatology Residents' Slide Collection.*

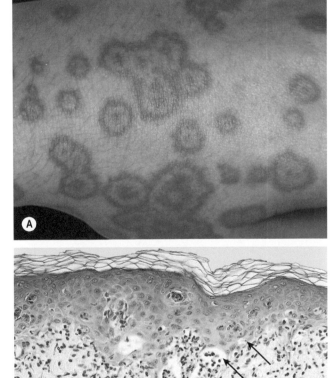

Fig. 1.36 Erythema multiforme. *A, Courtesy, Yale Dermatology Residents' Slide Collection. A, From Bolognia JL, Jorizzo JL, Schaffer JV. Dermatology, 3e. London: Saunders, 2012, with permission.*

ACUTE VS CHRONIC ECZEMATOUS/SPONGIOTIC

Acute Eczematous/Spongiotic Processes
Clinical:
Surface serum/crust ("weeping"/"boiling over") and/or vesicles (arrow), erythema (Figs. 1.37A, 1.38); can become impetiginized

Histopathologic:
Parakeratosis with serum/inflammatory cells and/or intraepidermal vesicles (arrow) and perivascular inflammation (Fig. 1.37B)

Chronic Eczematous/Spongiotic Processes
Clinical:
Thickened/lichenified (bar), scaly (arrow) plaques +/− erythema (Figs. 1.39A, 1.40)

Histopathologic:
Hyperkeratosis +/− parakeratosis (arrow), hypergranulosis, acanthosis (bar) and vertically streaked dermal collagen (asterisks), perivascular inflammation (Fig. 1.39B) Other eczematous processes are illustrated in Figs. 1.41–1.43.

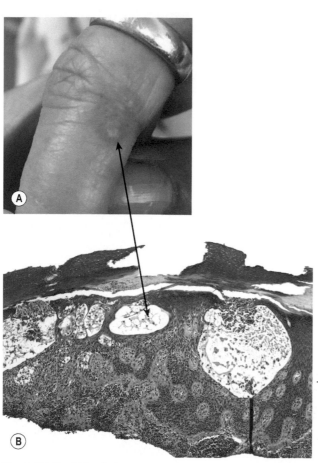

Fig. 1.37 Dyshidrotic eczema.

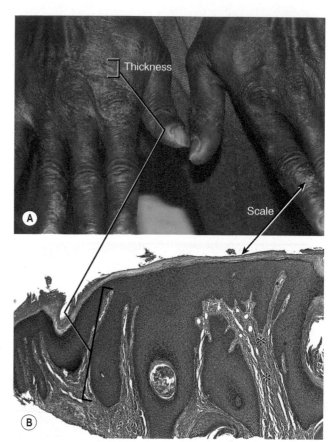

Fig. 1.39 Chronic dermatitis with lichenification. *A, Courtesy, Kalman Watsky, MD.*

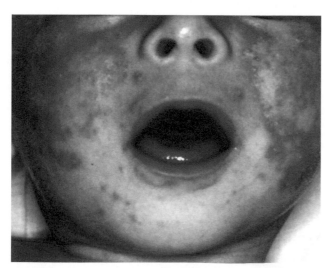

Fig. 1.38 Acute atopic dermatitis, infant. *Courtesy, Kalman Watsky, MD.*

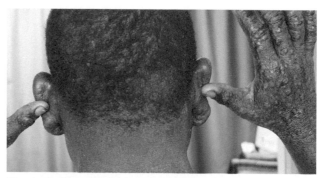

Fig. 1.40 Chronic atopic dermatitis. *Courtesy, Yale Dermatology Residents' Slide Collection.*

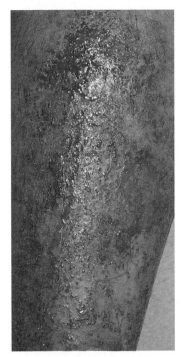

Fig. 1.41 Acute allergic contact dermatitis.

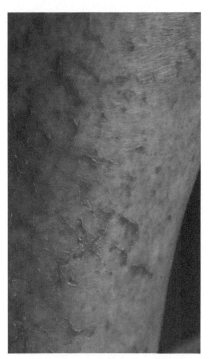

Fig. 1.42 Asteatotic eczema. *Courtesy, Yale Dermatology Residents' Slide Collection.*

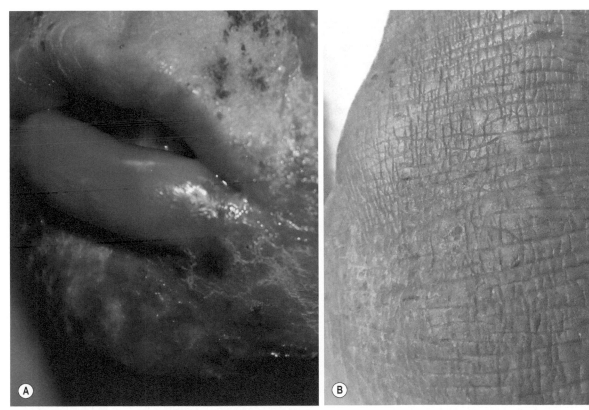

Fig. 1.43 Atopic dermatitis. **A** Acutely impetinized. **B** Chronically lichenified. *A, Courtesy, Yale Dermatology Residents' Slide Collection.*

INFLAMMATORY CELL TYPES – EPIDERMAL

Neutrophils – often associated with pustules clinically (Fig. 1.44; see Chapter 11)

Eosinophils – may be associated with blistering/erosions clinically (Fig. 1.45)

Lymphocytes (arrows) – often present in spongiotic processes but can also represent cutaneous T-cell lymphoma (Fig. 1.46)

Langerhans cells (circle) – the prototype is Langerhans cell histiocytosis; small collections of Langerhans cells are also present in spongiotic processes (Fig. 1.47; see Chapter 20)

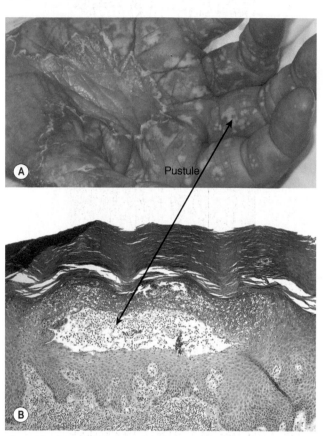

Fig. 1.44 Pustular psoriasis. *Courtesy, Yale Dermatology Residents' Slide Collection.*

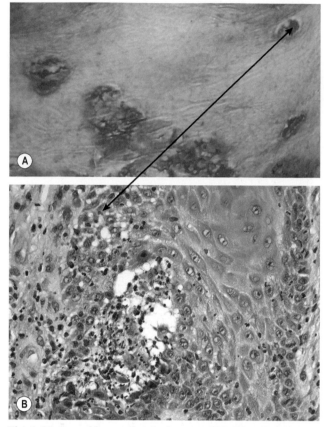

Fig. 1.45 Pemphigus vulgaris. *Courtesy, Yale Dermatology Residents' Slide Collection.*

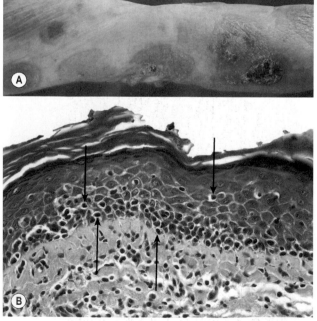

Fig. 1.46 Mycosis fungoides. *Courtesy, Yale Dermatology Residents' Slide Collection.*

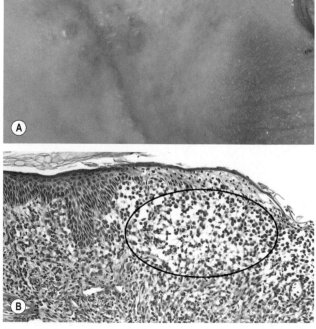

Fig. 1.47 Langerhans cell histiocytosis. *A, Courtesy, Irwin Braverman, MD.*

INFLAMMATORY CELL TYPES – DERMAL

The predominant type of dermal inflammatory cell can sometimes be predicted by the color of clinical lesions.

Langerhans cell histiocytosis – purpuric papules and plaques; Langerhans cells and extravasated erythrocytes in the dermis (see Fig. 1.47A,B; see Chapter 20)

Granulomatous disorders – classically red–brown to pink with a yellowish tinge if lesions are pressed firmly with a glass slide; collections of histiocytes (granulomas) are in the dermis (circles) (Fig. 1.48A,B; see Chapter 20)

Mast cells – pink to red–brown and may blister with manipulation; mast cells classically have central nuclei with abundant slightly granular cytoplasm (Fig. 1.48C,D)

Dense pan-dermal neutrophilic infiltrates – deep, hot red to vesicular/translucent when acute and untreated (Fig. 1.48E,F; see Chapter 16)

Dense pan-dermal lymphocytic or leukemic infiltrates – pink–red to purple firm papulonodule (Fig. 1.48G–L)

Sparse dermal lymphocytic infiltrates (may be admixed with neutrophils and/or eosinophils) – light pink (Fig. 1.48M,N)

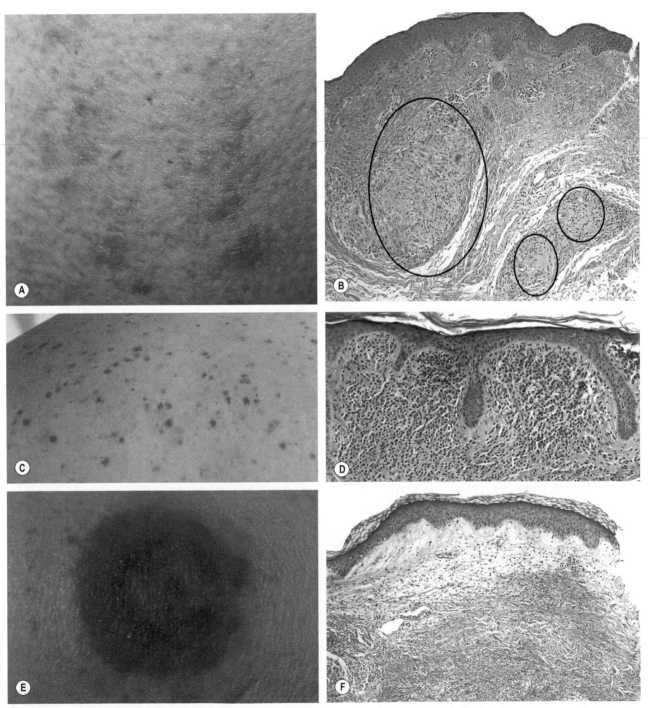

Fig. 1.48 Dermal inflammatory processes. **A,B** Sarcoidosis. **C,D** Mastocytosis. **E,F** Sweet syndrome.

Continued

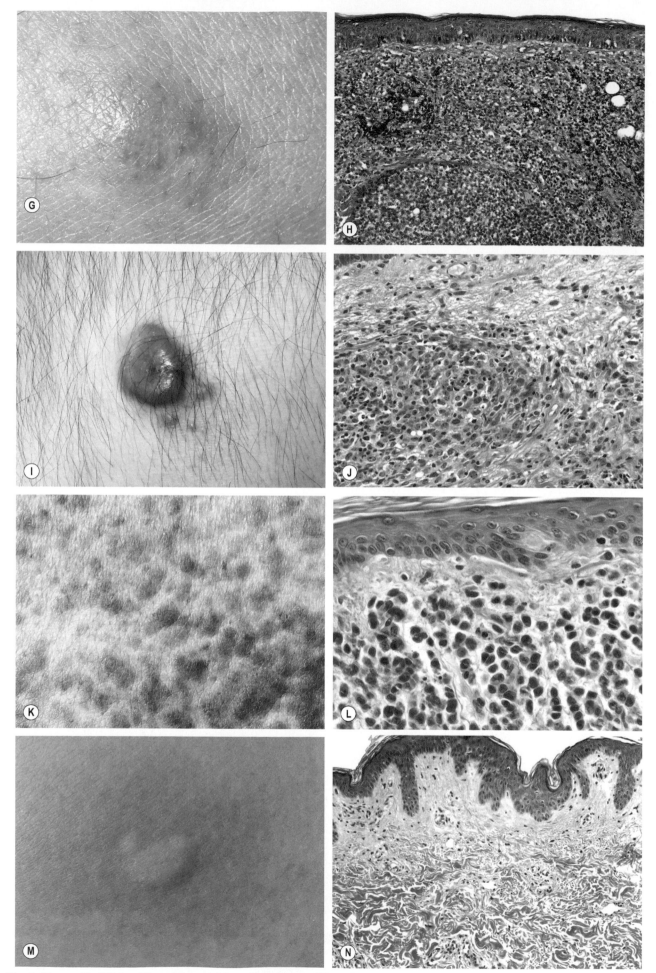

Fig. 1.48, cont'd G,H B-cell lymphoma. **I,J** Anaplastic large cell lymphoma. **K,L** Acute myelogenous leukemia. **M,N** Urticaria. *A,E–L, Courtesy, Yale Dermatology Residents' Slide Collection.*

CLASSIC MORPHOLOGY

(Figs. 1.49, 1.50)

Term	Clinical features	Clinical example	Microscopic example
Macule	• Flat, circumscribed, non-palpable • <1 cm in diameter • Often hypo- or hyperpigmented • Also other colors (e.g. pink, red, violet) • It can be round, oval, or irregular in shape • May be sharply marginated or blend into the surrounding skin	 Solar lentigines	
Patch	• Flat, circumscribed • >1 cm in diameter • Often hypo- or hyperpigmented • Also other colors (e.g. blue, violet)	 Vitiligo	
Papule	• Elevated, circumscribed • <1 cm in diameter • Elevation due to increased thickness of the epidermis and/or cells or deposits within the dermis • May have secondary changes (e.g. scale, crust) • Need to distinguish from vesicle or pustule • When viewed in profile, it may be flat-topped, dome-shaped, filiform, pedunculated, smooth, verrucous, or umbilicated	 Seborrheic keratoses	
Plaque	• Elevated, circumscribed • >1 cm in diameter • Elevation due to increased thickness of the epidermis and/or cells or deposits within the dermis • May have secondary changes (e.g. scale, crust, erosion) • May be a distinct lesion or formed by confluence of papules	 Psoriasis	
Nodule	• Elevated, circumscribed • Larger volume than papule, often >1.5 cm in diameter • Involves the dermis and may extend to the subcutis • Greatest mass may be beneath the skin surface • Can be compressible, soft, rubbery, or firm to palpation	 Epidermal inclusion cysts	 *Continued*

Related by size

Related by size

Fig. 1.49 Classic lesions. *Adapted from Bolognia JL, Schaffer JV, Duncan KO, Ko CJ. Dermatology Essentials, 1e. Philadelphia: Saunders, 2014, with permission.*

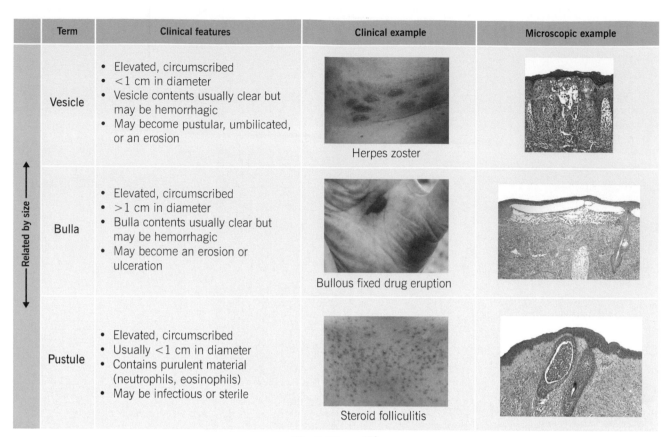

Term	Clinical features	Clinical example	Microscopic example
Vesicle	• Elevated, circumscribed • <1 cm in diameter • Vesicle contents usually clear but may be hemorrhagic • May become pustular, umbilicated, or an erosion	Herpes zoster	
Bulla	• Elevated, circumscribed • >1 cm in diameter • Bulla contents usually clear but may be hemorrhagic • May become an erosion or ulceration	Bullous fixed drug eruption	
Pustule	• Elevated, circumscribed • Usually <1 cm in diameter • Contains purulent material (neutrophils, eosinophils) • May be infectious or sterile	Steroid folliculitis	

Related by size

Fig. 1.49, cont'd

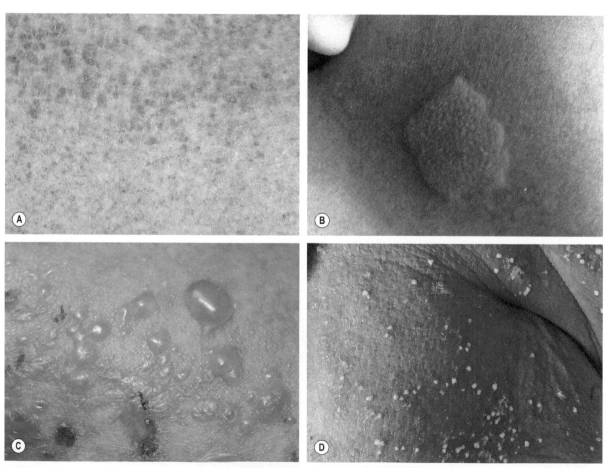

Fig. 1.50 Descriptive terms for primary morphology. **A** Macules (flat lesions <1 cm) in lower half of **A** versus papules (raised lesions <1 cm) in upper half of this example of biphasic amyloidosis. **B** Patch (flat lesion >1 cm) of erythema surrounding a plaque (raised lesion >1 cm) in this hive with a flare of erythema. **C** Vesicles (<1 cm in diameter) and bullae (>1 cm in diameter) in bullous pemphigoid. **D** Pustules in acute generalized exanthematous pustulosis. *C, D Courtesy, Yale Dermatology Residents' Collection.*

ZONATION OF COLOR

- **Typical target** – the prototype is erythema multiforme; three zones of color (middle zone is often edematous and pale; arrows) (Fig. 1.51A)
- **Atypical target** – papular (raised) atypical targets can be seen in erythema multiforme, but macular (flat) atypical targets should raise suspicion for a drug eruption; classically only two zones of color; the center may blister (Fig. 1.51B)

- **Annular, nonscaly** – ring with relatively unaffected center (Fig. 1.51C,D,E)
- **Annular, scaly** – ring of scale (Fig. 1.51F) or with scale on a pink border; scale on outer border in tinea (Fig. 1.51G); scale on the inner border in erythema annulare centrifugum (Fig. 1.51H)

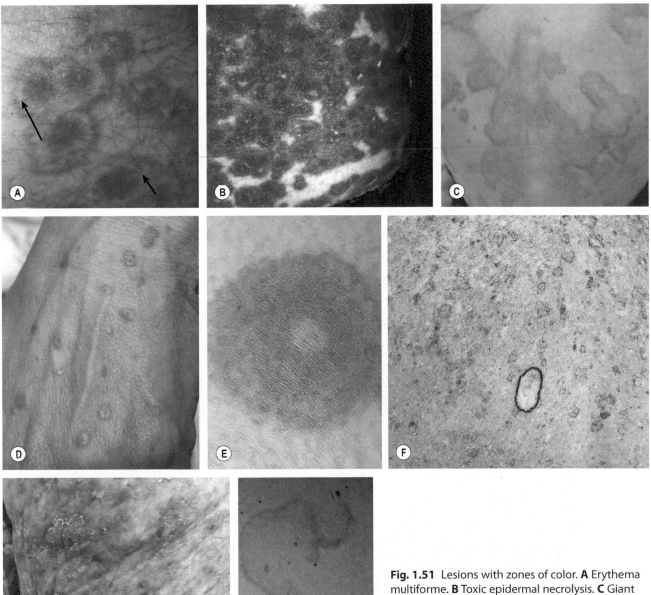

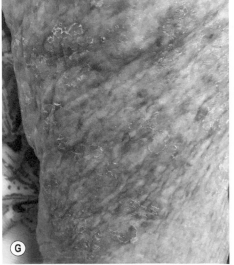

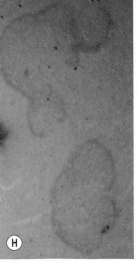

Fig. 1.51 Lesions with zones of color. **A** Erythema multiforme. **B** Toxic epidermal necrolysis. **C** Giant annular urticaria (urticaria multiforme). **D** Granuloma annulare. **E** Erythema chronicum migrans. **F** Pigmented porokeratosis. The area circled in black ink is the site of a biopsy-proven superficial basal cell carcinoma. **G** Tinea corporis. **H** Erythema annulare centrifugum. The center is losing the pink color, creating an annular lesion. *A, Courtesy, Kalman Watsky, MD; C–E,H Courtesy, Yale Dermatology Residents' Slide Collection. B, From Callen JP, Jorizzo JL. Dermatological Signs of Internal Disease, 4e. Philadelphia: Saunders, 2009.*

TOPOGRAPHY

(Fig. 1.52)

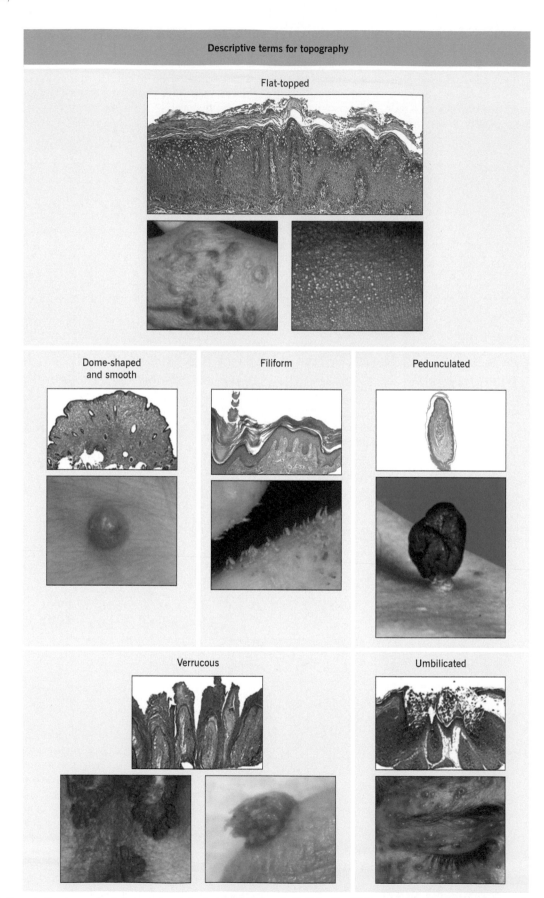

Fig. 1.52 Descriptive terms for topography. *Adapted from Bolognia JL, Schaffer JV, Duncan KO, Ko CJ. Dermatology Essentials, 1e. Philadelphia: Saunders, 2014, with permission.*

COLOR

(Fig. 1.53)

Color	Common causes		
	Endogenous		Exogenous
Pink to red to purple	• Erythrocytes • Inflammation • Vessels	Example: Kaposi sarcoma 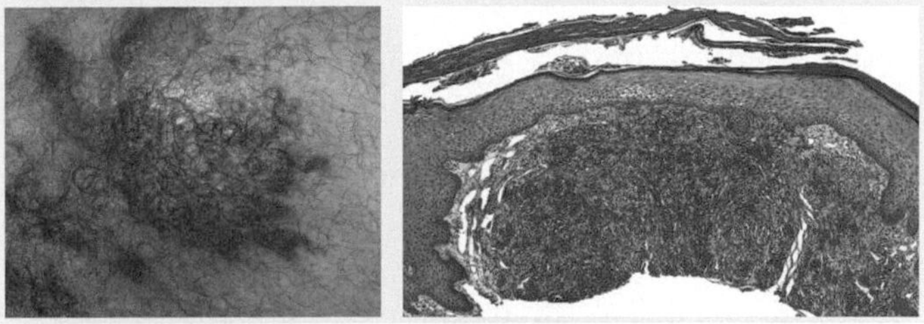	• Tattoo pigment
Black	• Necrosis • Melanin • Inflammation • Vessels (i.e. occlusion)	Example: Calciphylaxis 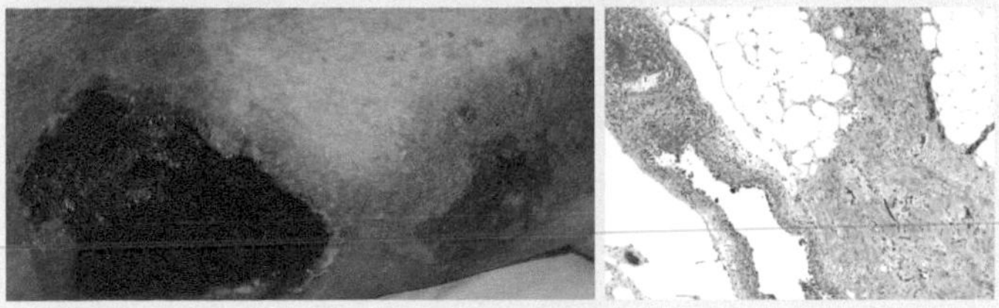	• Tattoo pigment • Poison ivy sap • Tick
Blue	• Vessels • Melanin	Example: Vascular malformation 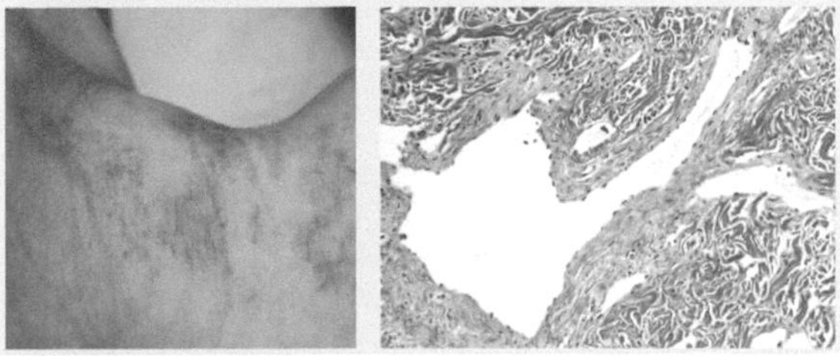	• Drug pigment (e.g. minocycline) • Heavy metals • Tattoo pigment
Yellow	• Lipid • Connective tissue (CT) • Deposition (e.g. urate in gout) • Keratin	Example: CT nevus 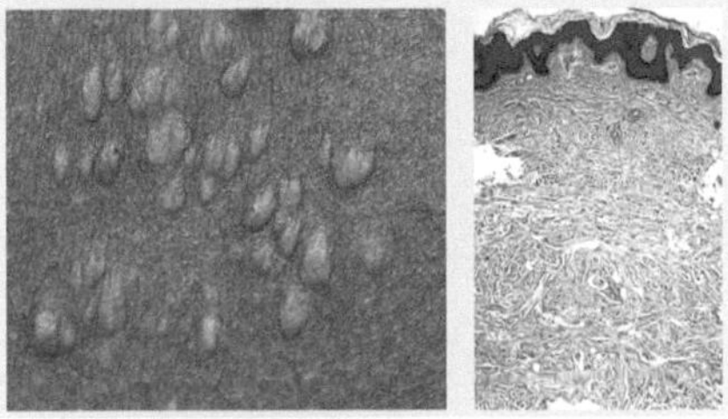	• Drug pigment
Brown	• Melanin • Hemosiderin • Cellular proliferation (e.g. dermatofibroma)	Example: Tinea nigra 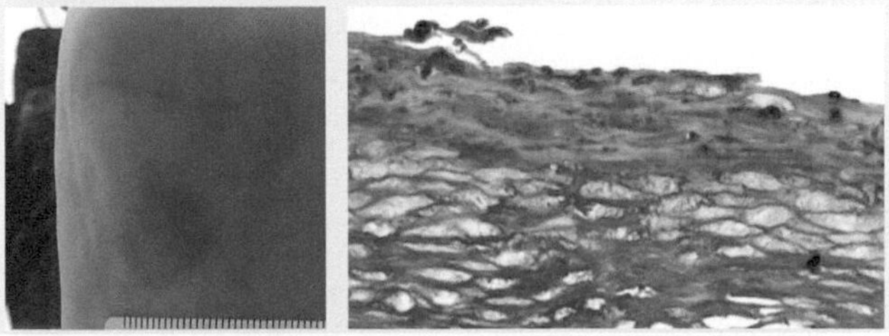	• Drug pigment • Pigmented fungus
White	• Decreased melanin • Vasospasm • Deposition (e.g. calcium) • Keratin • Cellular proliferation (e.g. scar)	Examples: Vitiligo and Nevus anemicus 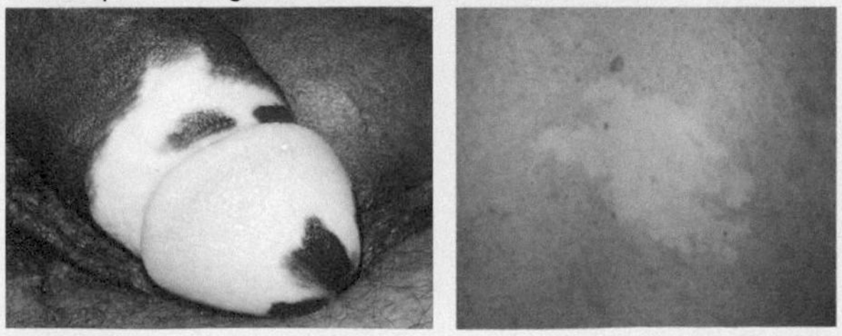	• Tattoo pigment

Fig. 1.53 Color as a clue to the clinical diagnosis. *Adapted from Bolognia JL, Jorizzo JL, Schaffer JV. Dermatology, 3e. London: Saunders, 2012, with permission.*

KERATODERMA

Diffuse – involving the entire palm or sole (Fig. 1.54A)
Focal – involving part of the palm or sole (Fig. 1.54B)

Punctate – small, discrete keratotic lesions on the palm or sole

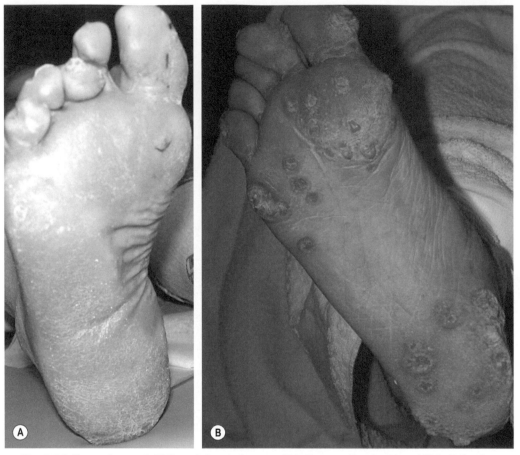

Fig. 1.54 Keratoderma. **A** Diffuse. **B** Focal. *Courtesy, Yale Dermatology Residents' Slide Collection.*

SCALE

Scale, Often Over Erythema

Key Differences (Fig. 1.55)

- Silvery to white–yellow or micaceous – e.g. psoriasis
- Collarettes +/− central fine scale – e.g. pityriasis rosea
- Wickham striae (linear scale) – lichen planus
- Greasy – e.g. seborrheic dermatitis
- Weeping – e.g. nummular dermatitis
- Lichenified – skin thickening with increased markings, e.g. lichen simplex chronicus
- Powdery (especially when lightly scraped) – e.g. tinea versicolor
- Cornflake-like – e.g. pemphigus foliaceus
- Trailing scale that is on the inner margin of the red, inflamed border – e.g. erythema annulare centrifugum
- Scale on the advancing, outer margin – e.g. tinea corporis

Scale, Often Without Erythema

Corrugated (arranged in parallel lines) – e.g. epidermolytic ichthyosis (Fig. 1.56A,B)
Rectangular shapes with overlying fine white scale – e.g. ichthyosis vulgaris (Fig. 1.56C,D)
Lamellar (plate-like, lifting at edges) – e.g. lamellar ichthyosis (Fig. 1.56E,F)
"Dirty" appearance, preferentially affects the posterior neck and spares the body folds – X-linked ichthyosis (Fig. 1.56G,H)

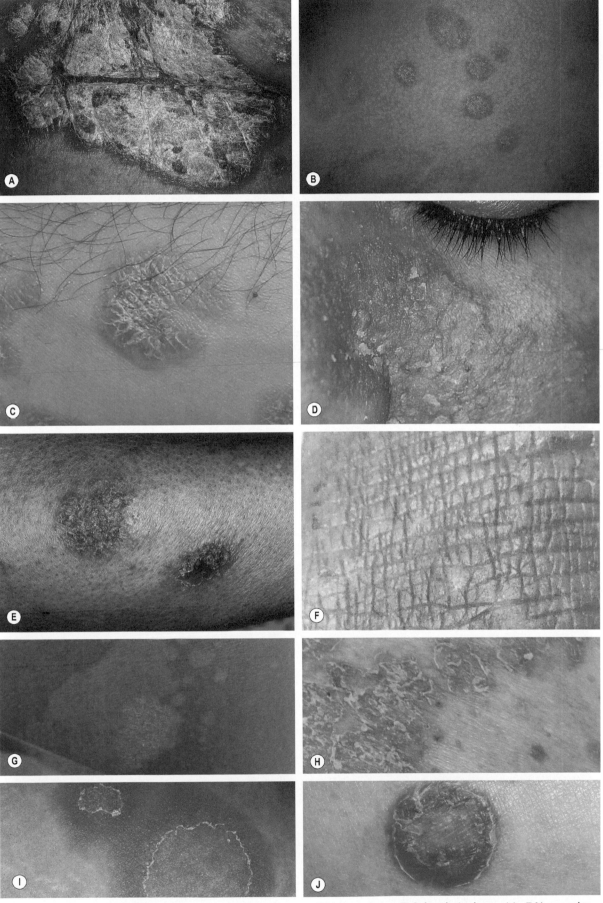

Fig. 1.55 Scale, often over erythema. **A** Psoriasis. **B** Pityriasis rosea. **C** Lichen planus. **D** Seborrheic dermatitis. **E** Nummular dermatitis. **F** Lichenification in chronic atopic dermatitis. **G** Tinea versicolor. **H** Pemphigus foliaceus. **I** Erythema annulare centrifugum. **J** Tinea corporis. *A,B,F, Courtesy, Yale Dermatology Residents' Slide Collection; E, Courtesy, Kalman Watsky, MD; H, Courtesy, NYU Slide Collection. A-F,H, From Bolognia JL, Jorizzo JL, Schaffer JV. Dermatology, 3e. London: Saunders, 2012, with permission. I, From Schwarzenberger K, Werchniak AE, Ko C. General Dermatology. London: Saunders, 2009.*

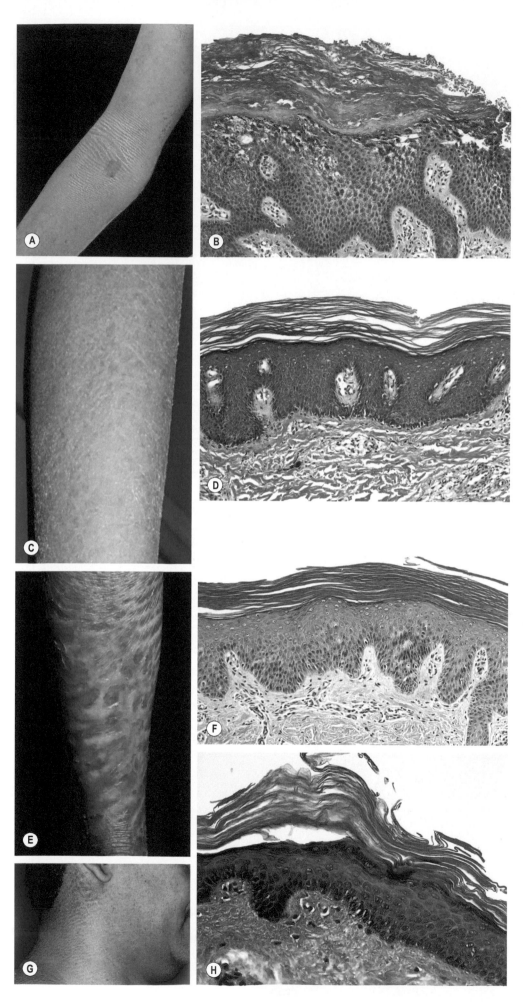

Fig. 1.56 Scale – often without erythema. **A,B** Epidermolytic ichthyosis. **C,D** Ichthyosis vulgaris. **E,F** Lamellar ichthyosis. **G,H** X-linked ichthyosis. *A,E Courtesy, Britt Craiglow, MD; C, Courtesy, Julie V Schaffer, MD; G, Courtesy, Gabriele Richard, MD and Franziska Ringpfeil, MD; H, From Fernandes NF, Janniger CK, Schwartz RA. X-linked ichthyosis: an oculocutaneous genodermatosis. J Am Acad Dermatol. 2010;62:480–85, © Elsevier.*

Differential Diagnosis for Given Body Sites and Morphology | 2

Although an elephant is easily recognizable given its distinctive features, larger cats may be harder to tell apart, especially because we see them infrequently and rarely, if ever, see them side by side. However, there are distinguishing features, even just in the morphology of their spots. Knowing the concept is aided by seeing the spots side by side (see Table 1.2). In this vein, this chapter addresses disorders that can present on a given body site with a particular morphology, emphasizing key differences and visually contrasting particular diseases side by side. Body sites covered include facial, body folds, acral, and truncal.

FACIAL

FACIAL: Multiple Papules, White–Yellow

Key Differences (Fig. 2.1)

- **Cowden syndrome** – verrucous (arrow) or smooth surfaced, may involve ears
- **Birt-Hogg-Dubé syndrome** – smooth, monomorphous, often on ears, neck, and central face
- **Syringomas** – often clustered over eyelids
- **Sebaceous hyperplasia** – often umbilicated, yellowish papules
- **Sebaceous tumors (especially sebaceous adenomas)** – yellow to pink or red papulonodules
- **Milia/comedones** – smooth, shiny papules; when punctured, keratin can be expressed
- **Trichoepitheliomas** – predilection for central face

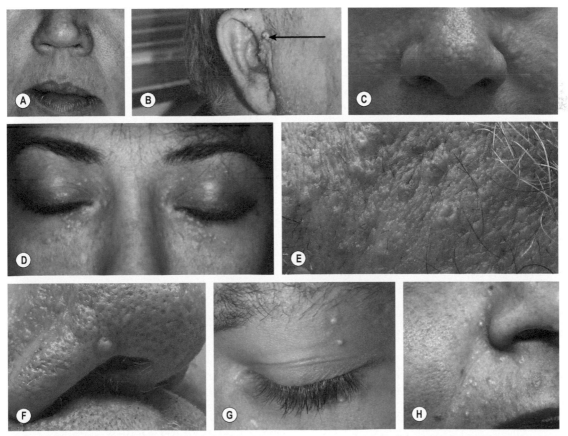

Fig. 2.1 Facial multiple papules, white–yellow. **A,B** Cowden syndrome. **C** Birt-Hogg-Dubé syndrome. **D** Syringomas. **E** Sebaceous hyperplasia. **F** Sebaceous adenomas in Muir–Torre syndrome. **G** Milia. **H** Multiple trichoepitheliomas. *A, Courtesy, Kalman Watsky, MD; B, Courtesy, Jennifer Choi, MD; C, Courtesy, Barry Goldberg, MD; D,G, Courtesy, Yale Dermatology Residents' Slide Collection; F, Courtesy, Dan Ring, MD; H, Courtesy, Sean Christensen, MD, PhD. A,F,G, From Bolognia JL, Jorizzo JL, Schaffer JV. Dermatology, 3e. London: Saunders, 2012, with permission.*

FACIAL: Multiple Papules, Red–Pink to Brown

- **Acne vulgaris** – comedones and/or pustules present as well
- **Acne rosacea** – absent comedones, telangiectasias often evident
- **Granulomatous rosacea** – brown–pink discrete papules

- **Angiofibromas** of tuberous sclerosis – firm papules clustered near nose/nasolabial folds
- **Trichoepitheliomas** and/or **cylindromas** – nose/nasolabial folds or other parts of face, other stigmata of tuberous sclerosis absent

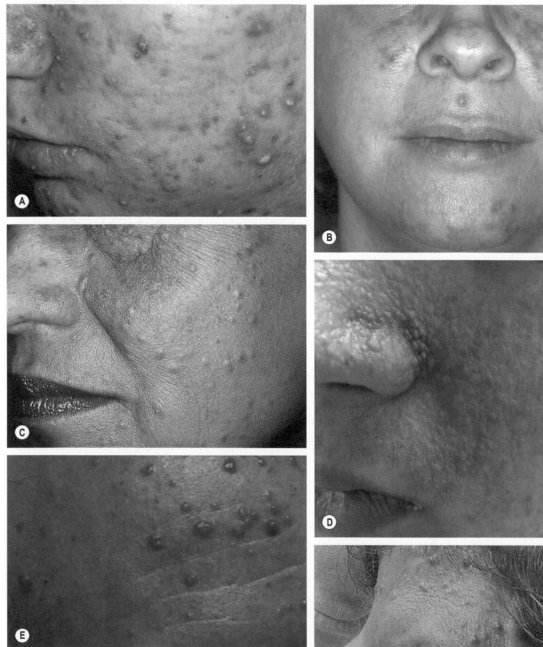

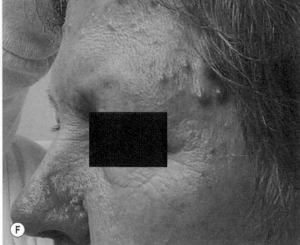

Fig. 2.2 Facial multiple papules, red–pink to brown.
A Acne vulgaris. **B** Acne rosacea. **C** Granulomatous rosacea.
D Angiofibromas of tuberous sclerosis. **E** Multiple familial
trichoepitheliomas. **F** Multiple cylindromas. *A, Courtesy,
Andrea L Zaenglein, MD and Diane Thiboutot, MD; B,C,
Courtesy, Yale Dermatology Residents' Slide Collection; D,
Courtesy, Brian Shuch, MD. A,C, From Bolognia JL, Jorizzo JL,
Schaffer JV. Dermatology, 3e. London: Saunders, 2012, with
permission.*

FACIAL: Acneiform Lesions

Key Differences (Fig. 2.3)

- **Acne vulgaris** – presence of open and closed comedones
- **Steroid-induced rosacea** – erythematous papules and papulopustules, absent comedones
- **Periorificial dermatitis** – monomorphous papules, confluent around the mouth
- **Keratosis pilaris rubra** – "grain-like" follicular papules on a background of erythema
- **Trichostasis spinulosa** – often on the nose; follicular orifices contain vellus hairs and keratinous debris that can be extruded with pressure
- **Pseudofolliculitis barbae** – follicular-based papules over the beard area

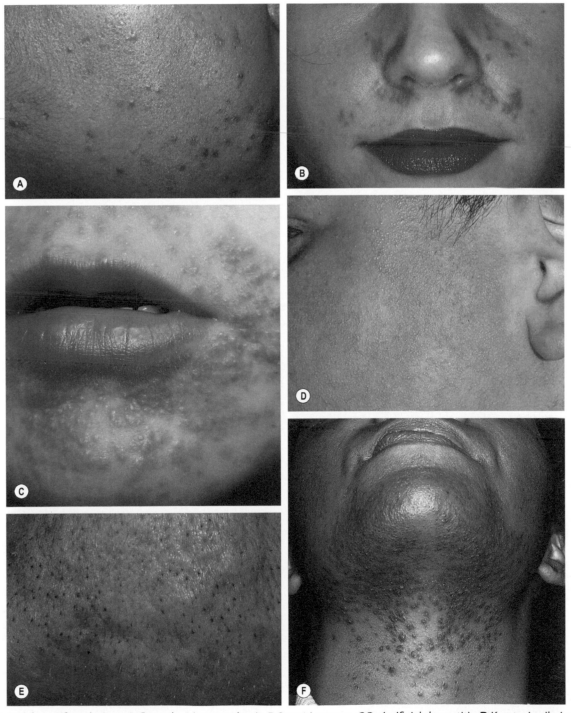

Fig. 2.3 Facial acneiform lesions. **A** Comedonal acne vulgaris. **B** Steroid rosacea. **C** Periorificial dermatitis. **D** Keratosis pilaris rubra. **E** Trichostasis spinulosa. **F** Pseudofolliculitis barbae. *A, Courtesy, Andrea L Zaenglein, MD and Diane Thiboutot, MD; B, Courtesy, Kalman Watsky, MD; C, Courtesy, Yale Dermatology Residents' Slide Collection; D, Courtesy, Julie V Schaffer, MD; E, Courtesy, Judit Stenn, MD; F, Courtesy, A Paul Kelly, MD. A,B,D–F, From Bolognia JL, Jorizzo JL, Schaffer JV. Dermatology, 3e. London: Saunders, 2012, with permission.*

FACIAL: Pustules

Pustules (see Chapter 11) may be sterile or caused by an infectious agent, in which case culture studies and/or biopsy may be necessary for a definitive diagnosis.

- **Acne vulgaris** – comedones often present
- **Acne rosacea** – absent comedones, background erythema/telangiectasias
- **Fungal or bacterial infection** – erythematous plaque studded with pustules

- **Herpes virus infection** – clustered vesicles and/or pustules; base may be erythematous

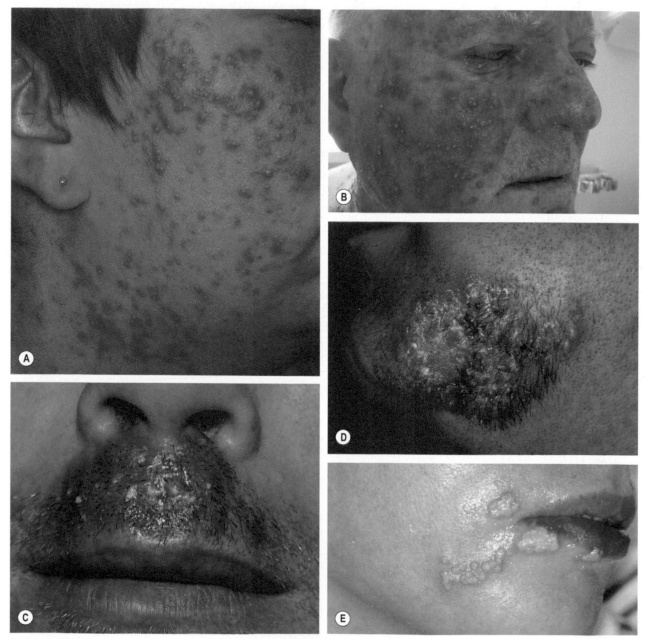

Fig. 2.4 Facial pustules. **A** Acne vulgaris. **B** Acne rosacea. **C** Fungal infection. **D** Staphylococcal folliculitis. **E** Herpes simplex virus infection. *A,C, Courtesy, Kalman Watsky, MD; B, Courtesy Uwe Wollina, MD; D, Courtesy, Yale Dermatology Residents' Slide Collection; E, Courtesy, Dirk Elston, MD. A,C,D, From Bolognia JL, Jorizzo JL, Schaffer JV. Dermatology, 3e. London: Saunders, 2012, with permission. B, From Wollina U. Rosacea and rhinophyma in the elderly. Clin Dermatol. 2011;29:61–8. E, From Elston D. Clinical image collection. Dermatopathology, 2e. London: Saunders, 2014.*

FACIAL: "Telangiectasia"

Key Differences (Fig. 2.5)

- **CREST syndrome (limited systemic sclerosis)** – mat-like (squared-off) telangiectasias
- **Osler–Weber–Rendu disease** – papular lesions (caused by arteriovenous malformations), affecting mucosal surfaces (lips, tongue, nasal)
- **Rosacea, erythematotelangiectatic** – overlaps with dermatoheliosis
- **Dermatoheliosis** – telangiectasias and erythema over facial prominences

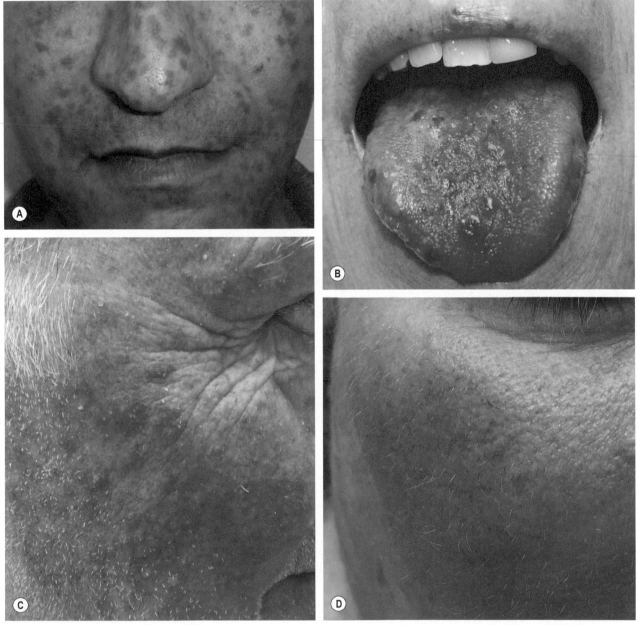

Fig. 2.5 Facial "telangiectasia." **A** CREST syndrome (limited systemic sclerosis). **B** Hereditary hemorrhagic telangiectasia (Osler–Weber–Rendu disease). **C** Erythematotelangiectatic rosacea. **D** Dermatoheliosis. *A, Courtesy, M Kari Connolly, MD; B, Courtesy, Yale Dermatology Residents' Slide Collection; C, From Two AM, Wu W, Gallo RL. Hata TR Rosacea : Part I. Introduction, categorization, histology, pathogenesis, and risk factors. J Am Acad Dermatol 2015; 72: 749–758, with permission. A, From Bolognia JL, Jorizzo JL, Schaffer JV. Dermatology, 3e. London: Saunders, 2012, with permission.*

Key Differences (Fig. 2.6)

- **Rosacea** – erythema is often fixed; telangiectasias in more advanced disease
- **Acute lupus erythematosus** – sparing of nasolabial folds, small erosions; scales may be present
- **Dermatomyositis** – involvement of eyelids and nasolabial folds
- **Allergic contact dermatitis** – edema and weeping lesions
- **Pemphigus erythematosus** – plaques with scale-crust that can lift at edges, like cornflakes, and obvious erosions
- **Seborrheic dermatitis** – greasy scale, often accentuated in nasolabial folds

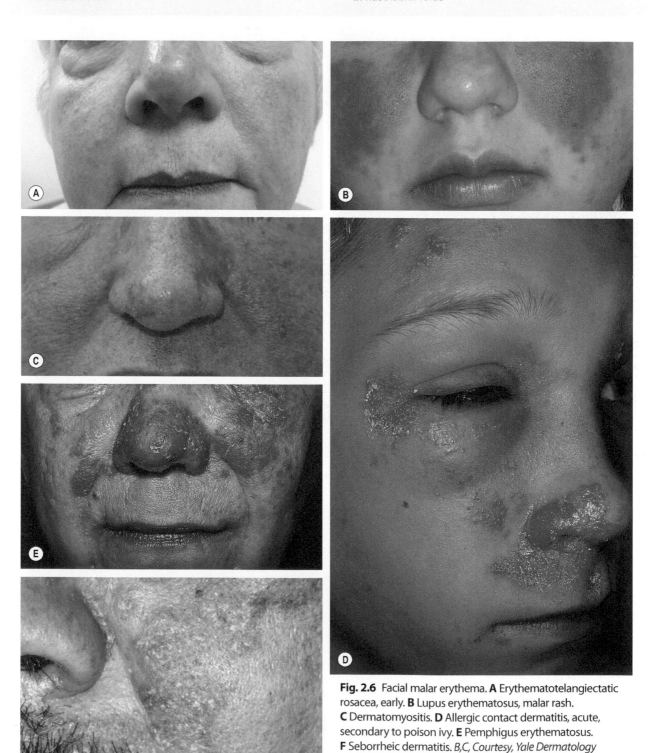

Fig. 2.6 Facial malar erythema. **A** Erythematotelangiectatic rosacea, early. **B** Lupus erythematosus, malar rash. **C** Dermatomyositis. **D** Allergic contact dermatitis, acute, secondary to poison ivy. **E** Pemphigus erythematosus. **F** Seborrheic dermatitis. *B,C, Courtesy, Yale Dermatology Residents' Slide Collection; D, Courtesy, Jean L Bolognia, MD; E, Courtesy, Ronald P Rapini, MD; F, Courtesy, Dirk Elston, MD. D,E, From Bolognia JL, Jorizzo JL, Schaffer JV. Dermatology, 3e. London: Saunders, 2012, with permission. F, From Elston D. Clinical image collection. Dermatopathology, 2e. London: Saunders, 2014.*

FACIAL: Juicy Papules/Plaques/Nodules

The infiltrate may be lymphocytic, mixed, neutrophilic, or granulomatous.

Key Differences (Fig. 2.7)

Lymphocytic
- Lymphoma:
- **Folliculotropic mycosis fungoides** – infiltrated plaque with loss of eyebrow hair
- **B-cell lymphoma** – pink–red to purple papulonodules
- **Lupus tumidus** – pink–violet plaques
- **Lymphocytic infiltrate of Jessner** – often annular, absent scale
- **Polymorphous light eruption** – edematous pink lesions, occur minutes to hours after sun exposure in spring and early summer

Mixed
- **Granuloma faciale** – red–brown plaque with prominent follicular orifices

Neutrophilic
- **Sweet syndrome** – crusted bright red papulonodules

Granulomatous
- **Sarcoidosis** – often affects the nose, infiltrated violaceous to red–brown plaque

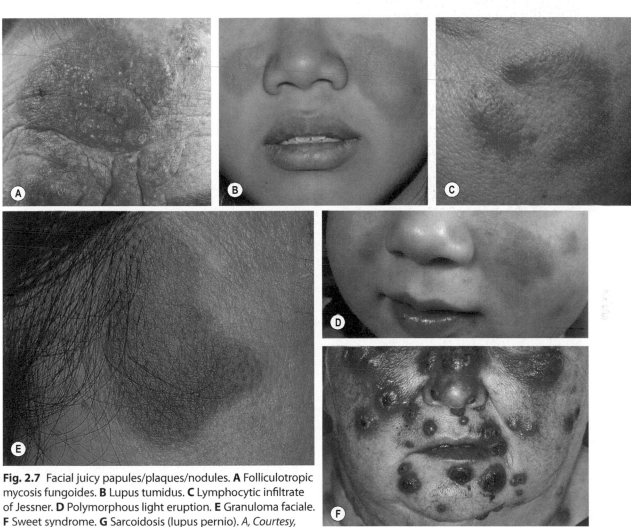

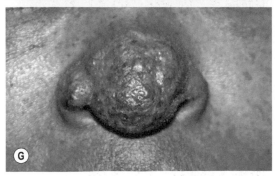

Fig. 2.7 Facial juicy papules/plaques/nodules. **A** Folliculotropic mycosis fungoides. **B** Lupus tumidus. **C** Lymphocytic infiltrate of Jessner. **D** Polymorphous light eruption. **E** Granuloma faciale. **F** Sweet syndrome. **G** Sarcoidosis (lupus pernio). *A, Courtesy, Rein Willemze, MD; B, Courtesy, Julie V Schaffer, MD; C, E, G, Courtesy, Yale Dermatology Residents' Slide Collection; D, NYU Slide Collection; F, Courtesy, Kalman Watsky, MD. A–G, From Bolognia JL, Jorizzo JL, Schaffer JV. Dermatology, 3e. London: Saunders, 2012, with permission.*

FACIAL: Flat Brown Patch

May be secondary to increased melanocytes, increased melanin, and/or dermal pigment.

- **Lentigo maligna (melanoma *in situ*)** – irregular, with color variation
- **Melasma** – evenly light brown, with an irregular border
- **Hori nevus** – light brown to blue–gray macules clustering into patches, on cheeks, typically in Asian women

- **Ochronosis** – brown to black patches secondary to topical hydroquinone

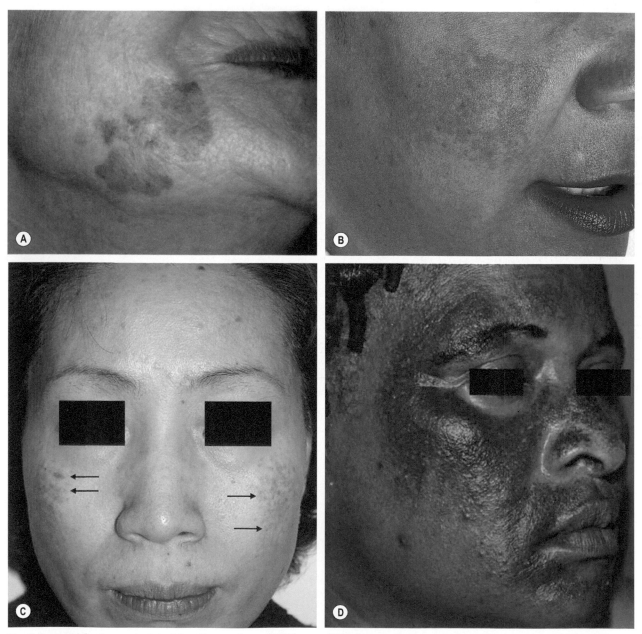

Fig. 2.8 Facial flat brown patch. **A** Lentigo maligna. **B** Melasma. **C** Hori nevus. **D** Ochronosis. *A, Courtesy, Yale Dermatology Residents' Slide Collection. B, Courtesy, NYU Slide Collection. D, Courtesy, Regional Dermatology Training Centre, Moshi, Tanzania. A,B, From Bolognia JL, Jorizzo JL, Schaffer JV. Dermatology, 3e. London: Saunders, 2012, with permission. C From, Park JM, Tsao H, Tsao S. Acquired bilateral nevus of Ota-like macules (Hori nevus). J Am Acad Dermatol. 2009;61:88–93. D, From Bolognia JL, Schaffer JV, Duncan KO, Ko CJ. Dermatology Essentials, 1e. Philadelphia: Saunders, 2014, with permission.*

FACIAL: Annular or Serpiginous

Key Differences (Fig. 2.9)

- **Tinea faciei** – scales may be minimal; pustules may be present; annular shape may be irregular
- **Seborrheic dermatitis, petaloid** – fine scales over regular, annular rings
- **Annular elastolytic giant cell granuloma** – central clearing, pink–red rim with minimal scale

- **Neonatal lupus erythematosus** – pink rings around eyes ("raccoon eyes"); circular pink macules and patches on the forehead and cheeks
- **Lymphocytic infiltrate of Jessner** – absent scale (see Fig. 2.7C)

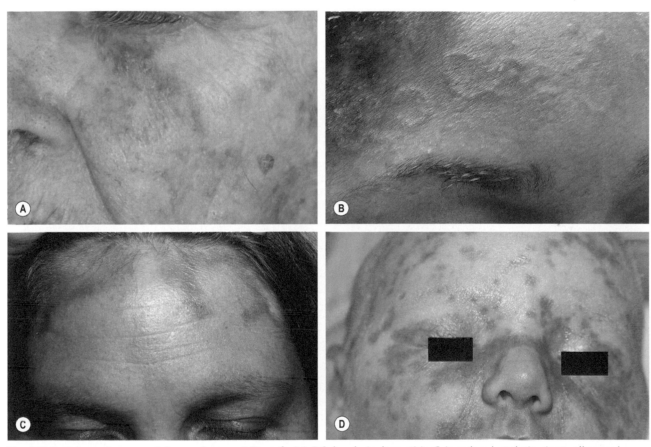

Fig. 2.9 Facial annular or serpiginous plaques. **A** Tinea faciei. **B** Seborrheic dermatitis. **C** Annular elastolytic giant cell granuloma (actinic granuloma). **D** Neonatal lupus erythematosus. *A, Courtesy, Jean L Bolognia, MD. From Bolognia JL, Jorizzo JL, Schaffer JV. Dermatology, 3e. London: Saunders, 2012, with permission. C, From James WD, Berger T, Elston D. Andrews' Diseases of the Skin, 11e. Edinburgh: Saunders, 2011, with permission. D, Courtesy, Yale Dermatology Residents' Slide Collection.*

FACIAL: Lip Swelling

May be secondary to edema, an infiltrative process, or a tumor.

- **Angioedema** – swelling of lips, often the periorbital region as well; absent erythema
- **Granulomatous cheilitis** – swelling of lip (lower > upper or both), ultimately becomes persistent; may be

associated with scrotal tongue and/or facial nerve palsy (Melkersson–Rosenthal syndrome)
- **Squamous cell carcinoma** – hyperkeratosis and induration of the lower lip

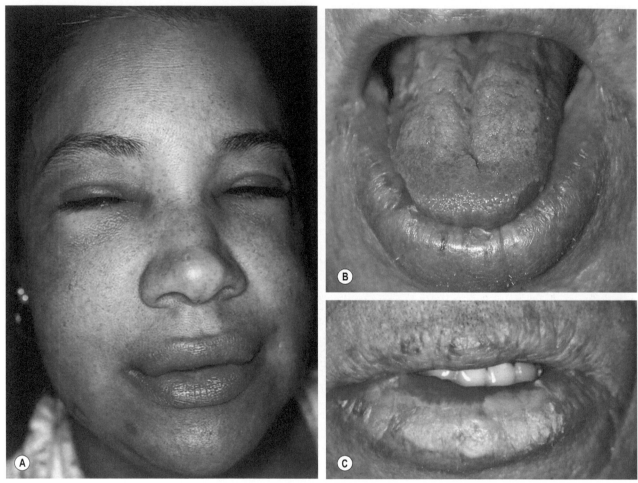

Fig. 2.10 Lip swelling and/or crusting. **A** Angioedema. **B** Granulomatous cheilitis. **C** Squamous cell carcinoma.

FACIAL: Lip Crusting

- **Erythema multiforme** or **Stevens–Johnson syndrome** – crusting and slight swelling of vermilion lips with slight extension beyond vermilion
- *Mycoplasma pneumoniae*–**induced rash and mucositis** – crusting and slight swelling, generally limited to the vermilion lips
- **Staphylococcal scalded skin syndrome** – child with a wrinkled, "old" appearance of the cutaneous lip around focal crusting on the vermilion lip

- **Irritant contact dermatitis** – irritation from a contactant, which mainly affected the lower lip in this case, with severe crusting of the lower > upper vermilion
- **Primary herpetic gingivostomatitis** – numerous discrete vesicles, some crusted, that are focally confluent on the vermilion lips and chin; there are scattered pink–red vesicles on the face surrounding the lips

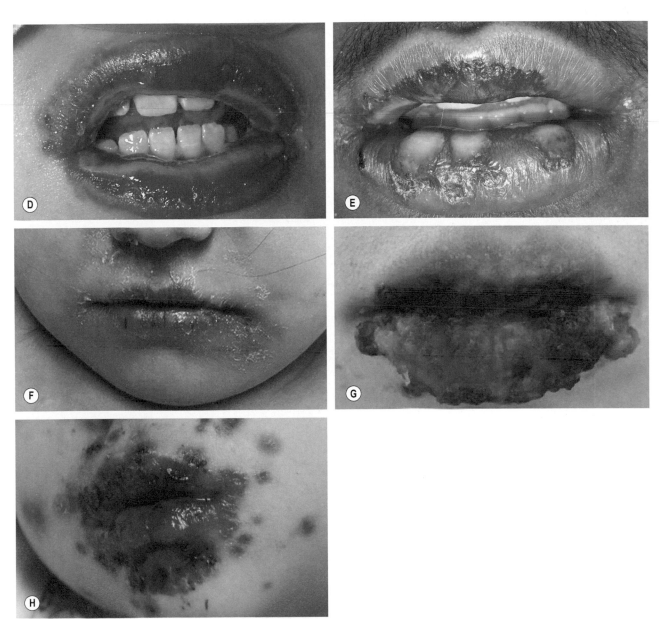

Fig. 2.10, cont'd   D Erythema multiforme. **E** *Mycoplasma pneumoniae*-induced rash and mucositis. **F** Staphylococcal scalded skin syndrome. **G** Irritant contact dermatitis. **H** Primary herpetic gingivostomatitis. *A, Courtesy, Clive E H Grattan, MD; B,D-H Courtesy, Yale Dermatology Residents' Slide Collection; C, Courtesy, H Peter Sawyer, MD. A,C, From Bolognia JL, Jorizzo JL, Schaffer JV. Dermatology, 3e. London: Saunders, 2012, with permission.*

FACIAL: Tongue

Key Differences (Fig. 2.11)

- **Geographic tongue** – well-delineated erythema with white serpiginous borders
- **Fissured (scrotal) tongue** – furrows and grooves
- **Amyloidosis** – macroglossia (impressions of teeth may be evident on lateral borders)
- **Hairy tongue** – elongated, discolored papillae
- **Median rhomboid glossitis** – diamond to oval area of erythema and atrophy, often caused by local overgrowth of *Candida*

- **Thrush** – solid white plaques in random distribution
- **Oral hairy leukoplakia** – shaggy white plaques on lateral tongue
- **Lichen planus** – erosions, lacy white plaques, and/or scarring

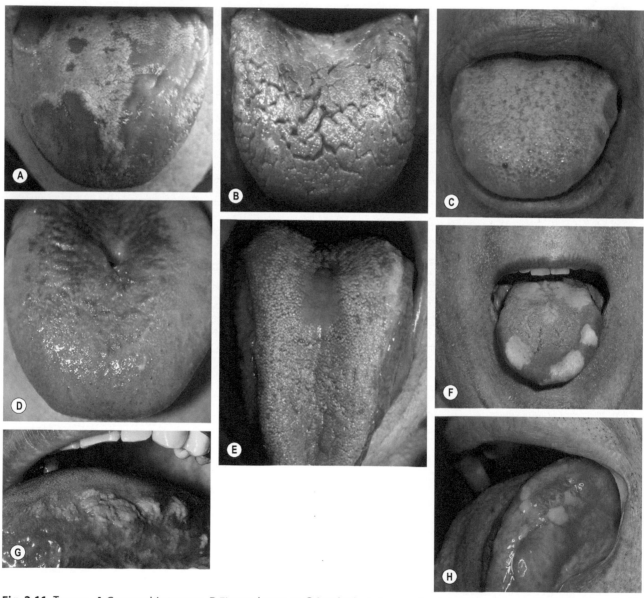

Fig. 2.11 Tongue. **A** Geographic tongue. **B** Fissured tongue. **C** Amyloidosis (macroglossia). **D** Hairy tongue. **E** Median rhomboid glossitis. **F** Thrush. **G** Oral hairy leukoplakia. **H** Lichen planus. *A–D, Courtesy, Yale Dermatology Residents' Slide Collection; E, Courtesy, NYU Slide Collection; G, Courtesy, Carl M Allen, MD, and Charles Camisa, MD; H, Courtesy, Louis A Fragola, Jr, MD. E,G, From Bolognia JL, Schaffer JV, Duncan KO, Ko CJ. Dermatology Essentials, 1e. Philadelphia: Saunders, 2014, with permission. F,H, From Bolognia JL, Jorizzo JL, Schaffer JV. Dermatology, 3e. London: Saunders, 2012, with permission.*

FACIAL: Gingiva

Key Differences (Fig. 2.12)

- **Desquamative (erosive) gingivitis** – erythema and erosions, associated with blistering disorders, such as cicatricial pemphigoid and pemphigus vulgaris
- **Gingival hyperplasia** – caused by medications (e.g. phenytoin, cyclosporine), mouth breathing, poor hygiene, infiltrative processes

- **Strawberry gums** – red–purple gingiva, resembling strawberries
- **Cobblestoning** – numerous papules

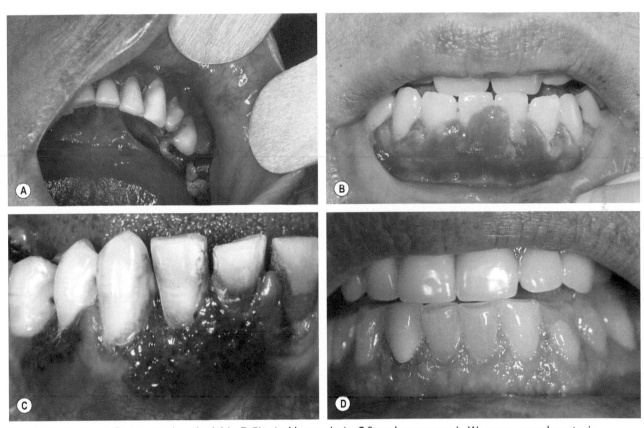

Fig. 2.12 Gingiva. **A** Desquamative gingivitis. **B** Gingival hyperplasia. **C** Strawberry gums in Wegener granulomatosis. **D** Gingival cobblestoning in Cowden syndrome. *A,B, Courtesy, Yale Dermatology Residents' Slide Collection; C, Courtesy Carl M Allen, MD, and Charles Camisa, MD. D, Courtesy, Jeffrey Callen, MD. A,C,D, From Bolognia JL, Jorizzo JL, Schaffer JV. Dermatology, 3e. London: Saunders, 2012, with permission.*

FACIAL: Buccal Mucosa

- **Morsicatio buccarum** – shaggy white plaque along bite line
- **Lichen planus** – lacy white plaques; erosions may be evident
- **Thrush** – cottage cheese–like white papules
- **Koplik spots of measles** – pinpoint white papules near molars

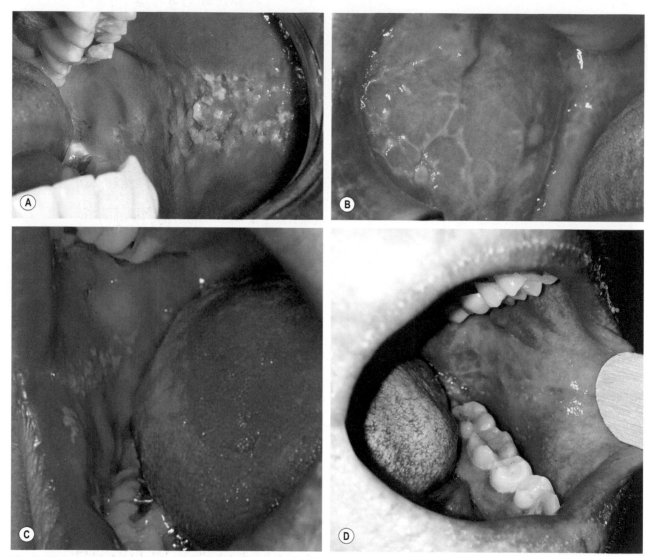

Fig. 2.13 Buccal mucosa. **A** Morsicatio buccarum. **B** Lichen planus. **C** Thrush. **D** Koplik spots of measles. *A, Courtesy Carl M Allen, MD, and Charles Camisa, MD; B,D Courtesy, Yale Dermatology Residents' Slide Collection; C, Courtesy, Judit Stenn, MD. A–C, From Bolognia JL, Jorizzo JL, Schaffer JV. Dermatology, 3e. London: Saunders, 2012, with permission.*

BODY FOLDS

BODY FOLDS: Diaper Area (Infants)

Key Differences (Fig. 2.14)

- **Irritant contact dermatitis** – spares folds
- **Candidiasis** – bright red erythema, satellite papulopustules (arrows)
- **Seborrheic dermatitis** – moist/scaly plaques, involving folds
- **Psoriasis** – well-demarcated, uniformly pink plaques, psoriatic lesions outside of body folds
- **Langerhans cell histiocytosis** – petechiae, erosions/ulcers

BODY FOLDS: Perineum/Groin of Adults

Key Differences (Fig. 2.15)

- **Intertrigo** – moist appearance
- **Inverse psoriasis** – well-demarcated, uniformly pink–red patches
- **Tinea** – often spares scrotum, annular border
- **Candidiasis** – often involves scrotum, satellite papulopustules
- **Erythrasma** – pink to brown scaly patches, pink fluorescence under Wood's lamp
- **Hailey–Hailey disease** – irregularly cracked appearance of linear erosions
- **Extramammary Paget disease** – white hyperkeratosis intermixed with red eroded foci
- **Langerhans cell histiocytosis** – petechiae and erosions

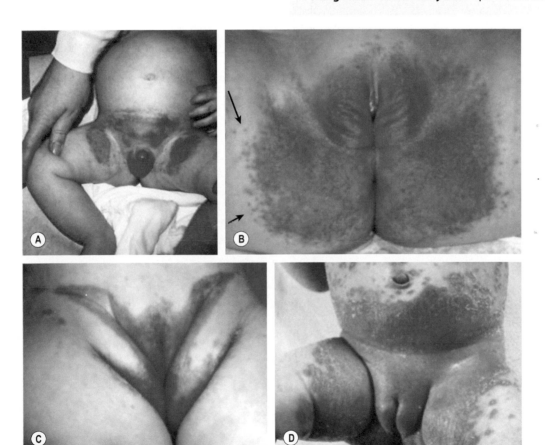

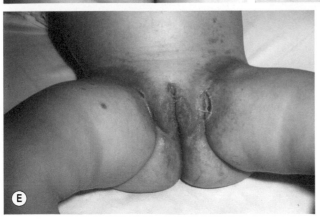

Fig. 2.14 Diaper area (infants). **A** Irritant contact dermatitis. **B** Candidiasis. **C** Seborrheic dermatitis. **D** Psoriasis. **E** Langerhans cell histiocytosis. *A–D, From Schachner LA, Hansen RE. Pediatric Dermatology, 4e. London: Mosby, 2011, with permission. E, Courtesy, Irwin Braverman, MD.*

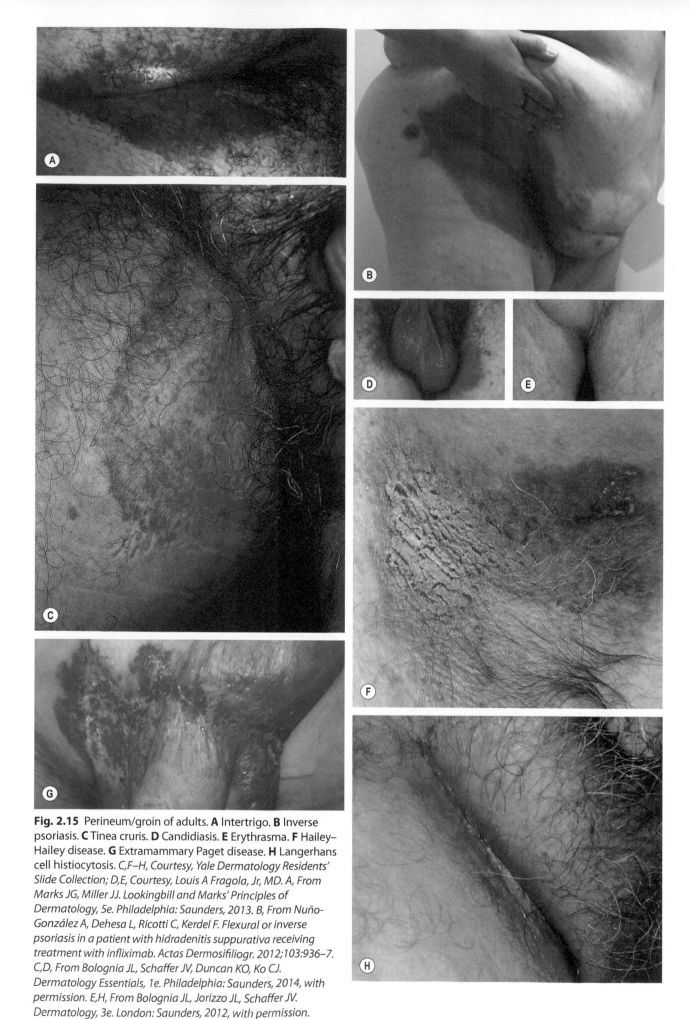

Fig. 2.15 Perineum/groin of adults. **A** Intertrigo. **B** Inverse psoriasis. **C** Tinea cruris. **D** Candidiasis. **E** Erythrasma. **F** Hailey–Hailey disease. **G** Extramammary Paget disease. **H** Langerhans cell histiocytosis. *C,F–H, Courtesy, Yale Dermatology Residents' Slide Collection; D,E, Courtesy, Louis A Fragola, Jr, MD. A, From Marks JG, Miller JJ. Lookingbill and Marks' Principles of Dermatology, 5e. Philadelphia: Saunders, 2013. B, From Nuño-González A, Dehesa L, Ricotti C, Kerdel F. Flexural or inverse psoriasis in a patient with hidradenitis suppurativa receiving treatment with infliximab. Actas Dermosifiliogr. 2012;103:936–7. C,D, From Bolognia JL, Schaffer JV, Duncan KO, Ko CJ. Dermatology Essentials, 1e. Philadelphia: Saunders, 2014, with permission. E,H, From Bolognia JL, Jorizzo JL, Schaffer JV. Dermatology, 3e. London: Saunders, 2012, with permission.*

BODY FOLDS: Vulvar Rash

- **Lichen sclerosus** – initially affects the clitoral hood and the perineal body; petechiae may be evident; shiny ivory–white plaque is classic; late stage with scarring
- **Lichen planus** – lacy white hyperkeratosis (arrow) may be evident; erosions often present on mucosal surfaces; late stage with scarring
- **Lichen simplex chronicus** – thickening (lichenification) +/– erythema
- **Psoriasis** – red plaques that may be well demarcated
- **Hailey–Hailey disease** – irregularly cracked appearance of linear erosions

BODY FOLDS: Perianal Rash

- **Perianal streptococcal disease** – sharply demarcated bright, moist erythema extending from the anal verge
- **Lichen sclerosus** – ivory–white foci (arrow)
- **Psoriasis** – well-demarcated, uniformly pink–red
- **Irritant contact dermatitis (erosive perianal eruption)** – often caused by frequent stooling and/or diarrhea in young babies; favors convex surfaces
- **Hand, foot, and mouth disease** – circular erosions and papulovesicles (see also Fig. 12.17)
- **Zinc deficiency** – perianal weepy plaques with peripheral crusting (see also Fig. 8.16)

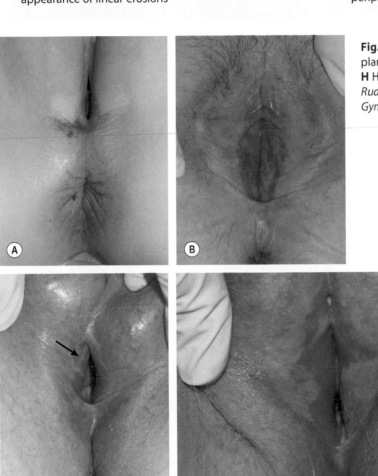

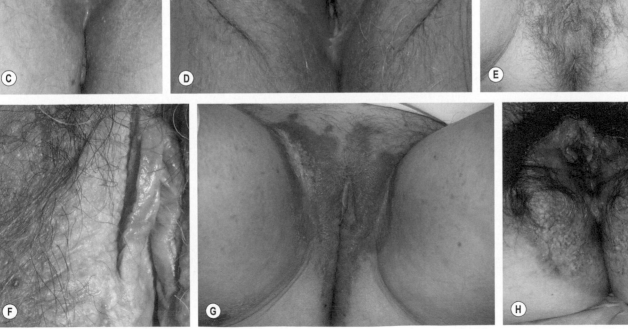

Fig. 2.16 Vulvar rash. **A,B** Lichen sclerosus. **C,D** Lichen planus. **E,F** Lichen simplex chronicus. **G** Psoriasis. **H** Hailey–Hailey disease. *A–H, From Black MM, Ambros-Rudolph C, Edwards L, Lynch PJ. Obstetric and Gynecologic Dermatology, 3e. London: Mosby, 2008.*

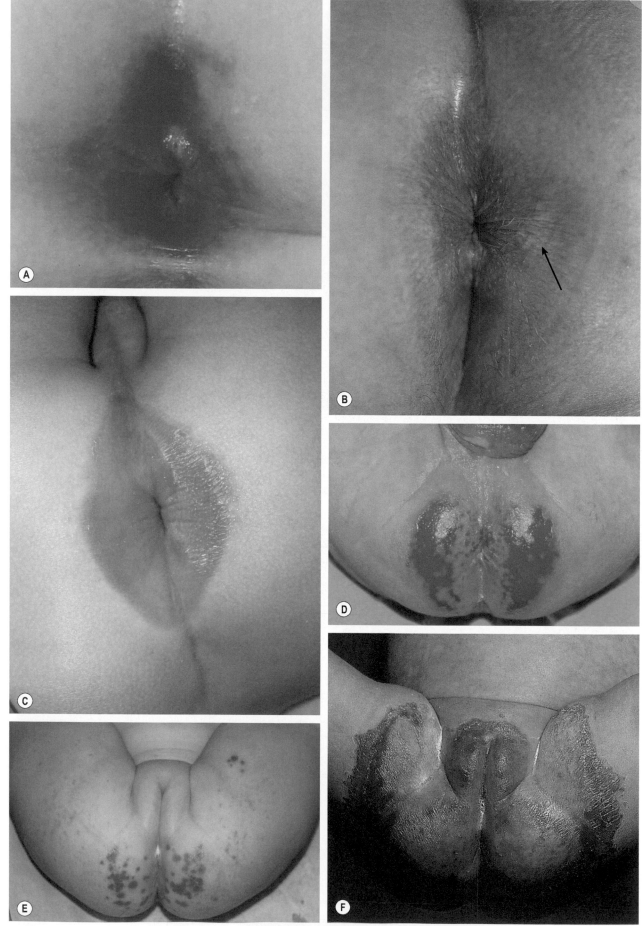

Fig. 2.17 Perianal rash. **A** Perianal streptococcal disease. **B** Lichen sclerosus. **C** Psoriasis. **D** Irritant contact dermatitis. **E** Hand, foot, and mouth disease. **F** Zinc deficiency. *B, Courtesy, Susan M Cooper, MD. A, Courtesy, Julie V Schaffer, MD. A,B, From Bolognia JL, Jorizzo JL, Schaffer JV. Dermatology, 3e. London: Saunders, 2012, with permission. C–F, From Eichenfield LF, Frieden IJ, Zaenglein AL, Mathes E. Neonatal and Infant Dermatology, 3e. London: Saunders, 2014.*

ACRAL: Palmar Rash

Key Differences (Fig. 2.18)

- **Eczematous dermatitis,** including **atopic dermatitis** and **contact dermatitis** – weeping, crusted lesions, often with foci of lichenification and fissuring; patch testing is important to differentiate allergic contact dermatitis from other eczematous processes, as clinical findings can be very similar
- **Dyshidrosis** – deep-seated vesicles on lateral surfaces of fingers

- **Psoriasis** – adherent, dry white–yellow scale over erythema
- **Tinea** – scales accentuated in creases; one hand may be spared
- **Crusted scabies** – prominent hyperkeratosis over hands and subungually

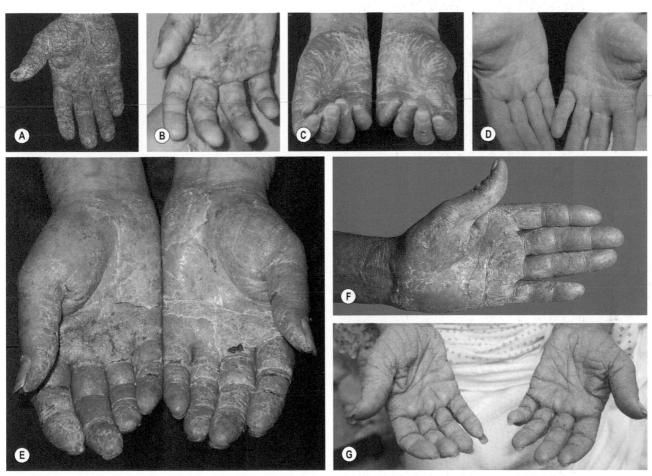

Fig. 2.18 Palmar rash. **A** Atopic dermatitis. **B** Dyshidrotic eczema. **C** Psoriasis. **D** Tinea manuum. **E** Irritant contact dermatitis. **F** Allergic contact dermatitis to chromate found in cement. **G** Crusted scabies. *A,D,G, Courtesy, Yale Dermatology Residents' Slide Collection; B, Courtesy, Dirk Elston, MD; C, Courtesy, Peter C M van de Kerkhof, MD; E, Courtesy, Kalman Watsky, MD; F, Courtesy, Peter S Friedmann, MD, and Mark Wilkinson, MD. A,C–F, From Bolognia JL, Jorizzo JL, Schaffer JV. Dermatology, 3e. London: Saunders, 2012, with permission. B, From Schachner LA, Hansen RE. Pediatric Dermatology, 4e. London: Mosby, 2011.*

CHAPTER

2

Differential Diagnosis for Given Body Sites and Morphology

ACRAL: Palmar Macules

- **Erythema multiforme** – target lesions with 3 zones; central zone may be vesicular
- **Syphilis, secondary** – brown–red macules, sometimes with a collarette of scale

ACRAL: Discrete Keratotic Lesions

- **Dyshidrotic eczema** – deep-seated vesicles (discrete spheres), often on the lateral fingers
- **Scabies** – linear burrows
- **Keratolysis exfoliativa** – annular collarettes of white scale

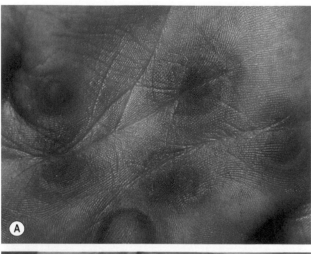

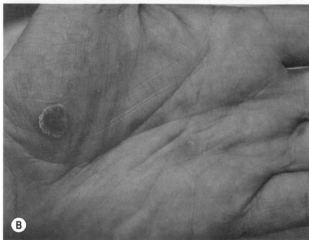

Fig. 2.19 Palmar macules. **A** Erythema multiforme.
B Secondary syphilis. *A, Courtesy, William Weston, MD; B, Courtesy, Yale Dermatology Residents' Slide Collection. A, From Bolognia JL, Jorizzo JL, Schaffer JV. Dermatology, 3e. London: Saunders, 2012, with permission.*

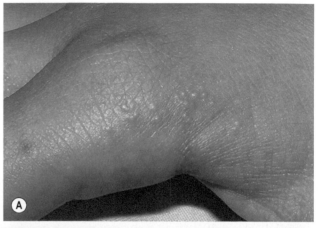

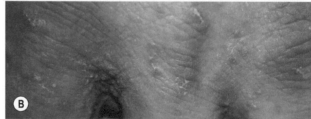

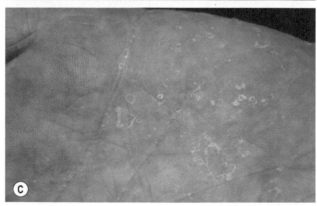

Fig. 2.20 Discrete keratotic lesions. **A** Dyshidrotic eczema.
B Scabies. **C** Keratolysis exfoliativa. *A, Courtesy, Anne Lucky, MD; B,C, Courtesy, Yale Dermatology Residents' Slide Collection. A, From Schachner LA, Hansen RE. Pediatric Dermatology, 4e. London: Mosby, 2011.*

ACRAL: Lower Leg Rash

Key Differences (Fig. 2.21)

- **Stasis dermatitis** – erythema, wet scale, often bilateral
- **Lipodermatosclerosis** – warm erythema when acute; tight skin; begins above the medial malleolus
- **Cellulitis** – warm, tender, often unilateral; expansion without treatment; associated fever and elevated white blood cell count
- **Necrobiosis lipoidica** – yellowish center, often with telangiectasia

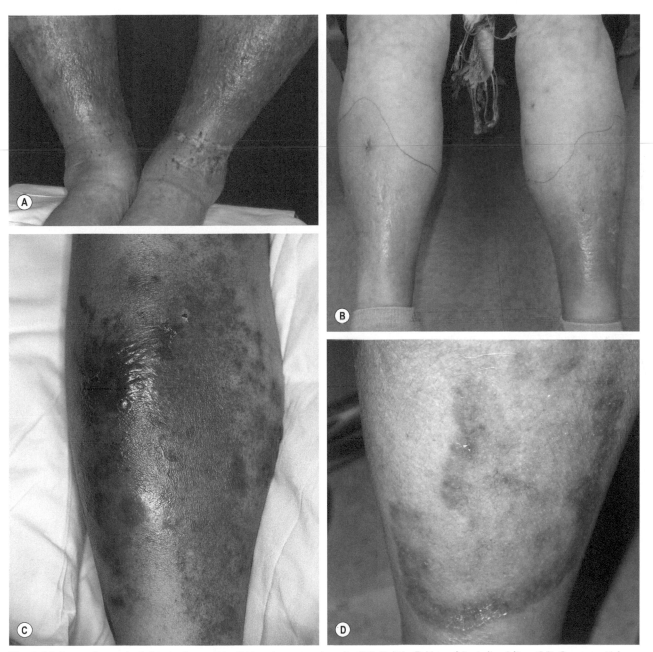

Fig. 2.21 Lower leg rash. **A** Stasis dermatitis. **B** Lipodermatosclerosis. **C** Cellulitis. **D** Necrobiosis lipoidica. *C,D, Courtesy, Yale Dermatology Residents' Slide Collection. A, From Elston D. Clinical image collection. Dermatopathology, 2e. London: Saunders, 2014. C, From Bolognia JL, Jorizzo JL, Schaffer JV. Dermatology, 3e. London: Saunders, 2012, with permission.*

ACRAL: Plantar Keratotic Lesions

Key Differences (Fig. 2.22)

- **Pitted keratolysis** – punched-out craters; favor pressure points
- **Punctate keratoderma** – discrete foci of hyperkeratosis

- **Plantar warts** – black dots, representing thrombosed capillaries

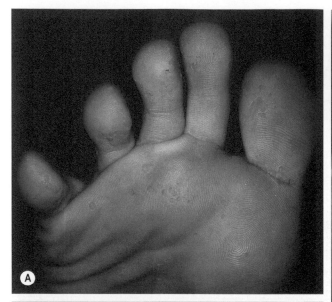

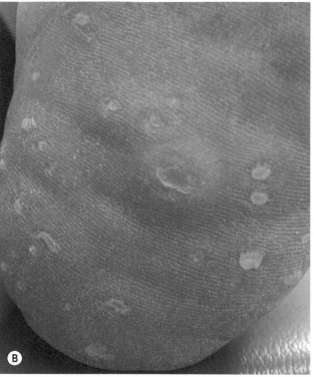

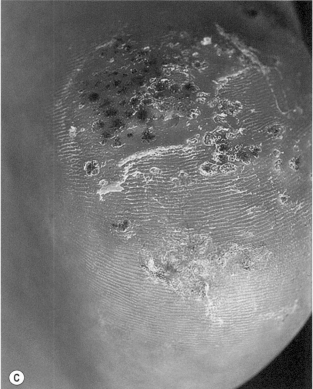

Fig. 2.22 Plantar keratotic lesions. **A** Pitted keratolysis. **B** Punctate keratoderma. **C** Plantar warts. *A, Courtesy, Kalman Watsky, MD; B, Courtesy, Yale Dermatology Residents' Slide Collection; C, Courtesy, Reinhard Kimabuer, MD, and Petra Lenz, MD. A,C, From Bolognia JL, Jorizzo JL, Schaffer JV. Dermatology, 3e. London: Saunders, 2012, with permission.*

ACRAL: Plantar Rash

Key Differences (Fig. 2.23)

- **Tinea pedis** – fine scale; hands or nails may be infected as well; pustules may be present
- **Psoriasis** – well-demarcated plaques with adherent thick scale
- **Contact dermatitis** – patch testing often necessary; distribution may give clue to the contactant
- **Juvenile plantar dermatosis** – glazed appearance

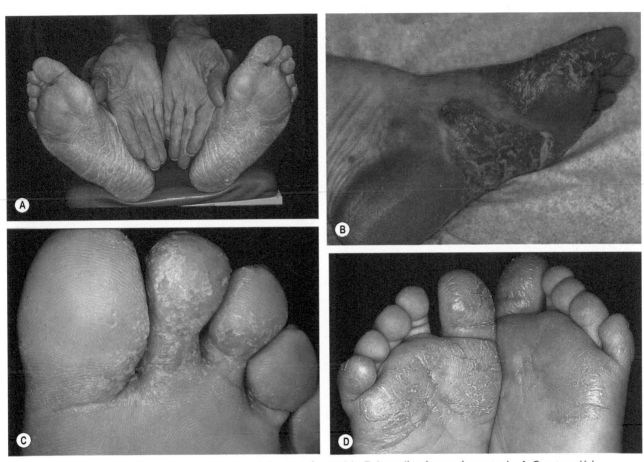

Fig. 2.23 Plantar rash. **A** Tinea pedis. **B** Psoriasis. **C** Contact dermatitis. **D** Juvenile plantar dermatosis. *A, Courtesy, Yale Dermatology Residents' Slide Collection; C, Courtesy, Louis A Fragola, Jr, MD; D, Courtesy, Kalman Watsky, MD. A,C,D, From Bolognia JL, Jorizzo JL, Schaffer JV. Dermatology, 3e. London: Saunders, 2012, with permission. B, From Menter A, Korman NJ, Elmets CA, et al. Guidelines of care for the management of psoriasis and psoriatic arthritis. J Am Acad Dermatol. 2011:65:137–74.*

TRUNCAL

TRUNCAL: Red–Brown to Pink Papules

Key Differences (Fig. 2.24)

- **Mastocytosis** – evenly pigmented red—brown papules that tend to be uniform; can blister with stroking
- **Histiocytosis** – discrete red–brown papules
- **Benign melanocytic nevi** – brown papules and macules that vary in size

- **Leiomyoma (pilar)** – pink to red–brown linear papules, often clustered
- **Neurofibromas** – soft, skin-colored to pinkish–tan, dome-shaped or polypoid, well-demarcated papules and nodules of various sizes, ill-defined violaceous lesions

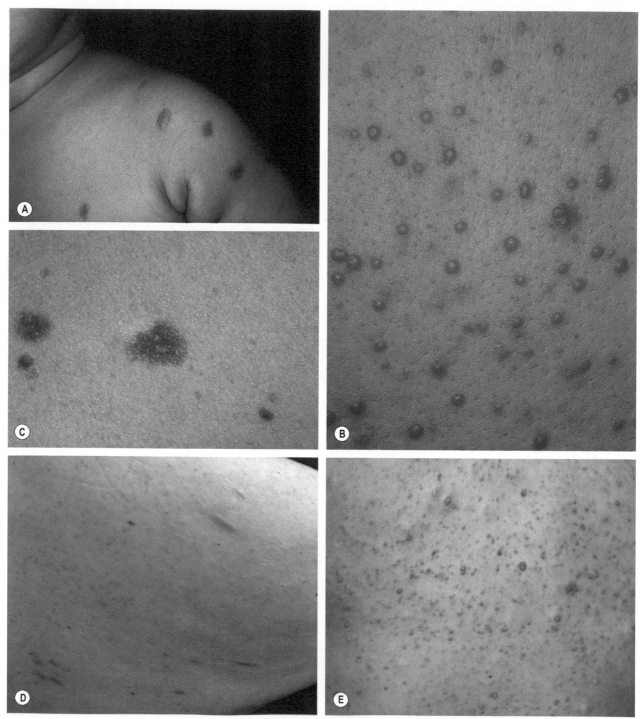

Fig. 2.24 Red–brown to pink papules on the trunk. **A** Mastocytosis. **B** Generalized eruptive histiocytoma. **C** Benign melanocytic nevi. **D** Pilar leiomyomas. **E** Neurofibromas. *A, Courtesy, Michael Tharp, MD; B, Courtesy, Yale Dermatology Residents' Slide Collection; C, Courtesy, Jean L Bolognia, MD; E, Courtesy, Julie V Schaffer, MD. A,B,E, From Bolognia JL, Jorizzo JL, Schaffer JV. Dermatology, 3e. London: Saunders, 2012, with permission.*

TRUNCAL: Rash on the Back, Hospitalized Patient

Key Differences (Fig. 2.25)

- **Drug eruption, maculopapular** – confluent pink macules and papules that extend beyond the back
- **Grover disease** – eroded pink papules, often sparing the buttocks

- **Folliculitis** – follicular papulopustules; often pustules are present

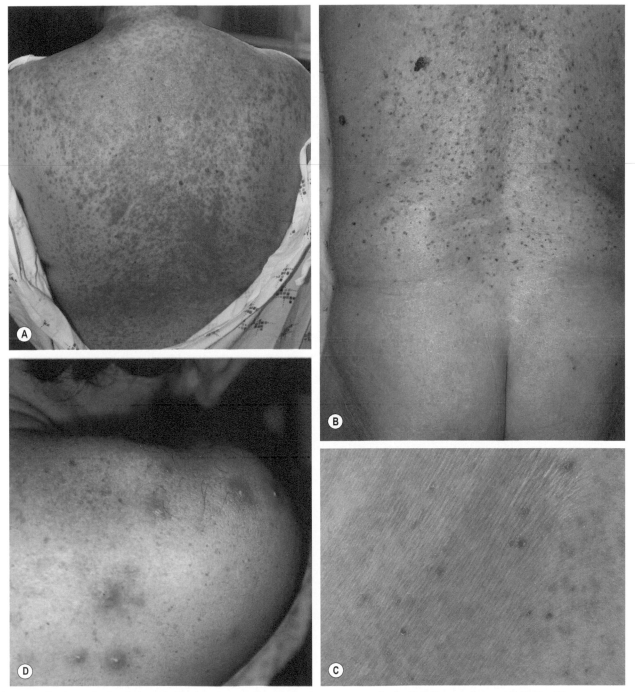

Fig. 2.25 Rash on the back, hospitalized patient. **A** Drug eruption to vemurafenib. **B,C** Grover disease. **D** Folliculitis. *A,D, Courtesy, Yale Dermatology Residents' Slide Collection; B, Courtesy, Jean L Bolognia, MD. B,D, From Bolognia JL, Jorizzo JL, Schaffer JV. Dermatology, 3e. London: Saunders, 2012, with permission.*

TRUNCAL: Pigment Change on Upper Back

- **Macular/biphasic amyloidosis** – rippled pattern of hyperpigmentation

- **Scleroderma (systemic sclerosis)** – salt and pepper pattern of pigment loss

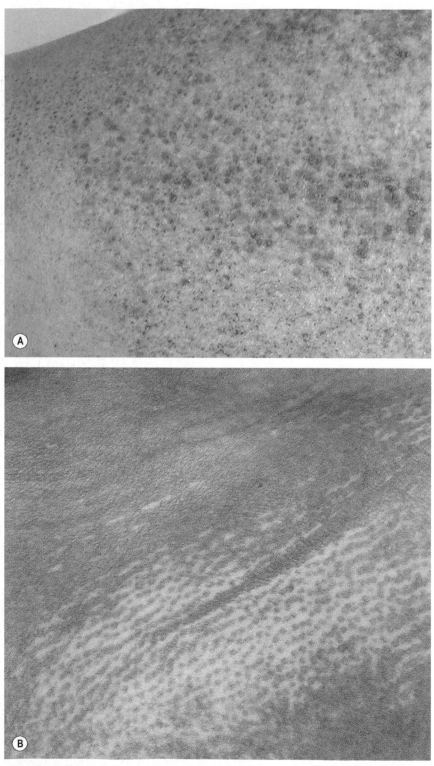

Fig. 2.26 Pigment change on upper back. **A** Biphasic amyloidosis. **B** Scleroderma.

Distribution – Specific Differentials | 3

This chapter covers three characteristic distributions: erythroderma, photodistribution, and mosaic (linear) lesions. Solitary pigmented lesions are also addressed because visual recognition of melanoma and its mimics is important.

ERYTHRODERMA (GENERALIZED ERYTHEMA)

Erythroderma (generalized erythema) can be caused by many different diseases. The color of the erythema, the presence/absence and quality of scales, and particular associated clues are helpful in separating these diseases (Table 3.1; Figs. 3.1–3.4). History and laboratory findings may also be useful.

Atopic dermatitis and other eczematous processes and other diseases can also present with erythroderma (Figs. 3.5–3.6).

Table 3.1 Erythroderma (generalized erythema)

Selected entities	Clinical	Salient clues, if present
Pityriasis rubra pilaris	• Salmon-pink to orange color • Fine scale	• Islands of sparing (Fig. 3.1A; see Fig. 5.12A) • Follicular papules (Fig. 3.1B) • Waxy palmoplantar keratoderma (Fig. 3.1C) • Nails: thickened • History of cephalocaudal spread
Psoriasis	• Pink–red color (Fig. 3.2A) • Silvery to white thick adherent scale, when present (Fig. 3.2B)	• Pustules • Nails: pitting or other changes • History of plaque-type psoriasis
Congenital ichthyosiform erythroderma (autosomal recessive congenital ichthyosis)	• Red–pink color (Fig. 3.3A–D) • Fine scale (may also have focal lamellar scales) (Fig. 3.3A–C)	• Ectropion • History of collodion membrane at birth
Erythrodermic mycosis fungoides	• Variable color • Variable scale • Variable atrophy or wrinkling	• Lymphadenopathy • History of mycosis fungoides
Sézary syndrome (Fig. 3.4)		• Distinguished from erythrodermic mycosis fungoides by circulating abnormal lymphocytes

Note: Not uncommonly, erythroderma can also be drug induced, of unknown cause (idiopathic), or caused by other disorders. (See also Figs 3.5, 3.6.)

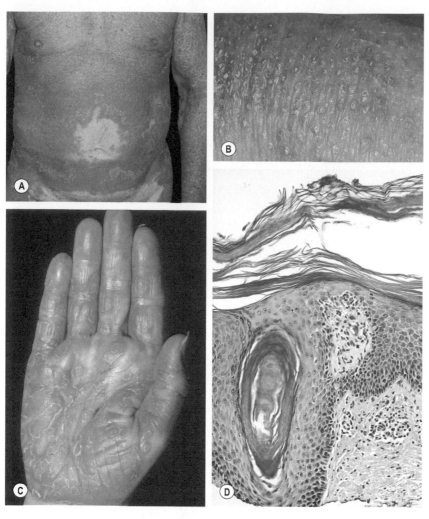

Fig. 3.1 Pityriasis rubra pilaris. **A** Islands of sparing. **B** Follicular prominence. **C** Waxy pink thickening of the palm. **D** Typical histopathologic findings include follicular plugging and hyperorthokeratosis alternating with parakeratosis in a checkerboard configuration. *A–C, From Schwarzenberger K, Werchniak AE, Ko C. General Dermatology. London: Saunders, 2009.*

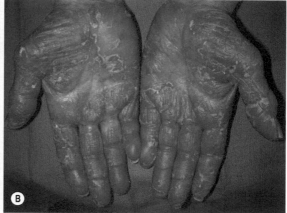

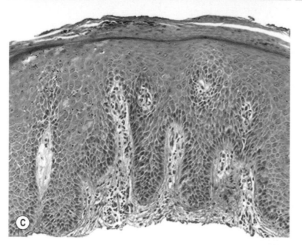

Fig. 3.2 Psoriasis, erythrodermic. **A** Red erythroderma. **B** Red palms with scale. **C** Histopathologic findings can include regular acanthosis and parakeratosis with discrete collections of neutrophils. *A, Courtesy, Yale Dermatology Residents' Slide Collection.*

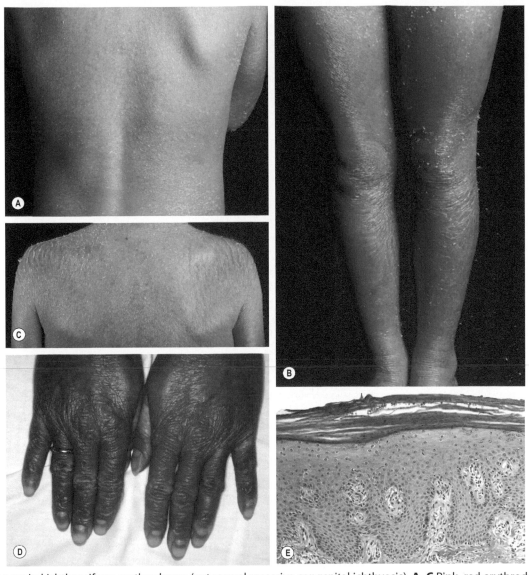

Fig. 3.3 Congenital ichthyosiform erythroderma (autosomal recessive congenital ichthyosis). **A–C** Pink–red erythroderma with fine scale. **D** Sometimes the erythema is more red. **E** Histopathologic findings include acanthosis and parakeratosis. *A–C, Courtesy, Britt Craiglow, MD; D, Courtesy, Leonard Milstone, MD.*

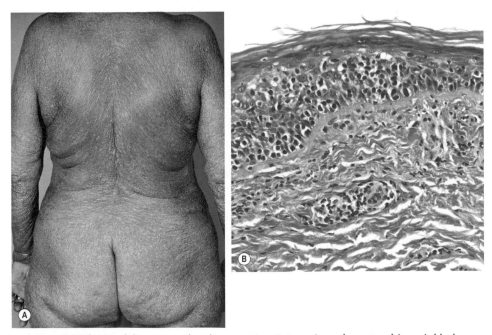

Fig. 3.4 Sézary syndrome. **A** Pink to red–brown erythroderma with subtle scale and an atrophic, wrinkled appearance in some areas. **B** Histopathologic findings can be nonspecific; helpful features would include atypical lymphocytes within the epidermis. *A, Courtesy, Rein Willemze, MD. From Bolognia JL, Jorizzo JL, Schaffer JV. Dermatology, 3e. London: Saunders, 2012, with permission.*

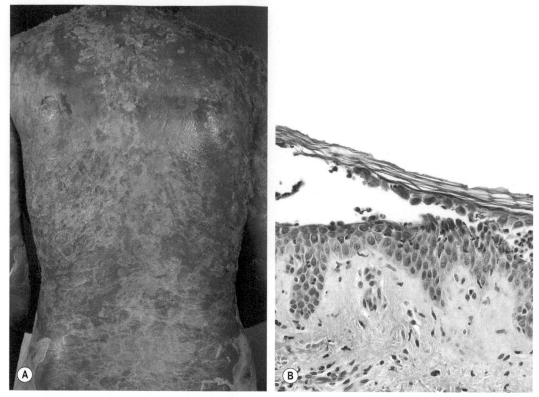

Fig. 3.5 Pemphigus foliaceus. **A** Focal erosions, red erythema, and thick scale. **B** Histopathologic findings include superficial acantholysis of the epidermis. *A, Courtesy, NYU Slide Collection. From Bolognia JL, Jorizzo JL, Schaffer JV. Dermatology, 3e. London: Saunders, 2012, with permission.*

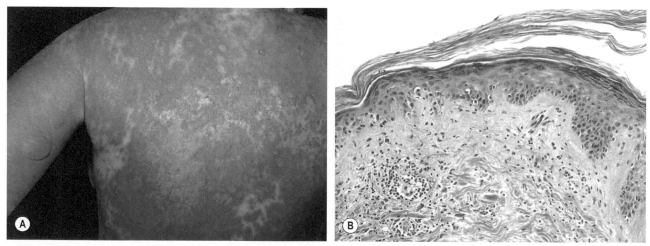

Fig. 3.6 Toxic epidermal necrolysis–like presentation of acute lupus erythematosus (acute syndrome of apoptotic pan-epidermolysis [ASAP]). **A** Blistering is focally present on the left arm. **B** Histopathologic findings would include interface change. *A, Courtesy, Yale Dermatology Residents' Slide Collection. From Bolognia JL, Jorizzo JL, Schaffer JV. Dermatology, 3e. London: Saunders, 2012, with permission.*

PHOTODISTRIBUTION

Once a photodistribution is determined (see Fig. 1.16A; Fig. 3.7), the primary involvement of the epidermis (Figs. 3.8, 3.9) vs dermis (Figs. 3.10, 3.11) and the morphology of primary lesions aid in narrowing the differential diagnosis; there are also histopathologic clues (Table 3.2).

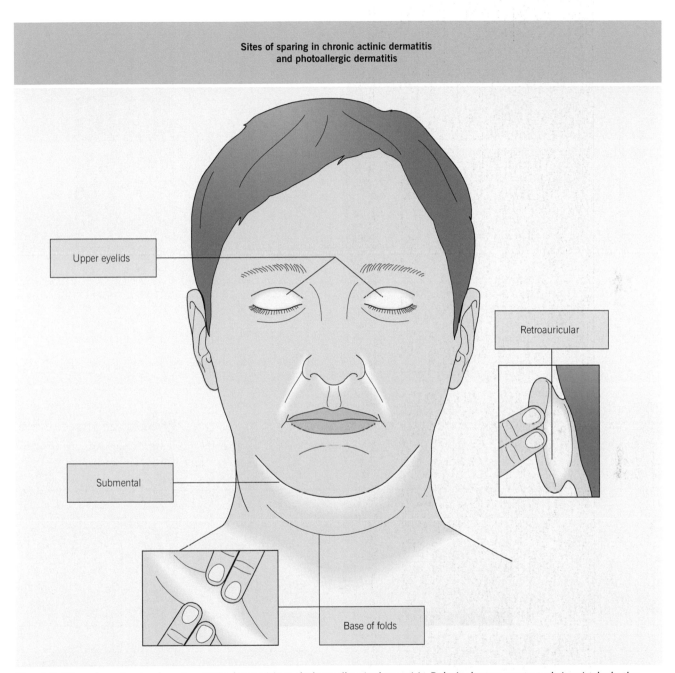

Sites of sparing in chronic actinic dermatitis and photoallergic dermatitis

Upper eyelids

Retroauricular

Submental

Base of folds

Fig. 3.7 Sites of sparing in chronic actinic dermatitis and photoallergic dermatitis. Relatively sun-protected sites include the upper eyelids, the nasolabial folds, the retroauricular areas, the submental region, and the deepest portion of skin furrows. *From Bolognia JL, Jorizzo JL, Schaffer JV. Dermatology, 3e. London: Saunders, 2012, with permission.*

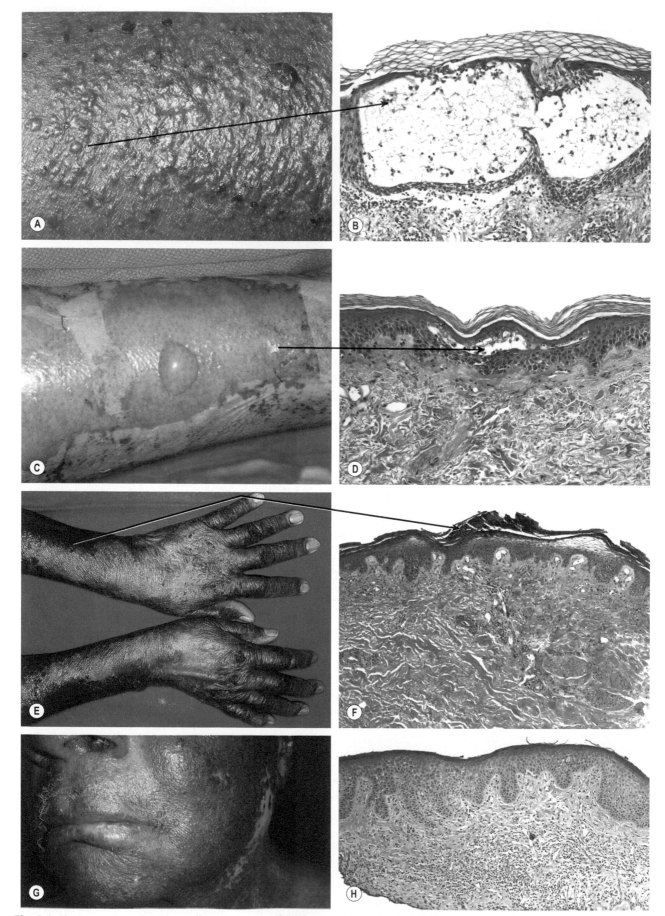

Fig. 3.8 Photoreactions. **A,B** Photoallergic reaction. **C,D** Phototoxic reaction. **E,F** Pellagra (niacin deficiency). **G,H** Chronic actinic dermatitis. *B, Courtesy, Lorrenzo Cerroni, MD; E, Courtesy, Yale Dermatology Residents' Slide Collection. G, Courtesy, Henry Lim, MD. A,C, From Schwarzenberger K, Werchniak AE, Ko C. General Dermatology. London: Saunders, 2009. B,E,G, From Bolognia JL, Jorizzo JL, Schaffer JV. Dermatology, 3e. London: Saunders, 2012, with permission.*

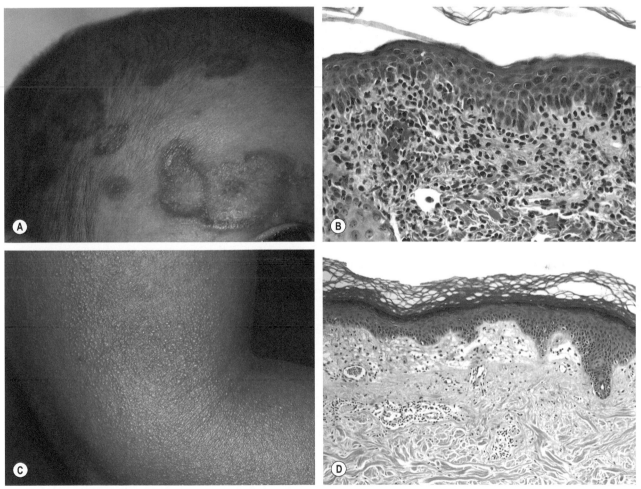

Fig. 3.9 Hydroa vacciniforme. *Courtesy, John L M Hawk, MD. From Bolognia JL, Jorizzo JL, Schaffer JV. Dermatology, 3e. London: Saunders, 2012, with permission.*

Vesiculation

Fig. 3.10 Erythematous papules and plaques. **A,B** Neonatal lupus erythematosus. **C,D** Polymorphous light eruption. *A, Courtesy, Julie V Schaffer, MD; C, Courtesy, Yale Dermatology Residents' Slide Collection. A,C, From Bolognia JL, Jorizzo JL, Schaffer JV. Dermatology, 3e. London: Saunders, 2012, with permission.*

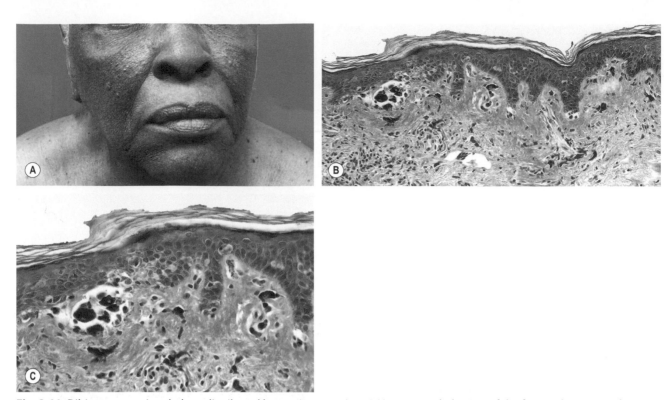

Fig. 3.11 Diltiazem-associated photodistributed hyperpigmentation. **A** New-onset darkening of the face with sparing of more photoprotected areas. **B,C** There is interface change and pigment incontinence.

Table 3.2 Photoreactions		
Entity	**Morphology**	**Histopathology**
Epidermal photoreactions		
Photoallergic reaction	• Acute spongiotic/eczematous process	• Vesicles • Eosinophils
Phototoxic reaction (e.g. sunburn)	• Depending on severity, erythema to blistering	• Necrotic keratinocytes
Pellagra	• Flaky paint-like scale and erythema	• Parakeratosis and/or necrosis of the upper epidermis
Chronic actinic dermatitis	• Lichenification and erythema	• Mild spongiosis, acanthosis, hyperkeratosis
Hydroa vacciniforme	• Vesicles and erythema	• Reticular degeneration
Dermal photoreactions		
Neonatal lupus erythematosus	• Annular erythematous plaques	• Interface vacuolar change • Dermal lymphocytes
Polymorphous light eruption	• Erythematous, edematous papules and plaques	• Papillary dermal edema • Perivascular lymphocytes
Drug-induced pigmentary alteration	• Pigment change in sun-exposed skin	• Dermal deposition of melanin pigment

MOSAIC DISTRIBUTION

A mosaic distribution of lesions (see Fig. 1.18B) can be specific for particular genodermatoses (Fig. 3.12); lesions may be caused by epidermal (Fig. 3.13) or dermal processes (Fig. 3.14).

- **Epidermal nevus** – brown papules, clustered in linear arrays (see Fig. 1.19)
- **Inflammatory linear verrucous epidermal nevus** – erythematous scaly papules and plaques, resembling psoriasis (see Fig. 1.28A)
- **Linear porokeratosis** – pink, linear lesions with raised, scaly borders on careful examination
- **Incontinentia pigmenti** – scalloped or reticulated arrangement of erythema and vesicles, sometimes admixed with verrucous lesions and/or hyperpigmented, lace-like patterns (see Fig. 1.29)

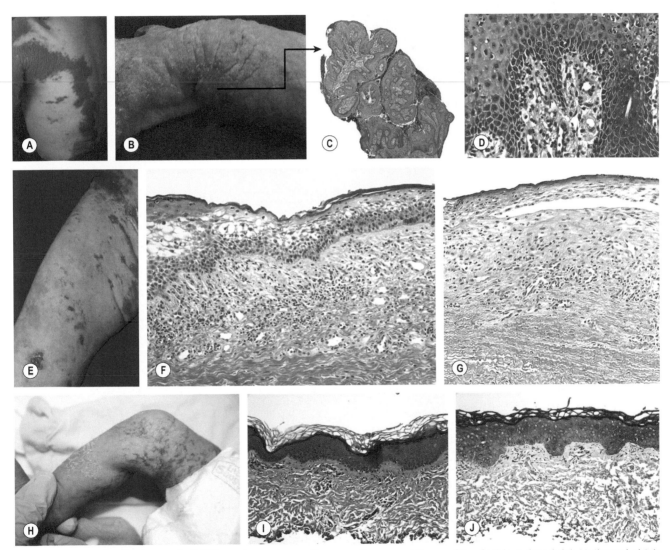

Fig. 3.12 Linear distribution. **A–D** CHILD syndrome (verruciform xanthoma on biopsy of the friable red nodule). Unilateral, thick pink plaques. **E-G** Goltz syndrome with characteristic atrophy and telangiectasias. Although classic microscopic findings include adipocytes high up in the dermis, biopsy of telangiectatic, atrophic areas may only show dermal atrophy and inflammation. **H–J** Incontinentia pigmenti, stage 3 (hyperpigmentation), with characteristic scalloped borders. Prominent pigment incontinence (I) highlighted with Fontana Masson staining (J). *A,B, Courtesy, Leonard Milstone, MD; E,G, Courtesy, Yale Dermatology Residents' Slide Collection. E, From Bolognia JL, Jorizzo JL, Schaffer JV. Dermatology, 3e. London: Saunders, 2012, with permission.*

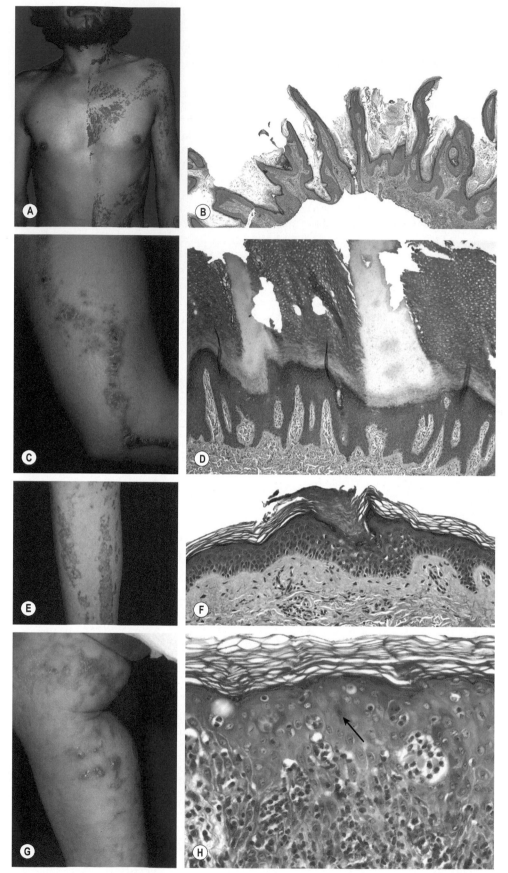

Fig. 3.13 Linear distribution. **A,B** Epidermal nevus. Acanthosis and hyperkeratosis resembling a seborrheic keratosis (B). **C,D** Inflammatory linear verrucous epidermal nevus. Alternating orthokeratosis and parakeratosis (D). **E,F** Linear porokeratosis. Cornoid lamella (column of parakeratosis; F). **G,H** Incontinentia pigmenti. Eosinophilic spongiosis with necrotic keratinocytes (arrow; H). *A,C,E, Courtesy, Yale Dermatology Residents' Slide Collection; H, Courtesy, Laura B Pincus, MD. A,E,G, From Bolognia JL, Jorizzo JL, Schaffer JV. Dermatology, 3e. London: Saunders, 2012, with permission. C, From Bolognia JL, Schaffer JV, Duncan KO, Ko CJ. Dermatology Essentials, 1e. Philadelphia: Saunders, 2014, with permission.*

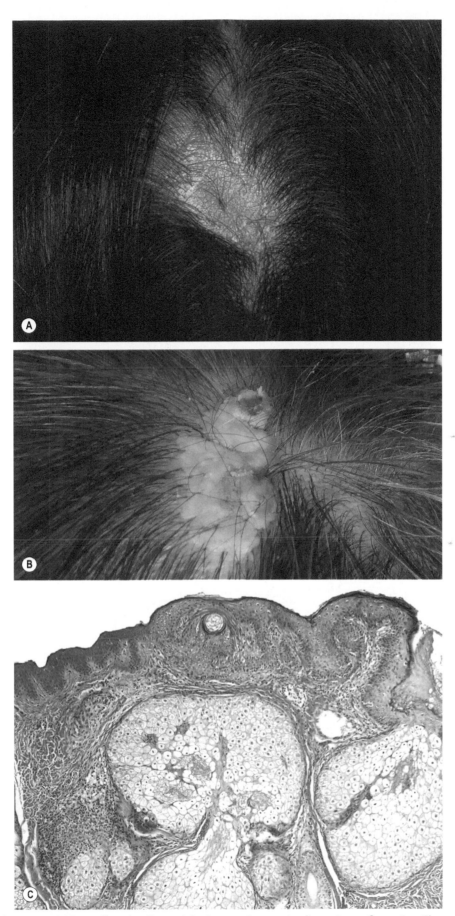

Fig. 3.14 Nevus sebaceus. **A,B** Mammillated, yellow–pink plaque, often oval or linear in configuration. The scalp is a typical site. **C** Histopathologic findings include acanthosis of the epidermis and sebaceous glands connecting to the epidermal surface.
A, Courtesy, Yale Dermatology Residents' Slide Collection. A, From Bolognia JL, Jorizzo JL, Schaffer JV. Dermatology, 3e. London: Saunders, 2012, with permission.

LOCALIZED PIGMENTED TUMORS

Key Differences (Fig. 3.15)

- **Angiokeratoma** – red–black lacunae clearly visible as well-demarcated roundish structures; histopathology: dilated vessels in the superficial dermis containing erythrocytes
- **Malignant melanoma** – asymmetry of color and structure, blue–white structures, and irregular streaks at the periphery; histopathology: asymmetric arrangement of melanocytic nests, with single melanocytes trailing off to one periphery
- **Nodular malignant melanoma** – predominant blue–white veil with irregular black to brown dots, globules,

and blotches; histopathology: prominent dermal collections of atypical melanocytes
- **Pigmented basal cell carcinoma** – leaf-like areas (islands of blue–gray color) at the periphery and a small erosion of reddish color; histopathology: basaloid islands containing melanin pigment
- **Seborrheic keratosis** –typical milia-like cysts (white shining globules) and comedo-like openings (black targetoid globules); histopathology: acanthosis of the epidermis with pseudohorn cysts

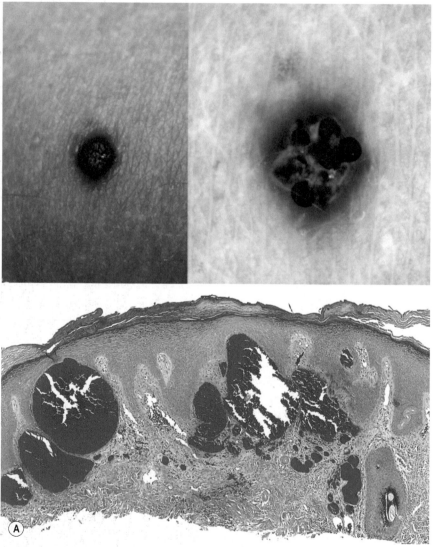

Fig. 3.15 Localized pigmented tumors. **A** Angiokeratoma.

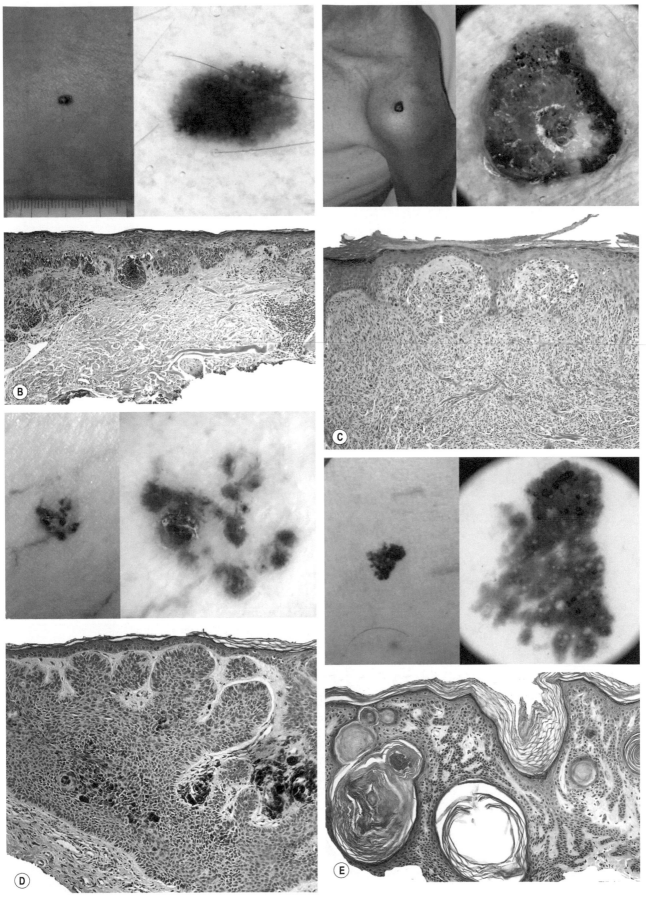

Fig. 3.15, cont'd **B** Malignant melanoma. **C** Nodular malignant melanoma. **D** Pigmented basal cell carcinoma. **E** Seborrheic keratosis. Clinical and dermoscopic photos, *Courtesy, Giuseppe Argenziano, MD, and Iris Zalaudek, MD. From Bolognia JL, Schaffer JV, Duncan KO, Ko CJ. Dermatology Essentials, 1e. Philadelphia: Saunders, 2014, with permission.*

Spongiotic/Eczematous Processes | 4

This chapter covers acute to subacute presentations of atopic dermatitis, seborrheic dermatitis, asteatotic eczema, stasis dermatitis, id reaction, nummular dermatitis, contact dermatitis, and tinea.

Clinical:
Acute lesions – weeping or oozing +/− crusting over edematous pink papules or plaques (see Fig. 1.33)
Subacute lesions – scaly or crusted pink patches or plaques

ATOPIC DERMATITIS

Clinical:
Infancy
Distribution: favors face and extensor surfaces (Figs. 4.1, 4.2)

Childhood
Distribution: favors flexural surfaces (see Fig. 5.18; Fig. 4.3)

Adult
(See Chapter 5; see Fig. 2.18A)

Chronic – thickened, lichenified plaques (see Figs. 1.39, 1.43 and Chapter 5)

Histopathologic:
Eczematous processes have epidermal spongiosis (interkeratinocytic edema) in common. Acute lesions can have larger spaces within the epidermis that correspond to vesicles (or occasionally bullae) clinically. The degree of spongiosis is variable but generally is greatest in acute lesions and can be very subtle in chronic lesions.

Atopic Dermatitis Clues
Keratosis pilaris, xerosis, ichthyosis, pityriasis alba – see Chapter 5

Histopathologic:
Eosinophils may be present within the epidermis and the dermal infiltrate

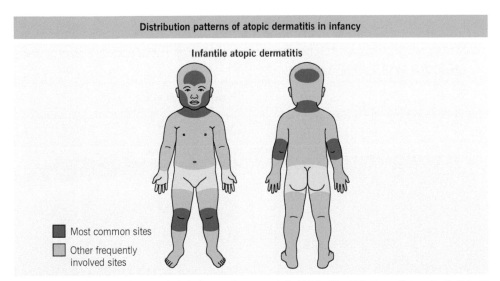

Fig. 4.1 Distribution patterns of atopic dermatitis in infancy. *Courtesy, Julie V Schaffer, MD. From Bolognia JL, Schaffer JV, Duncan KO, Ko CJ. Dermatology Essentials, 1e. Philadelphia: Saunders, 2014, with permission.*

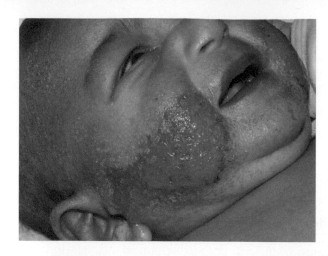

Fig. 4.2 Atopic dermatitis, infancy. Acute lesions involving the lower cheek. *Courtesy, Julie V Schaffer, MD. From Bolognia JL, Schaffer JV, Duncan KO, Ko CJ. Dermatology Essentials, 1e. Philadelphia: Saunders, 2014, with permission.*

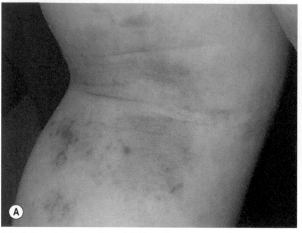

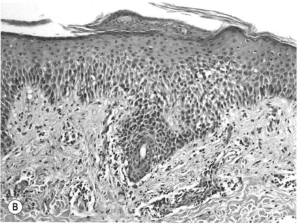

Fig. 4.3 A Atopic dermatitis, childhood. Acute to subacute lesions in the popliteal fossa. **B** Histopathologic findings include intercellular edema within the epidermis (spongiosis) and overlying parakeratosis with serum. *A, Courtesy, Julie V Schaffer, MD. From Bolognia JL, Schaffer JV, Duncan KO, Ko CJ. Dermatology Essentials, 1e. Philadelphia: Saunders, 2014, with permission.*

SEBORRHEIC DERMATITIS, INFANT

Clinical:
Moist, scaly plaques involving the folds (see Fig. 2.14C; Fig. 4.4)

Histopathologic:
There may be parakeratosis flanking the follicular infundibulum

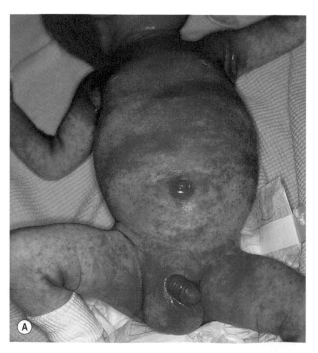

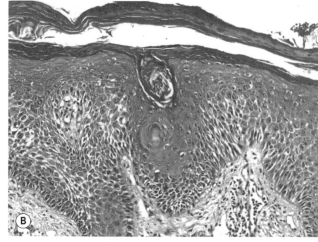

Fig. 4.4 Infantile seborrheic dermatitis. **A** Moist, ill-defined plaques favoring the body folds but also involving other sites in this case. **B** Intercellular edema within the epidermis with overlying parakeratosis. *A, Courtesy, Robert Hartman, MD. From Bolognia JL, Schaffer JV, Duncan KO, Ko CJ. Dermatology Essentials, 1e. Philadelphia: Saunders, 2014, with permission.*

SEBORRHEIC DERMATITIS, ADULT

Clinical:
Predilection for the scalp, posterior ears, central face, upper chest and back
Variably colored papules and plaques with flaking and/or greasy scale (Fig. 4.5; see Figs. 1.55D, 2.6F)
Lesions may be annular (see Fig. 2.9B)

Histopathologic:
There may be parakeratosis flanking the follicular infundibulum

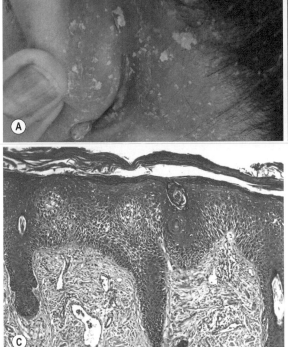

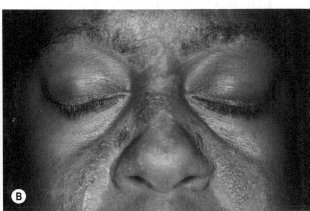

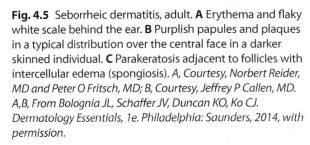

Fig. 4.5 Seborrheic dermatitis, adult. **A** Erythema and flaky white scale behind the ear. **B** Purplish papules and plaques in a typical distribution over the central face in a darker skinned individual. **C** Parakeratosis adjacent to follicles with intercellular edema (spongiosis). *A, Courtesy, Norbert Reider, MD and Peter O Fritsch, MD; B, Courtesy, Jeffrey P Callen, MD. A,B, From Bolognia JL, Schaffer JV, Duncan KO, Ko CJ. Dermatology Essentials, 1e. Philadelphia: Saunders, 2014, with permission.*

ASTEATOTIC ECZEMA (XEROTIC ECZEMA, ECZEMA CRAQUELÉ)

Clinical:
Favors the lower extremities, flanks, and lateral upper back
Pruritus may be present
Superficial cracking of the skin (Fig. 4.6)

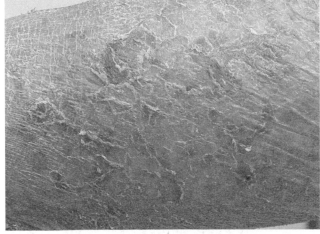

Fig. 4.6 Asteatotic eczema. *Courtesy, Kalman Watsky, MD.*

STASIS DERMATITIS

Clinical:
Predilection for the lower extremities, often bilateral
Associated lower extremity edema +/− signs of
venous hypertension: varicosities (Fig. 4.7), petechiae,
lipodermatosclerosis (see Fig. 2.21), ulceration above
medial malleolus (Fig. 4.8; see Chapter 10), livedoid
vasculopathy

Histopathologic:
Capillaries are often slightly thickened, somewhat
clustered vertically, and increased in number

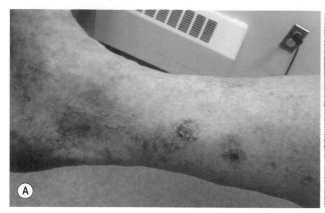
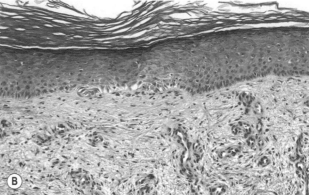

Fig. 4.7 Stasis dermatitis. **A,B** Vasculature is prominent.

ID REACTION

Clinical:
Relatively widespread (may be generalized); predilection
for extensor extremities (see Fig. 4.8)
Associated with another localized dermatitis that is
elsewhere on the body (i.e. allergic contact dermatitis,
stasis dermatitis, tinea)

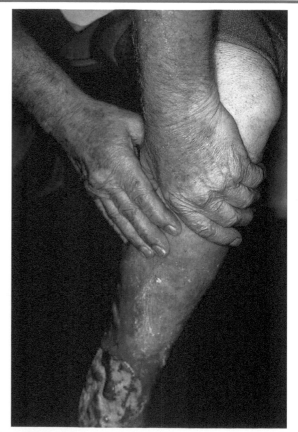

Fig. 4.8 Id reaction (autosensitization dermatitis). The extensor
forearms are involved. The patient had allergic contact dermatitis
to neomycin and stasis dermatitis. There is also a venous ulcer
over the medial malleolus. *Courtesy, Jean L Bolognia, MD. From
Bolognia JL, Schaffer JV, Duncan KO, Ko CJ. Dermatology Essentials,
1e. Philadelphia: Saunders, 2014, with permission.*

NUMMULAR DERMATITIS

Clinical:
Typically on the arms and legs
Coin-shaped 2- to 3-cm plaques (Fig. 4.9), classically
weeping or oozing (see Fig. 1.55E)

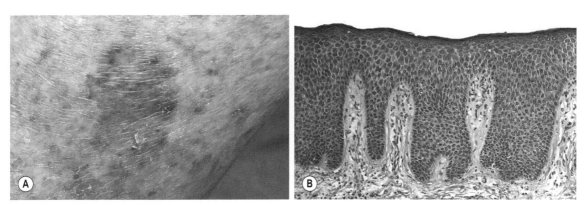

Fig. 4.9 Nummular dermatitis. **A** Circular thin plaque. **B** Histopathologic features of this case include acanthosis, spongiosis, and parakeratosis.

ALLERGIC CONTACT DERMATITIS

Clinical:
Delayed-type hypersensitivity reaction in a previously
sensitized person
Acute lesions with weeping and vesicles or blisters
(Fig. 4.10) are more common than chronic lesions
(Fig. 4.11), but the latter is not uncommon on the hands
(see Fig. 2.18F)

Histopathologic:
Eosinophils may be present within the epidermis and the
dermal infiltrate

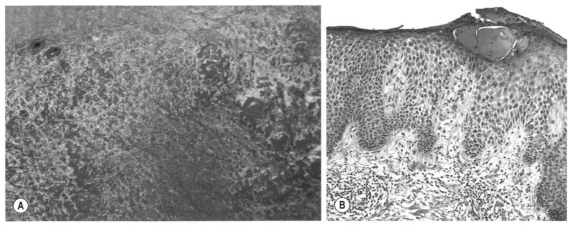

Fig. 4.10 Acute allergic contact dermatitis to chlorhexidine. **A** Acute, vesicular lesions. **B** There is spongiosis with eosinophils.
A, Courtesy, Yale Dermatology Residents' Slide Collection.

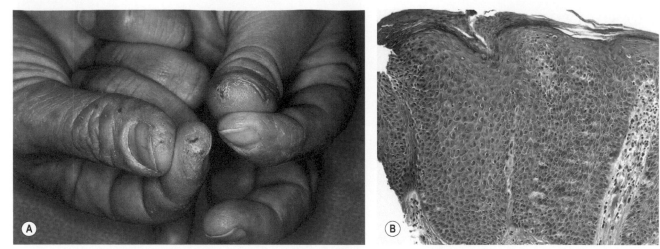

Fig. 4.11 A Chronic allergic contact dermatitis to glutaraldehyde in an optometrist. **B** Chronic eczematous processes have acanthosis, mild spongiosis, and focal parakeratosis as histopathologic findings. *A, Courtesy, Kalman Watsky, MD. From Bolognia JL, Schaffer JV, Duncan KO, Ko CJ. Dermatology Essentials, 1e. Philadelphia: Saunders, 2014, with permission.*

IRRITANT CONTACT DERMATITIS (FIGS. 4.12, 4.13)

Clinical:
Because of a local toxic (nonimmunologic) effect from a contactant (see Figs. 2.17D; 2.18E, 2.23C)
Chronic lesions with skin thickening +/− fissures are more common than acute lesions

Histopathologic:
There may be scattered superficial necrotic keratinocytes or superficial epidermal necrosis

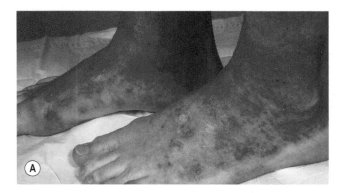

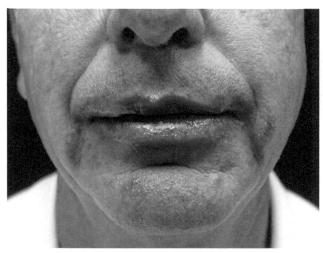

Fig. 4.13 Cheilitis and perioral involvement caused by irritant contact dermatitis (lip licking). *Courtesy, Jeffrey P Callen, MD. From Bolognia JL, Schaffer JV, Duncan KO, Ko CJ. Dermatology Essentials, 1e. Philadelphia: Saunders, 2014, with permission.*

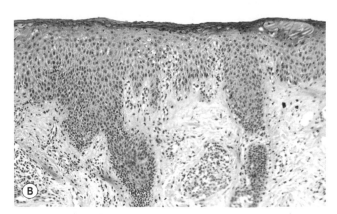

Fig. 4.12 Bilateral irritant contact dermatitis caused by chronic wearing of occlusive footwear. *Courtesy, David Cohen, MD. From Bolognia JL, Schaffer JV, Duncan KO, Ko CJ. Dermatology Essentials, 1e. Philadelphia: Saunders, 2014, with permission.*

TINEA

Clinical:
Annular, scaly border (potassium hydroxide [KOH] preparation of scale can confirm the diagnosis) (Figs. 4.14A,B; see Figs. 2.9A, 2.15C, 2.18D, 2.23A)

Histopathologic:
Fungal organisms (hyphae appear somewhat refractile; when cut in cross-section, resemble hollow circles) within the stratum corneum

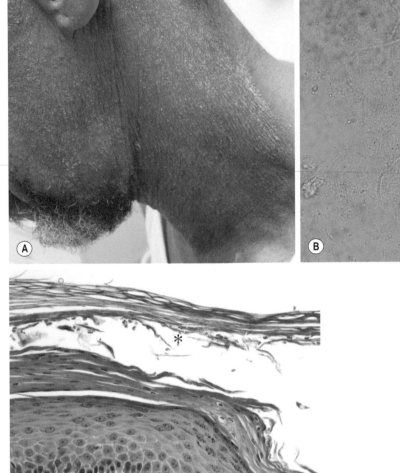

Fig. 4.14 Tinea corporis. **A** A rim of scale is evident on the posterior neck. **B** Potassium hydroxide (KOH) preparation of scale shows branching hyphae. **C** Histopathologic findings include mild spongiosis, parakeratosis, and hyphae within the stratum corneum (above asterisk).

BULLOUS PEMPHIGOID, ECZEMATOUS

Clinical:
Various atypical presentations of bullous pemphigoid have been described
One atypical presentation is eczematous (Fig. 4.15)

Histopathologic:
Subepidermal split with eosinophils (see Fig. 4.15C)

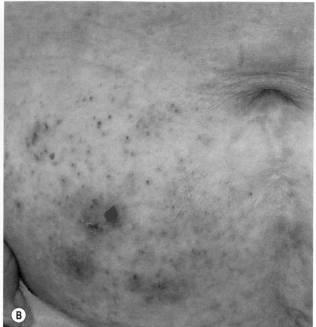

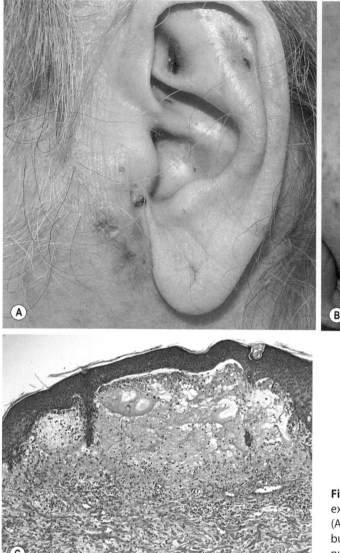

Fig. 4.15 Bullous pemphigoid, eczematous. **A,B** There are excoriated light pink papules and plaques on the face (A) and trunk (B). **C** Histopathologic features are typical of bullous pemphigoid, with a subepidermal split with numerous eosinophils. *A–C, Courtesy, Yale Dermatology Residents' Slide Collection.*

Papulosquamous/Psoriasiform Rashes | 5

The term "psoriasiform" is used to mean "psoriasis-like," and therefore psoriasis is the prototype for these disorders, which generally have dry scales over erythematous plaques and papules. Some experts use "papulosquamous" for similar lesions (see Fig. 8.10).

This chapter is not all-inclusive, and other rashes can be psoriasiform (e.g. drug eruptions). This chapter covers psoriasis, pityriasis rubra pilaris, chronic eczematous dermatitis, and pemphigus foliaceus.

PSORIASIS – CLASSIC PLAQUE TYPE

Clinical:
Often symmetric
Typically on the elbows/knees/scalp/lower back (Fig. 5.1)
May be more generalized (Fig. 5.2; see Fig. 6.1)
Well-demarcated erythematous plaques (bar) that are pink–red because of superficial vessels (circles) (Fig. 5.3A)
Well-developed adherent scales are silvery to yellow (arrow) (Fig. 5.4; see Fig. 1.55A)

Histopathologic:
Silvery scales correspond to dry parakeratosis lacking serum (arrow) (Fig. 5.3B)

Hyperplastic/thickened epidermis (bar) with a diminished granular cell layer
Prominent vessels in the papillary dermis (circles)

Psoriasis – Clues
Lesions may koebnerize (linear arrays) (Fig. 5.5)
Nail changes – distal onycholysis (blue arrows), pitting (orange arrows), subungual hyperkeratosis (green arrow) (Fig. 5.6), oil spots, thickening/yellow discoloration (Fig. 5.7)

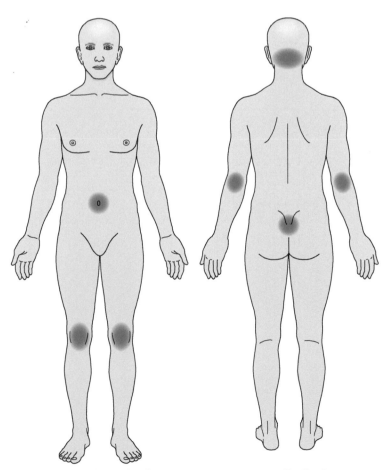

Fig. 5.1 Psoriasis, plaque type, most common distribution.

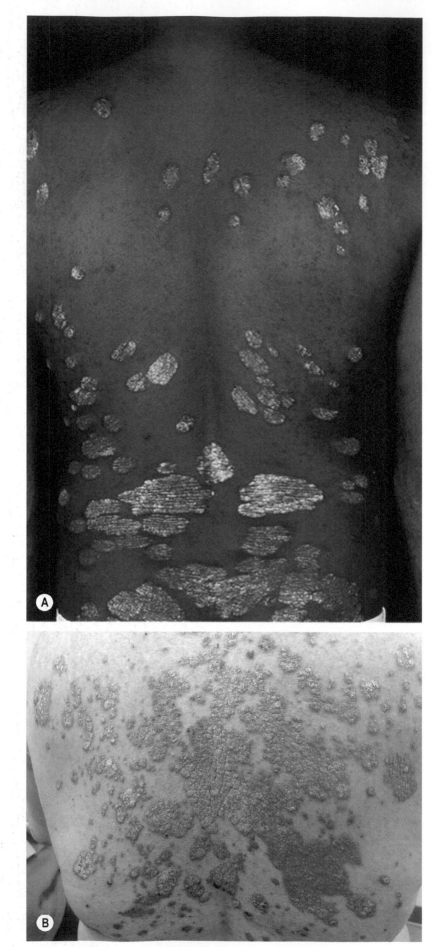

Fig. 5.2 Psoriasis, plaque type. *A, Courtesy, Peter C M van de Kerkhof, MD. From Bolognia JB, Jorizzo JL, Rapini RP. Dermatology, 2e. London: Saunders, 2008, with permission.*

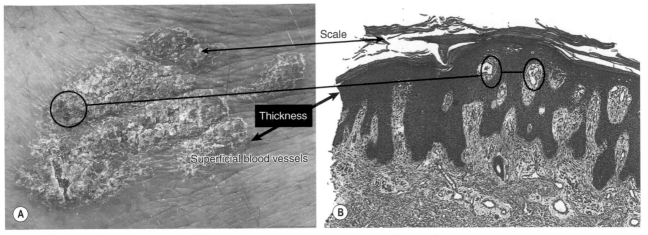

Scale

Thickness

Superficial blood vessels

Fig. 5.3 Psoriasis. Well-demarcated, pink–red plaque with adherent, white-yellow scales.

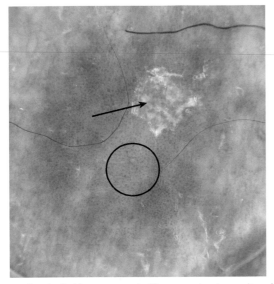

Fig. 5.4 Psoriasis (dermoscopy). Silvery scales (arrow) and prominent regular dotted vessels (circle). *Courtesy, Giuseppe Argenziano, MD, and Iris Zalaudek, MD. From Bolognia JL, Jorizzo JL, Schaffer JV. Dermatology, 3e. London: Saunders, 2012, with permission.*

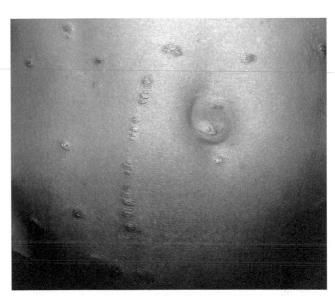

Fig. 5.5 Psoriasis, koebnerization. *Courtesy, Yale Dermatology Residents' Slide Collection. From Bolognia JL, Jorizzo JL, Schaffer JV. Dermatology, 3e. London: Saunders, 2012, with permission.*

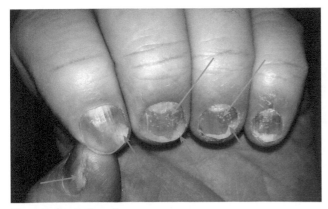

Fig. 5.6 Psoriatic nails.

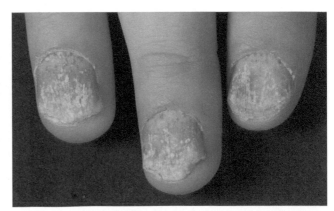

Fig. 5.7 Psoriatic nails. *Courtesy, Peter CM van de Kerkhof, MD, and Frank O Nestlé, MD. From Bolognia JL, Jorizzo JL, Schaffer JV. Dermatology, 3e. London: Saunders, 2012, with permission.*

PSORIASIS VARIANTS

Guttate (see Chapter 6) – small lesions with characteristic scales, generally <1 cm in size (Fig. 5.8, see Figs. 6.1, 6.21)

Palmoplantar (see Chapter 2) – lesions with typical scales; underlying skin in these sites may not be erythematous (Fig. 5.9; see Figs. 2.18C, 2.23B)

Inverse (see Chapter 2) – minimal scales over thin, pink plaques (Fig. 5.10; see Figs. 2.14–2.17)

Pustular (see Chapter 11) – erythema and pustules; pustules may form "lakes of pus" (Fig. 5.11; see Fig. 11.21)

Erythrodermic (see Fig. 3.2)

Linear (see Fig. 1.28A)

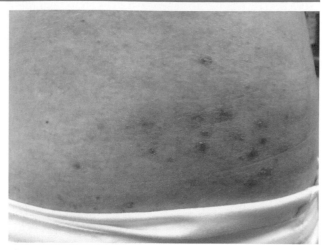

Fig. 5.8 Guttate psoriasis.

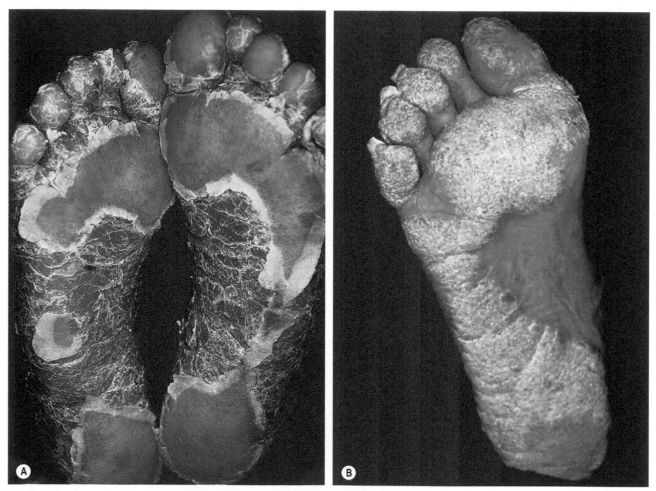

Fig. 5.9 Plantar psoriasis. *A, Courtesy, Peter CM van de Kerkhof, MD. B, Courtesy, Yale Dermatology Residents' Slide Collection. From Bolognia JL, Jorizzo JL, Schaffer JV. Dermatology, 3e. London: Saunders, 2012, with permission.*

Fig. 5.10 Inverse psoriasis. *Courtesy, Ronald P Rapini, MD. From Bolognia JL, Jorizzo JL, Schaffer JV. Dermatology, 3e. London: Saunders, 2012, with permission.*

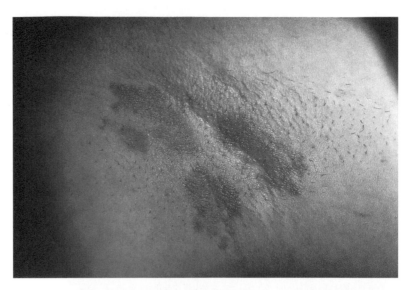

Fig. 5.11 Pustular psoriasis. On the finger, this is termed acrodermatitis continua of Hallopeau. *Courtesy, Yale Dermatology Residents' Slide Collection. From Bolognia JL, Schaffer JV, Duncan KO, Ko CJ. Dermatology Essentials, 1e. Philadelphia: Saunders, 2014, with permission.*

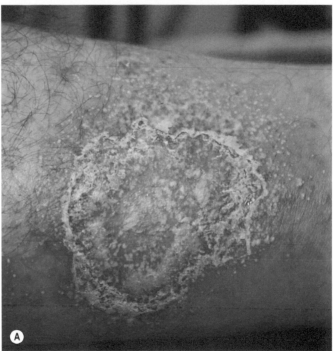

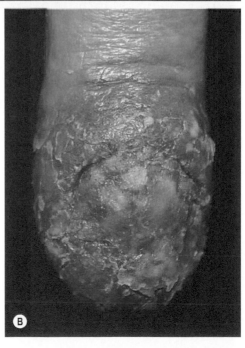

PITYRIASIS RUBRA PILARIS (CLASSIC TYPE)

Clinical:
Once well-developed, easily recognizable (Figs. 5.12, 5.13; see Fig. 3.1). Early lesions can resemble psoriasis (Fig. 5.14A; see Fig. 6.19A).
Classic adult/juvenile – salmon to orange erythroderma with islands of sparing (large or small in size) and follicular papules
The atypical juvenile subtype is associated with *CARD14* mutations, and the term *CARD14-associated papulosquamous eruption* has been proposed for such cases

Histopathologic:
Checkerboard pattern of orthokeratosis and parakeratosis, acanthosis, and perivascular lymphocytes; follicular plugging (see Fig. 5.14; arrow)

Pityriasis Rubra Pilaris – Clues
Orange (arrow) to pink waxy keratoderma (Fig. 5.15)
Thickened nails
Islands of sparing (arrows) (Fig. 5.16)
Follicular papules (Fig. 5.17)

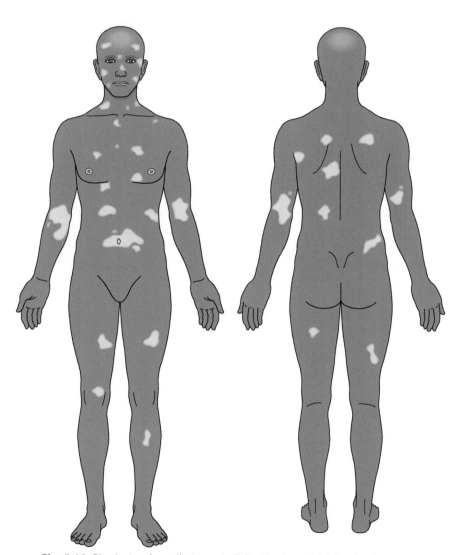

Fig. 5.12 Pityriasis rubra pilaris, typical distribution with islands of sparing.

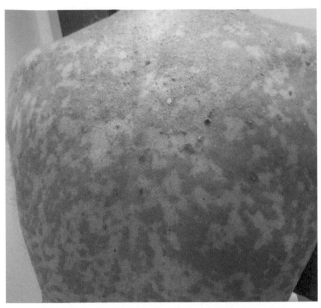

Fig. 5.13 Pityriasis rubra pilaris. *Courtesy, Brett King, MD.*

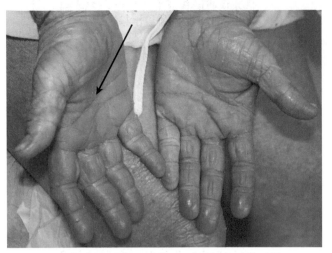

Fig. 5.15 Waxy keratoderma. *Courtesy, Evelyn Lilly, MD.*

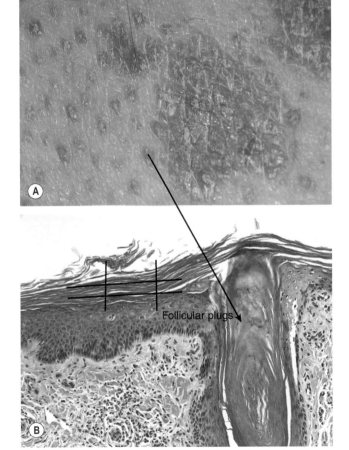

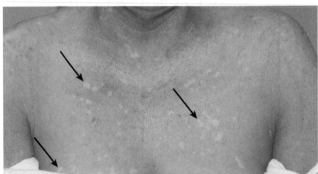

Fig. 5.16 Islands of sparing. *Courtesy, Evelyn Lilly, MD.*

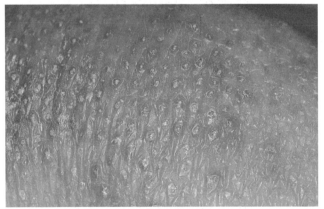

Fig. 5.14 Pityriasis rubra pilaris. Follicular prominence corresponds to follicles plugged with keratin. Checkboard alternating orthokeratosis and parakeratosis is a classic feature that is not always present.

Fig. 5.17 Follicular hyperkeratosis. *From Schwarzenberger K, Werchniak AE, Ko C. General Dermatology. London: Saunders, 2009.*

CHRONIC ECZEMATOUS DERMATITIS

Clinical:

Atopic dermatitis typically shows chronic changes after infancy, in typical sites (Fig. 5.18).

Thickened skin with accentuated skin markings (lichenification) (Figs. 5.19, 5.20)

Excoriations are common

Histopathologic:

Parakeratosis, minimal spongiosis, acanthosis, preserved granular layer (Fig. 5.20B)

There are many clues and associated features of atopic dermatitis (Figs. 5.21–5.27).

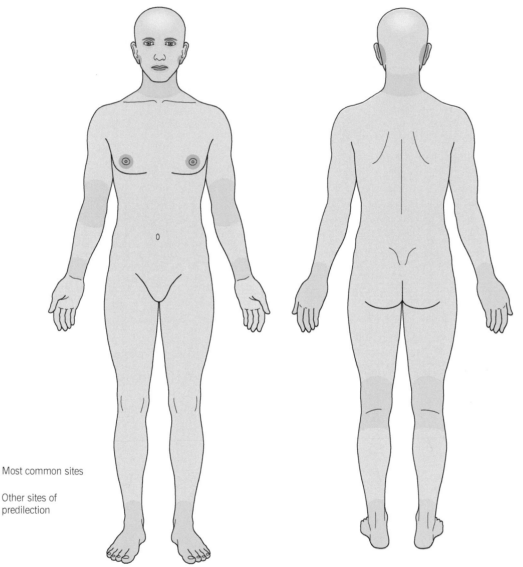

Most common sites

Other sites of predilection

Fig. 5.18 Atopic dermatitis, common sites affected after infancy. *From Bolognia JL, Schaffer JV, Duncan KO, Ko CJ. Dermatology Essentials, 1e. Philadelphia: Saunders, 2014, with permission.*

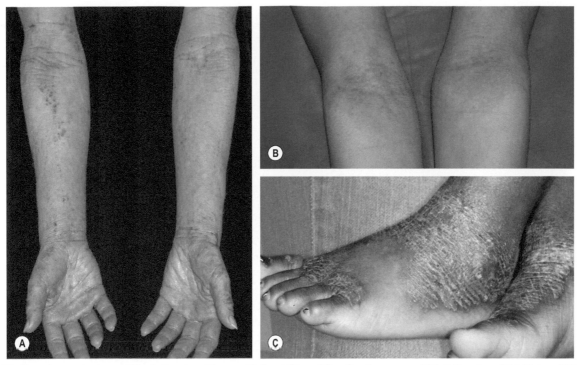

Fig. 5.19 Chronic atopic dermatitis. *A, Courtesy, Thomas Bieber, MD, and Caroline Bussmann, MD. B, Courtesy, Dirk Elston, MD; C, Courtesy Anne Lucky, MD. A, From Bolognia JL, Jorizzo JL, Schaffer JV. Dermatology, 3e. London: Saunders, 2012, with permission. B, From Elston D. Clinical image collection. Dermatopathology, 2e. London: Saunders, 2014. C, From Schachner LA, Hansen RE. Pediatric Dermatology, 5e. London: Mosby, 2011.*

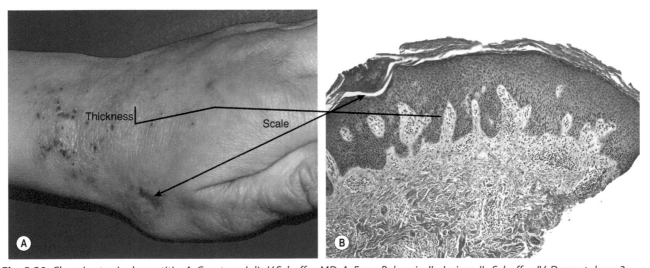

Fig. 5.20 Chronic atopic dermatitis. *A, Courtesy, Julie V Schaffer, MD. A, From Bolognia JL, Jorizzo JL, Schaffer JV. Dermatology, 3e. London: Saunders, 2012, with permission.*

ATOPIC DERMATITIS – CLUES

Associated features of atopic dermatitis

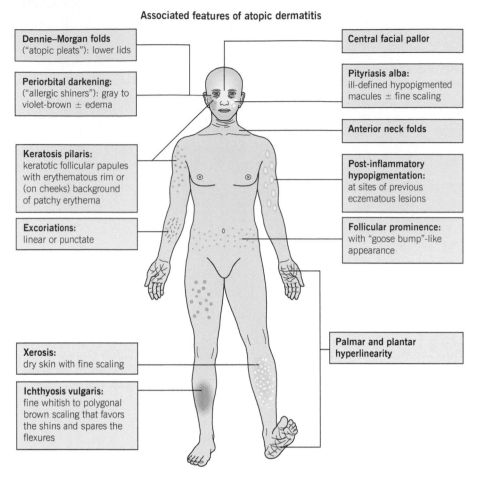

Dennie–Morgan folds ("atopic pleats"): lower lids

Periorbital darkening: ("allergic shiners"): gray to violet-brown ± edema

Keratosis pilaris: keratotic follicular papules with erythematous rim or (on cheeks) background of patchy erythema

Excoriations: linear or punctate

Xerosis: dry skin with fine scaling

Ichthyosis vulgaris: fine whitish to polygonal brown scaling that favors the shins and spares the flexures

Central facial pallor

Pityriasis alba: ill-defined hypopigmented macules ± fine scaling

Anterior neck folds

Post-inflammatory hypopigmentation: at sites of previous eczematous lesions

Follicular prominence: with "goose bump"-like appearance

Palmar and plantar hyperlinearity

Fig. 5.21 Associated features of atopic dermatitis. *From Bolognia JL, Schaffer JV, Duncan KO, Ko CJ. Dermatology Essentials, 1e. Philadelphia: Saunders, 2014, with permission.*

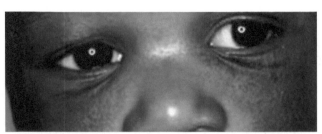

Fig. 5.22 Dennie–Morgan folds on the lower lids. *From Bolognia JL, Schaffer JV, Duncan KO, Ko CJ. Dermatology Essentials, 1e. Philadelphia: Saunders, 2014, with permission.*

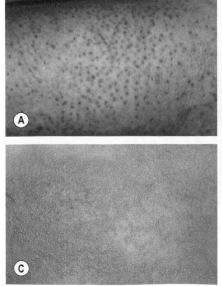

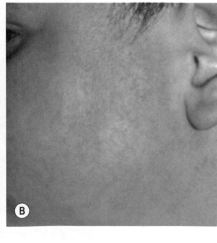

Fig. 5.23 A Keratosis pilaris. **B,C** Keratosis pilaris rubra on the face. *A, Courtesy, Yale Dermatology Residents' Slide Collection; B,C, Courtesy, Julie V Schaffer, MD. From Bolognia JL, Schaffer JV, Duncan KO, Ko CJ. Dermatology Essentials, 1e. Philadelphia: Saunders, 2014, with permission.*

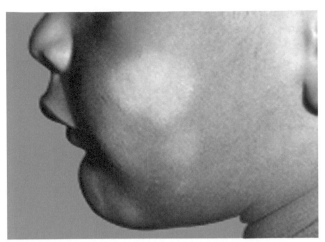

Fig. 5.24 Pityriasis alba. *Courtesy, Anthony J Mancini, MD. From Bolognia JL, Schaffer JV, Duncan KO, Ko CJ. Dermatology Essentials, 1e. Philadelphia: Saunders, 2014, with permission.*

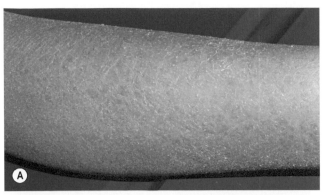

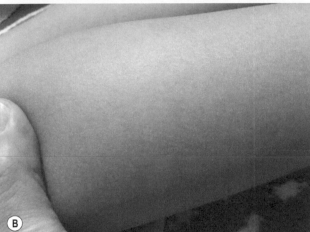

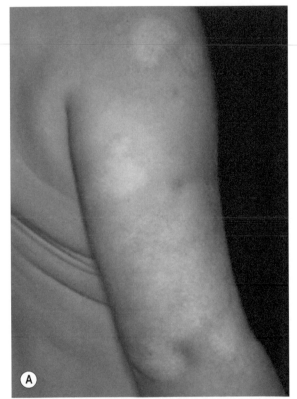

Fig. 5.26 Ichthyosis vulgaris versus mild xerosis. **A** Ichthyosis vulgaris. **B** Xerosis, mild. *A, Courtesy, Julie V Schaffer, MD. A, From Bolognia JL, Schaffer JV, Duncan KO, Ko CJ. Dermatology Essentials, 1e. Philadelphia: Saunders, 2014, with permission.*

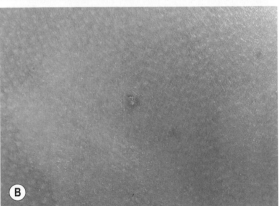

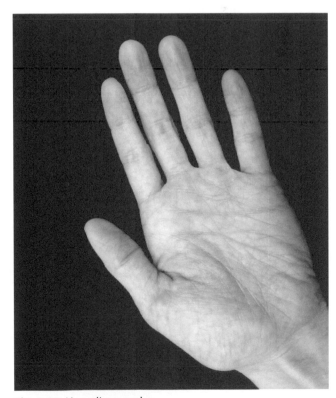

Fig. 5.25 Postinflammatory hypopigmentation. *A, Courtesy, Thomas Bieber, MD and Caroline Bussman, MD. From Bolognia JL, Schaffer JV, Duncan KO, Ko CJ. Dermatology Essentials, 1e. Philadelphia: Saunders, 2014, with permission.*

Fig. 5.27 Hyperlinear palm.

PEMPHIGUS FOLIACEUS

Clinical:

Favors the scalp/face/upper trunk (Fig. 5.28; see Fig. 6.19B) but may become generalized (see Chapter 3)
Erosions are a major clue (arrows; Fig. 5.29)

Histopathologic:

Individual lesions are thickened (bar), red, with cornflake-like scales (arrow; Fig. 5.30A)
Scales and erosions correlate with subcorneal blistering (arrow; Fig. 5.30B)

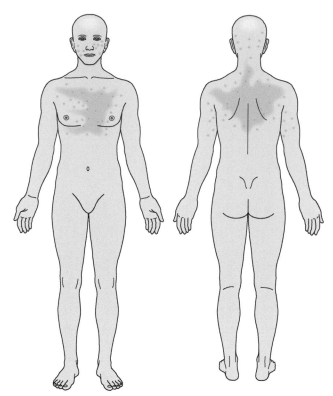

Fig. 5.28 Pemphigus foliaceus. The distribution often favors the central face, scalp, and upper trunk.

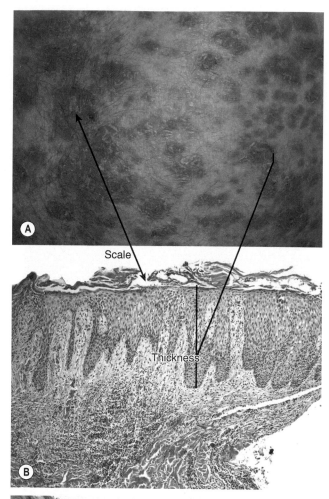

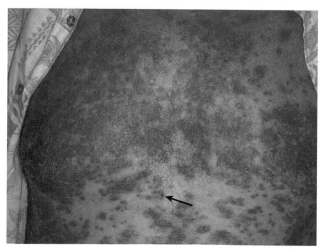

Fig. 5.29 Pemphigus foliaceus.

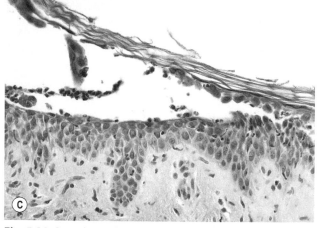

Fig. 5.30 Pemphigus foliaceus. **A,B** Superficial erosions overlying pink plaques of thickened epidermis. **C** Superficial acantholysis is more obvious in this example.

PSORIASIFORM RASHES

Key Differences (Fig. 5.31)

- **Psoriasis** – adherent, white to silvery scales over bright red erythematous, well-demarcated papules and plaques
- **Pityriasis rubra pilaris** – fine scales over pink–orange erythema, follicular papules
- **Subacute cutaneous lupus erythematosus** – pink–red plaques, generally with fewer scales than in psoriasis, often on the upper trunk
- **Pemphigus foliaceus** – erosions and cornflake-like scales
- **Psoriasiform drug reaction to a TNF-inhibitor** — pink–red papules and plaques that can look identical to psoriasis

- **Graft-versus-host disease** – pink–red papules with adherent white scales resembling guttate psoriasis; a history of a stem cell transplant is important, and biopsy findings (necrotic keratinocytes) may be helpful
- **Chronic atopic dermatitis** (not shown; see Fig. 5.20A) – may be psoriasiform microscopically; clinically, lesions are not well-demarcated with accentuated skin markings (thickening), excoriations

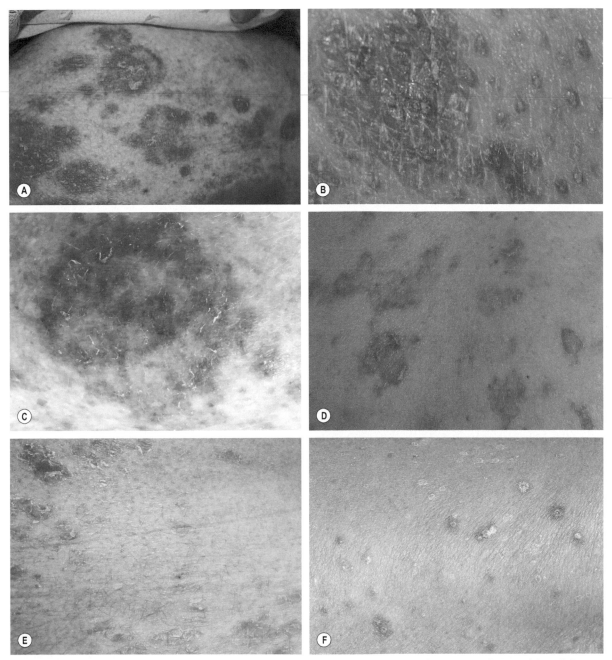

Fig. 5.31 Psoriasiform rashes. **A** Psoriasis. **B** Pityriasis rubra pilaris. **C** Subacute lupus erythematosus. **D** Pemphigus foliaceus. **E** Psoriasiform drug reaction to a TNF-inhibitor. **F** Graft-versus-host disease. *C, Courtesy, Julie V Schaffer, MD. D,E, Courtesy, Yale Dermatology Residents' Collection; F, Courtesy, Julia Lehman, MD. C, From Bolognia JL, Jorizzo JL, Schaffer JV. Dermatology, 3e. London: Saunders, 2012, with permission.*

Small, Scaly Lesions | 6

This chapter includes guttate psoriasis, pityriasis rosea, lichen planus, pityriasis lichenoides, tinea versicolor, secondary syphilis, small plaque parapsoriasis, and Darier disease. The characteristic lesion is a papule with overlying scale.

GUTTATE PSORIASIS

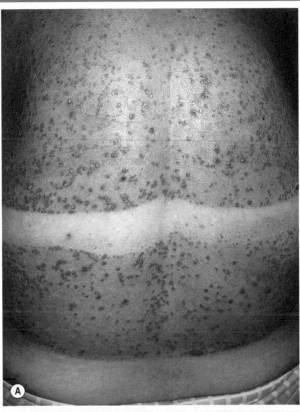

Clinical:
Pink to red papules (Fig. 6.1) with adherent white scales (arrow; Fig. 6.2), generally <1 cm in diameter scattered over the trunk and extremities

Histopathologic:
Slight acanthosis and mounds of parakeratosis that often contain neutrophils (arrow; see Fig. 6.2)
Mild spongiosis may be evident
Dilated papillary dermal vessels may be present (circles; see Fig. 6.2)

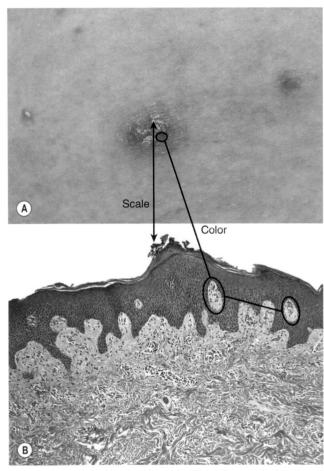

Fig. 6.2 Guttate psoriasis. Mounds of parakeratosis, often with neutrophils.

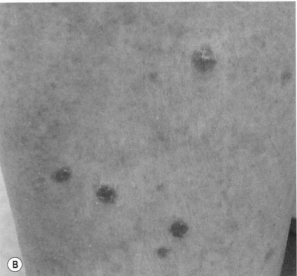

Fig. 6.1 Guttate psoriasis. Lesions in (**A**) developed after a sunburn (Koebner phenomenon). *A, Courtesy, Ronald Rapini, MD. A, From Bolognia JL, Jorizzo JL, Schaffer JV. Dermatology, 3e. London: Saunders, 2012, with permission.*

PITYRIASIS ROSEA

Clinical:

Classically, starts with a herald patch (often the largest lesion)

- Precedes development of a widespread, symmetric eruption (see below)

Once well developed, widespread and symmetric (Fig. 6.3)

- Proximal extremities and trunk
- Follow Langer's lines, forming a "Christmas tree" pattern on the back

Fine white central scale (arrow) (Figs. 6.4, 6.5; see Fig. 1.55B) sometimes with collarettes (Fig. 6.6) overlying round to oval thin salmon-colored (circle) papules/plaques

Histopathologic:

Mounds of parakeratosis (arrow; see Fig. 6.4), generally without neutrophils

Mild spongiosis, mild perivascular lymphocytic infiltrate with extravasated erythrocytes (circle; see Fig. 6.4)

Pityriasis Rosea – Variants
Inverse (see Fig. 6.6A)
- Tends to affect body folds (axillae, groin)
- Long axis of lesions along Langer's lines (see Fig. 6.3)

In Pigmented Skin (see Fig. 6.6B)
- May have follicular prominence
- May be hyperpigmented centrally

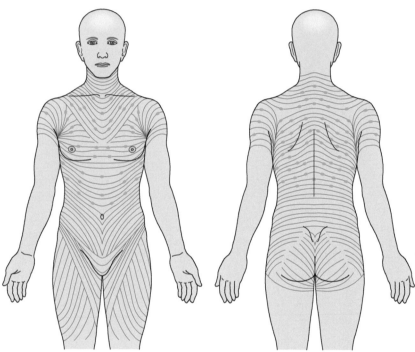

Fig. 6.3 Pityriasis rosea. The typical distribution, with lesions oriented with long axes parallel to the red lines (Langer's lines). *From Bolognia JL, Schaffer JV, Duncan KO, Ko CJ. Dermatology Essentials, 1e. Philadelphia: Saunders, 2014, with permission.*

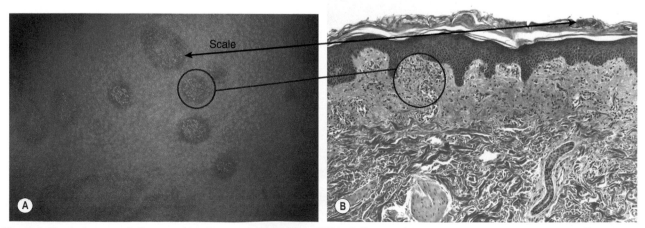

Fig. 6.4 Pityriasis rosea. *A, Courtesy, Yale Dermatology Residents' Slide Collection. A,B, From Bolognia JL, Jorizzo JL, Schaffer JV. Dermatology, 3e. London: Saunders, 2012, with permission.*

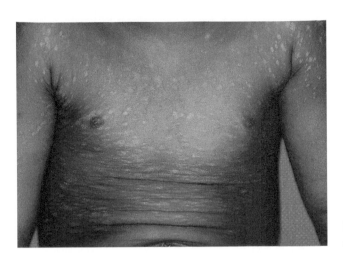

Fig. 6.5 Pityriasis rosea. *From James WD, Berger T, Elston D. Andrews' Diseases of the Skin, 11e. Edinburgh: Saunders, 2011.*

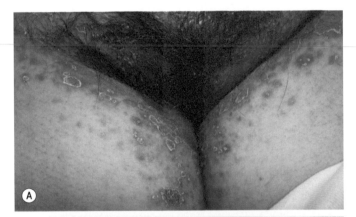

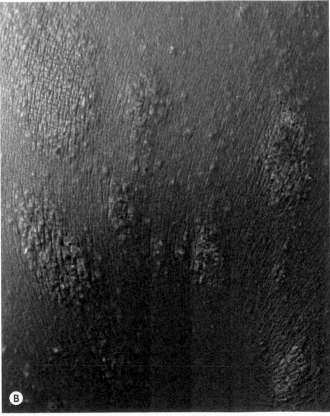

Fig. 6.6 Pityriasis rosea. **A** Inverse pityriasis rosea. **B** Pityriasis rosea in dark skin. *A, Courtesy, Yale Dermatology Residents' Slide Collection. B, Courtesy, Aisha Sethi, MD. B, From Bolognia JL, Schaffer JV, Duncan KO, Ko CJ. Dermatology Essentials, 1e. Philadelphia: Saunders, 2014, with permission.*

LICHEN PLANUS

Often Symmetric

- Classically on the wrists/forearms, ankles/shins, dorsal hands/feet, genital area (Fig. 6.7)
- May be more generalized

Flat-topped violaceous (circle) papules/plaques (Figs. 6.8, 6.9A)

Classic scales are interconnecting white lines (Wickham's striae) (arrow) (see Fig. 1.55C), possibly corresponding to hyperkeratosis/hypergranulosis (arrow) (see Fig. 6.9; Fig. 6.10)

Histopathologic:

Hyperplastic epidermis (hyperkeratotic and hypergranulotic) and lichenoid inflammation (circle) with pigment incontinence (orange arrows) (Fig. 6.9B)

Lichen Planus – Clues

Nail changes (Fig. 6.11) – atrophy and loss of nails, longitudinal fissuring, violaceous color periungually, pterygium (extension of skin onto nail bed), trachyonychia

Oral findings – lacy white plaques (arrows; Fig. 6.12), erosions/ulcers (see Figs. 2.11H, 2.13B)

Koebnerization – lesions secondary to trauma, often in a linear configuration (Fig. 6.13A)

Thicker lesions or bullous lesions, particularly on the shins (see Figs. 6.13A,B; see Figs. 12.13, 24.16)

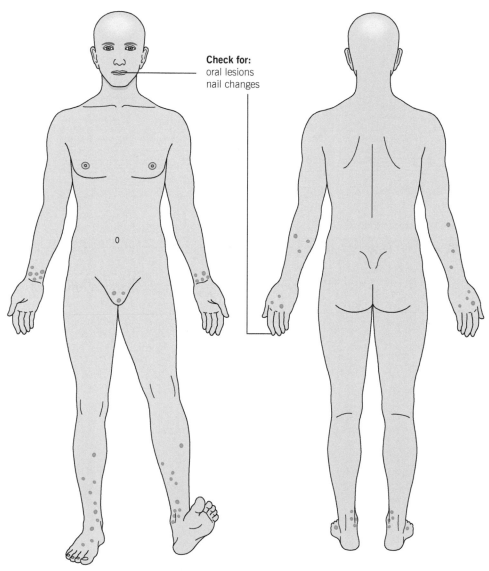

Check for:
oral lesions
nail changes

Fig. 6.7 Lichen planus, typical distribution.

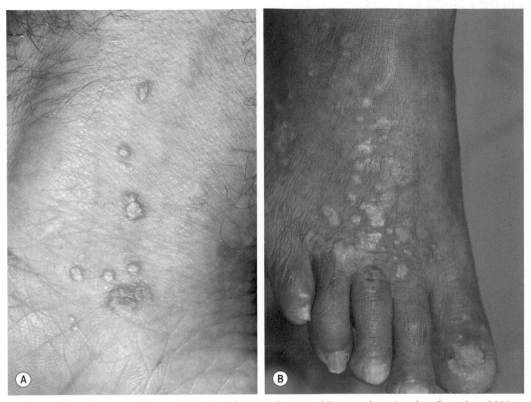

Fig. 6.8 Lichen planus. *From Schwarzenberger K, Werchniak AE, Ko C. General Dermatology. London: Saunders, 2009.*

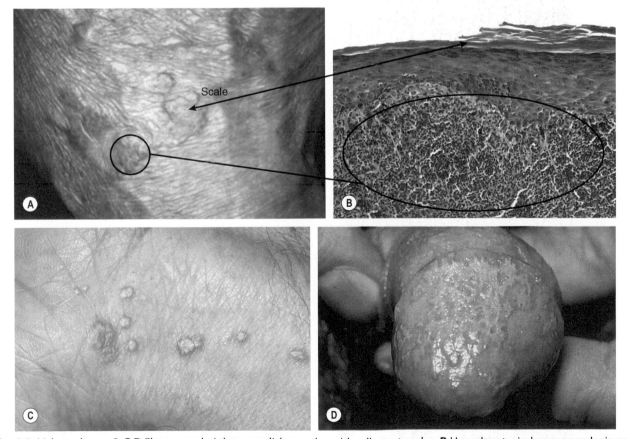

Scale

Fig. 6.9 Lichen planus. **A,C,D** Flat-topped pink to purplish papules with adherent scales. **B** Hyperkeratosis, hypergranulosis, and lichenoid inflammation are present. *A,B, Courtesy, Yale Dermatology Residents' Slide Collection.*

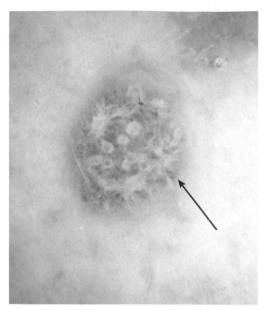

Fig. 6.10 Lichen planus, dermoscopy. *Courtesy, Iris Zalaudek, MD. From Bolognia JL, Jorizzo JL, Schaffer JV. Dermatology, 3e. London: Saunders, 2012, with permission.*

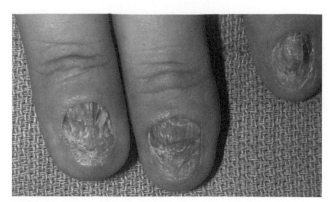

Fig. 6.11 Lichen planus of the nails. *Courtesy, Yale Dermatology Residents' Slide Collection.*

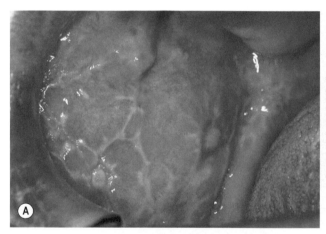

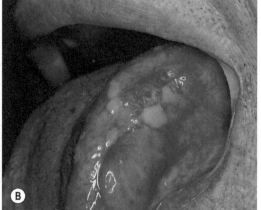

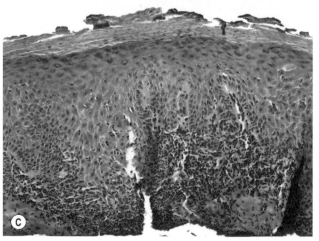

Fig. 6.12 Lichen planus, oral. Oral lesions include lacy white plaques (**A**) and erosions (**B**). Histopathologic findings are similar to those seen in Fig. 6.9. *A, Courtesy, Yale Dermatology Residents' Slide Collection; B, Courtesy, Louis A Fragola, Jr, MD. A,B, From Bolognia JL, Jorizzo JL, Schaffer JV. Dermatology, 3e. London: Saunders, 2012, with permission.*

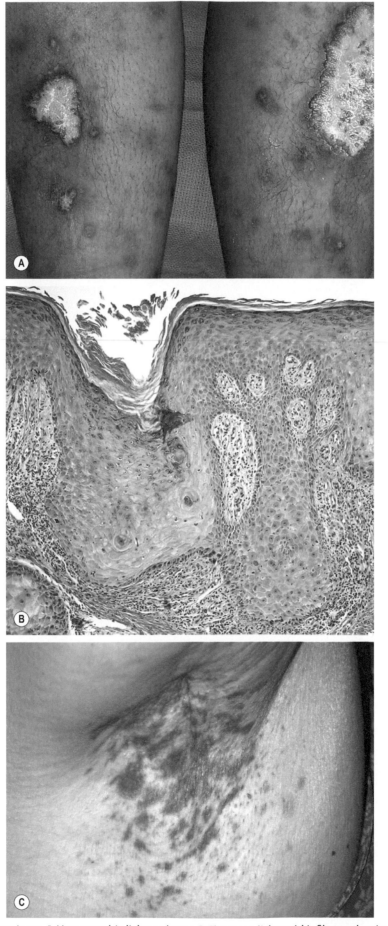

Fig. 6.13 Lichen planus – variants. **A** Hypertrophic lichen planus. **B** There is a lichenoid infiltrate that is concentrated at the bases of the acanthotic rete. **C** Lichen planus pigmentosus inversus. *Courtesy, Yale Dermatology Residents' Slide Collection.*

PITYRIASIS LICHENOIDES

Acute and chronic forms exist on a spectrum

Pityriasis Lichenoides et Varioliformis Acuta (Fig. 6.14A,B)
Clinical:
Pink to red papules with scale, some eroded or crusted, and vesicles
Lesions appear in crops and heal with scarring

Histopathologic:
Parakeratosis above the epidermis, with exocytosis of lymphocytes, interface change, and superficial and deep perivascular inflammation

Pityriasis Lichenoides Chronica (Fig. 6.14C-E)
Clinical:
Red–brown to pink papules, sometimes with scale
Lesions may be hypopigmented
Lesions appear in crops

Histopathologic:
Exocytosis of lymphocytes with sparse perivascular inflammation

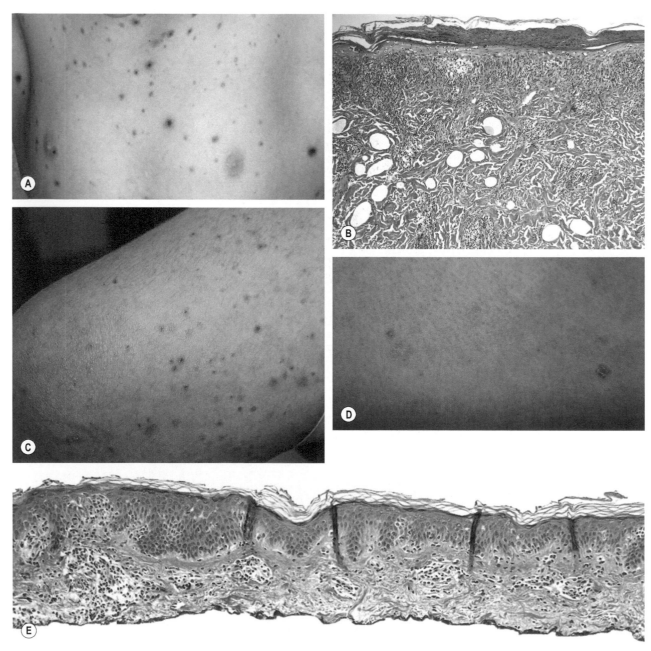

Fig. 6.14 Pityriasis lichenoides. **A,B** Pityriasis lichenoides et varioliformis acuta. **C–E** Pityriasis lichenoides chronica. *A, Courtesy, Julie V Schaffer, MD. C,D, Courtesy, Yale Dermatology Residents' Slide Collection. A, From Bolognia JL, Schaffer JV, Duncan KO, Ko CJ. Dermatology Essentials, 1e. Philadelphia: Saunders, 2014, with permission.*

TINEA VERSICOLOR

Clinical:
Superficial infection (*Malassezia* spp.)
Symmetric round to oval macules/patches to thin papules/plaques; color is variable (pink to brown or hypopigmented in dark skin); subtle powdery scale (arrow; Fig. 6.15; see Fig. 1.55G)

Histopathologic:
Round yeast and elongated pseudo hyphal forms in clusters in the stratum corneum (short arrows; see Fig. 6.15E); epidermis otherwise appears normal

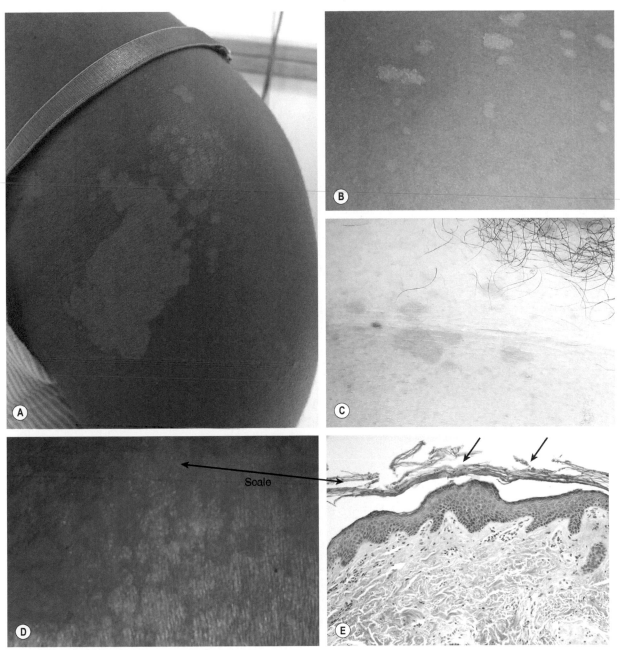

Fig. 6.15 Tinea versicolor. **A,B,C** Hypopigmented thin papules and plaques. **D,E** Fine, powdery scales containing yeast and pseudo hyphal forms.

SYPHILIS, SECONDARY

Clinical:
Thin pink or red–brown papules and plaques with scale, often on the trunk (Fig. 6.16)

Histopathologic:
Psoriasiform hyperplasia with lichenoid and perivascular lymphoplasmacytic inflammation (see Fig. 6.16)

Syphilis – Clues
Red–brown papules/plaques, sometimes with collarettes of scale, on palms/soles (Fig. 6.17; see Fig. 2.19B)

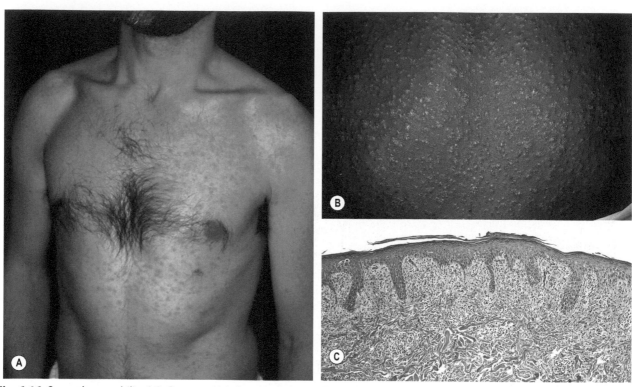

Fig. 6.16 Secondary syphilis. *A,B, Courtesy, Yale Dermatology Residents' Slide Collection. A,B, From Bolognia JL, Schaffer JV, Duncan KO, Ko CJ. Dermatology Essentials, 1e. Philadelphia: Saunders, 2014, with permission.*

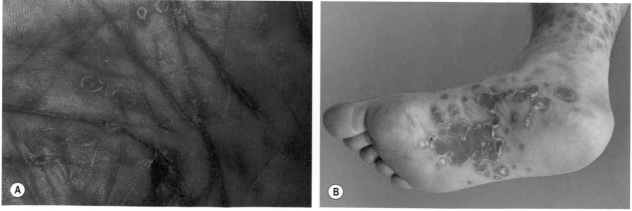

Fig. 6.17 Secondary syphilis, acral lesions. *A, Courtesy, Yale Dermatology Residents' Slide Collection. B, Courtesy, Angelika Stary, MD. A,B, From Bolognia JL, Schaffer JV, Duncan KO, Ko CJ. Dermatology Essentials, 1e. Philadelphia: Saunders, 2014, with permission.*

SMALL PLAQUE PARAPSORIASIS

Clinical:
Lesions <5 cm in diameter (Fig. 6.18A); lesions in digitate dermatosis may be longer than 5 cm

Digitate Dermatosis (a Type of Small Plaque Parapsoriasis)
Clinical:
Brown to pink thin plaques with subtle scale
Lesions arranged like "fingerprints" (Fig. 6.18B)

Histopathologic:
Subtle spongiosis and scattered lymphocytes within the epidermis (Fig. 6.18C)

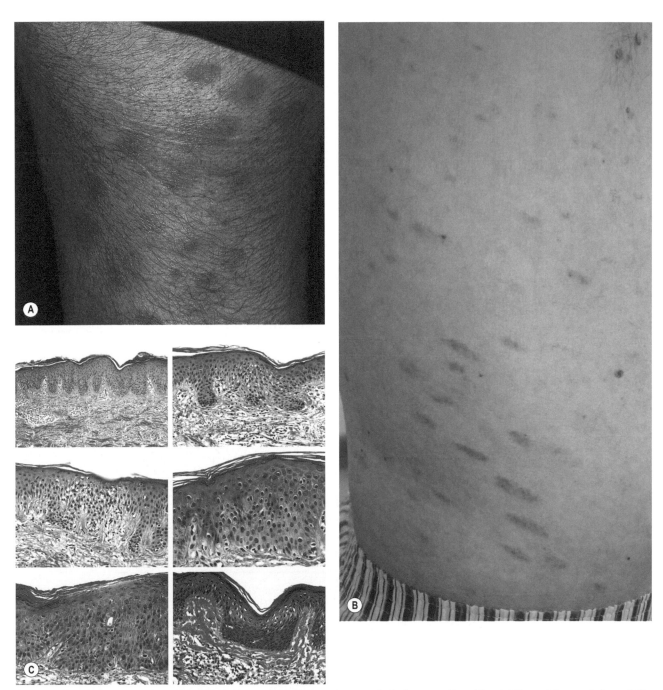

Fig. 6.18 Small plaque parapsoriasis. **(B)** is also termed *digitate dermatosis*. *A, Courtesy, Gary Wood, MD, and George Reizner, MD; B, Courtesy, Yale Dermatology Residents' Slide Collection. A, From Bolognia JL, Schaffer JV, Duncan KO, Ko CJ. Dermatology Essentials, 1e. Philadelphia: Saunders, 2014, with permission. C, From Belousova IE, Vanecek T, Samtsov AV, et al. A patient with clinicopathologic features of small plaque parapsoriasis presenting later with plaque-stage mycosis fungoides: report of a case and comparative retrospective study of 27 cases of "nonprogressive" small plaque parapsoriasis. J Am Acad Dermatol. 2008;59:474–82, © Elsevier.*

OTHER DISORDERS THAT CAN PRESENT WITH SCALY PAPULES/PLAQUES

Scabies
Clinical:
Lesions of different morphology, including eczematous thin plaques and inflammatory papules (see Fig. 23.5)
Linear burrows are an important clue (see Fig. 23.6A,B; see Figs.2.20B and 13.5)

Histopathologic:
Spongiosis with mites, scybala, and/or egg casings in the stratum corneum (see Fig. 23.7)

Pityriasis Rubra Pilaris (see also Chapter 5)
Clinical:
Classically, erythroderma that descends from the head to the feet (see Figs. 3.1, 5.12–17)
Early lesions on the trunk can be discrete and scaly (Fig. 6.19A)

Histopathologic:
Checkerboard pattern of parakeratosis, irregular acanthosis, follicular plugging

Pemphigus foliaceus
Clinical:
Crusted, scaly, or eroded papules (Fig. 6.19B; see Fig. 5.30)

Histopathologic:
Acantholysis below the stratum corneum

Lupus erythematosus
Clinical:
Papulosquamous lesions, sometimes annular, on the trunk or extremities (Fig. 6.19C; see Figs. 5.31C. 8.10)

Histopathologic:
Necrotic cells in basal and suprabasal layers, superficial perivascular lymphocytic inflammation

Darier Disease (Keratosis Follicularis)
Clinical:
Autosomal dominant genodermatosis; *ATP2A2* mutations
Predilection for the scalp, face, chest, back (seborrheic areas) (Fig. 6.20A); sometimes intertriginous
Crusted pink to brown papules that become confluent (Fig. 6.20B,C)

Histopathologic:
Acantholytic dyskeratosis capped by hyperkeratosis (Fig. 6.20D)

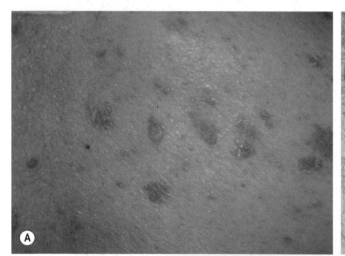

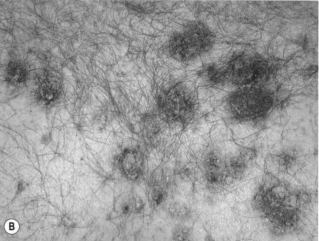

Fig. 6.19 A Pityriasis rubra pilaris. Early papulosquamous lesions on the chest. **B** Pemphigus foliaceus. Crusted and eroded lesions on the trunk. **C** Subacute cutaneous lupus erythematosus. Scaly papules on the trunk. *B,C, Courtesy, Yale Dermatology Residents' Collection.*

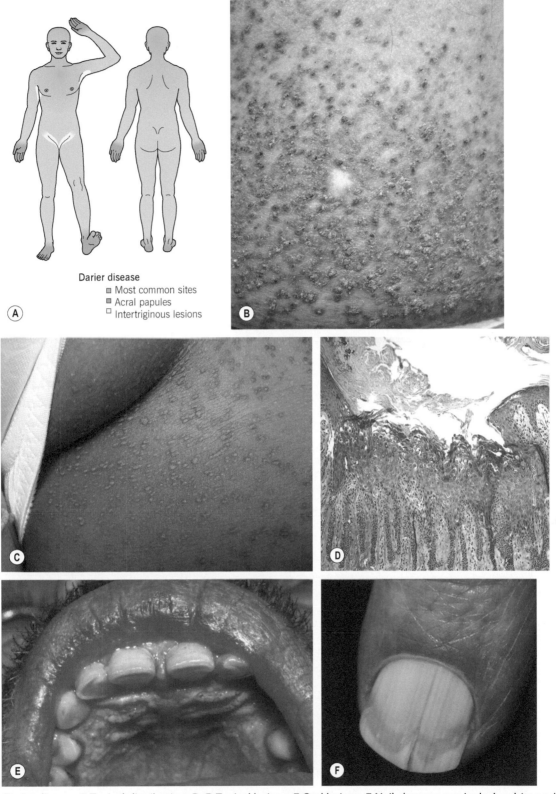

Darier disease
■ Most common sites
■ Acral papules
▢ Intertriginous lesions

Fig. 6.20 Darier disease. **A** Typical distribution. **B–D** Typical lesions. **E** Oral lesions. **F** Nail changes can include white and red streaks (shown) and V-shaped notches. *B,F, Courtesy, Yale Dermatology Residents' Slide Collection. A, From Bolognia JL, Schaffer JV, Duncan KO, Ko CJ. Dermatology Essentials, 1e. Philadelphia: Saunders, 2014, with permission. E, Courtesy, Daniel Hohl, MD. E, From Bolognia JL, Jorizzo JL, Schaffer JV. Dermatology, 3e. London: Saunders, 2012, with permission.*

SMALL, SCALY LESIONS WITH ERYTHEMA

Key Differences (Fig. 6.21)

Guttate psoriasis – silvery scales over pink–red erythema
Pityriasis rosea – central or collarette scale over pink–red erythema
Lichen planus – linear, interconnecting scale (Wickham's striae) over violaceous, flat papules

Pityriasis lichenoides (chronica) – red–brown papules, some scaly
Digitate dermatosis – dull pink–brown, elongated ovals
Syphilis – red–brown to violaceous papules

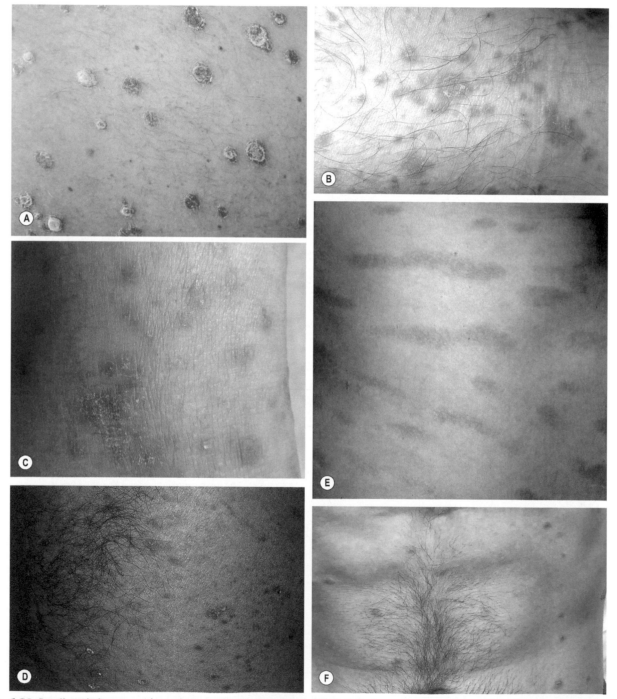

Fig. 6.21 Small, scaly lesions with erythema. **A** Guttate psoriasis. **B** Pityriasis rosea. **C** Lichen planus. **D** Pityriasis lichenoides (chronica). **E** Digitate dermatosis. **F** Syphilis. *D,F Courtesy, Yale Dermatology Residents' Slide Collection; B,E, From Schwarzenberger K, Werchniak AE, Ko C. General Dermatology. London: Saunders, 2009. D,F, From Bolognia JL, Jorizzo JL, Schaffer JV. Dermatology, 3e. London: Saunders, 2012, with permission.*

UMBILICATED OR CRUSTED PAPULES

Key Differences (Fig. 6.22)

Molluscum contagiosum – Pink–red to white papules with central dell, can be crusted

Cryptococcosis – pink–purple papules with central crusted dell

Histoplasmosis – pink papules, some umbilicated

Varicella – pink papules, some crusted; vesicles on a light pink–red base ("dewdrop on a rose petal") may be present

Eczema herpeticum – monomorphous punched out appearing crusted papules

Herpes folliculitis – punched out papules; centering of lesions over follicles can be a helpful clue

Coxsackie virus infection – vesicles, some crusted

Langerhans cell histiocytosis – crusted red–brown papules; typically on scalp, in groin

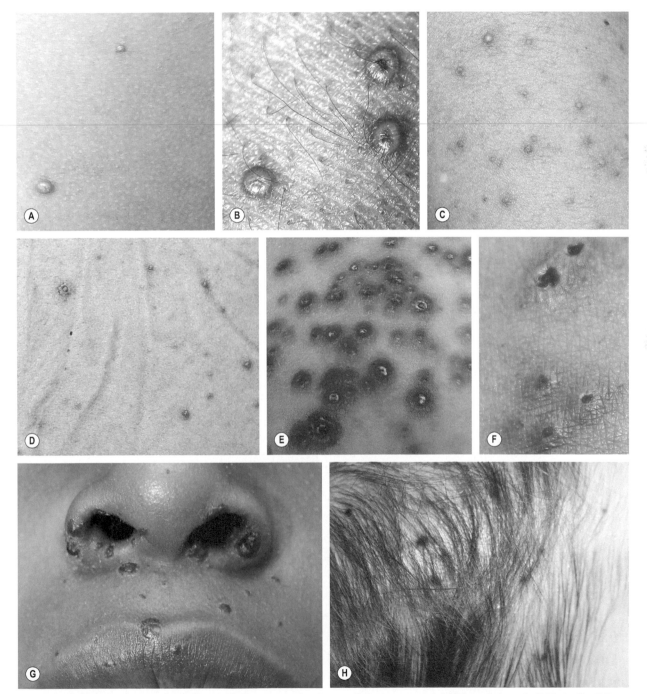

Fig. 6.22 Umbilicated or crusted papules. **A** Molluscum contagiosum. **B** Cryptococcosis. **C** Histoplasmosis. **D** Varicella. **E** Eczema herpeticum. **F** Herpes folliculitis. **G** Coxsackie virus infection. **H** Langerhans cell histiocytosis. *B-H, Courtesy, Yale Dermatology Residents' Slide Collection.*

Epidermal-Based Lesions | 7

Epidermal-based lesions generally have a characteristic morphology and/or color (Tables 7.1–7.4). Thickness of the tumor is reflected in the microscopic appearance (acanthosis). Other characteristic features are marked.

Table 7.1 Epidermal-based lesions: color – brown

Lesion	Appearance	Histopathology	Other clues
Seborrheic keratosis	• Various colors (Fig. 7.1A) but commonly tan to dark brown plaque • Horn cysts (arrows; Fig. 7.1B,C; see Fig. 3.15) • Stuck on appearance	• Several different subtypes, commonly acanthosis with pseudohorn cysts	**Dermoscopy** • Multiple milia-like cysts • Comedo-like openings
Solar lentigo (Fig. 7.2)	Uniform macules Sun-exposed skin	Pigmented basal cell layer	**Dermoscopy** • Moth-eaten borders • Fingerprinting • Short, interrupted thin lines
Junctional melanocytic nevus (Fig. 7.3)	• Brown macule	• Regular distribution of melanocytes, often in nests	**Dermoscopy** • Regular pigment network
Melanoma *in situ*	• Asymmetry • Irregular borders • Variegate pigment (Fig. 7.4; see Fig. 2.8A)	• Irregular confluent melanocytes	• On acral surfaces, pigment on the ridges is an important clue (Fig. 7.5) **Dermoscopy** • Asymmetry of color and structure • Atypical network • Blue–white structures • Black dots and globules

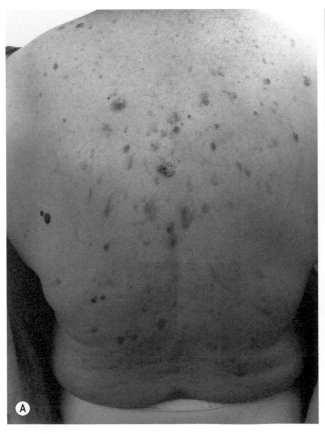

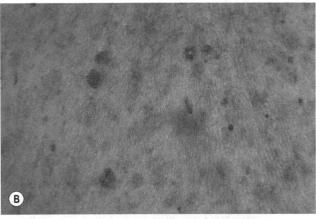

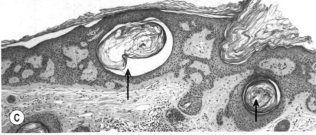

Fig. 7.1 Seborrheic keratosis.

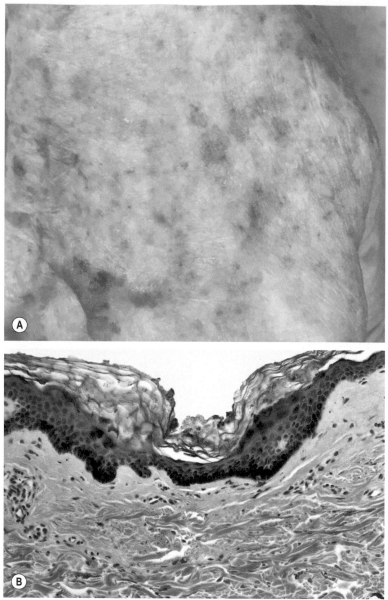

Fig. 7.2 Solar lentigo.

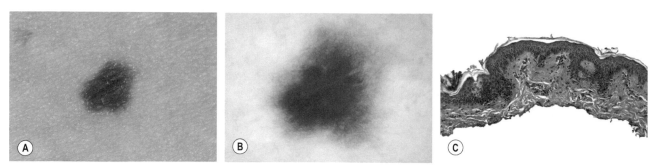

Fig. 7.3 Junctional melanocytic nevus. *A,B, Courtesy, Giuseppe Argenziano, MD, and Iris Zalaudek, MD. A,B, From Bolognia JL, Jorizzo JL, Schaffer JV. Dermatology, 3e. London: Saunders, 2012, with permission.*

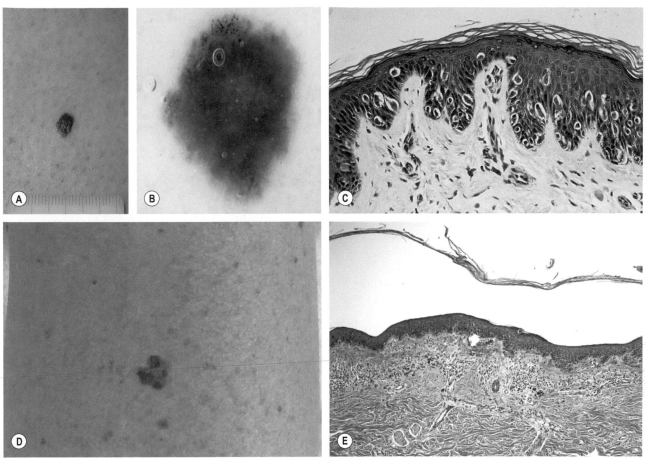

Fig. 7.4 Melanoma *in situ. A,B, Courtesy, Giuseppe Argenziano, MD, and Iris Zalaudek, MD. C, Courtesy, Helmut Kerl, MD. A–C, From Bolognia JL, Jorizzo JL, Schaffer JV. Dermatology, 3e. London: Saunders, 2012, with permission.*

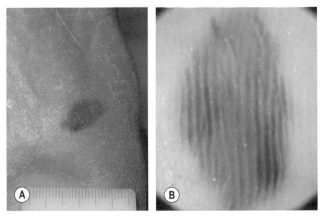

Fig. 7.5 Melanoma *in situ*, acral. *A,B, Courtesy, Giuseppe Argenziano, MD, and Iris Zalaudek, MD. C, Courtesy, Helmut Kerl, MD. A,B, Bolognia JL, Schaffer JV, Duncan KO, Ko CJ. Dermatology Essentials, 1e. Philadelphia: Saunders, 2014, with permission. C, From Bolognia JL, Jorizzo JL, Schaffer JV. Dermatology, 3e. London: Saunders, 2012, with permission.*

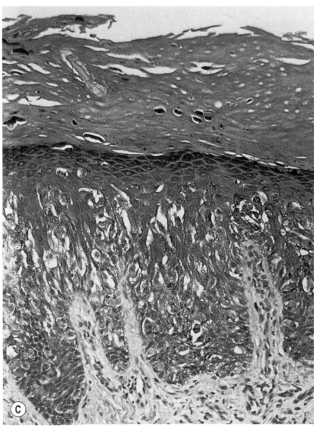

Table 7.2 Epidermal-based lesions: color – pink–red to tan

Lesion	Appearance	Histopathology	Other clues
Actinic keratosis (Fig. 7.6)	• Gritty white–yellow scale, may be subtle • Papule or plaque	• Atypical keratinocytes underlying parakeratosis	
Lichenoid keratosis (Fig. 7.7)	• Flat-surfaced pink plaque	• Band of dermal lymphocytes	
Disseminated superficial actinic porokeratosis	• Thin skin-colored to tan–pink papule or plaque • Raised, sharp rim (arrow; Fig. 7.8)	• Tiered parakeratosis above an abnormal granular layer	
Large cell acanthoma	• Thin pink to tan plaque (Fig. 7.9)	• Enlarged keratinocytes	
Squamous cell carcinoma *in situ* (Fig. 7.10)	• Irregular to hyperkeratotic scale over a red–pink flat-surfaced (occasionally more elevated) papule or plaque	• Atypical cells throughout the entire epidermis	**Dermoscopy** • Glomerular vessels • Superficial scales
Superficial basal cell carcinoma (Fig. 7.11)	• Scaly pink plaque	• Basaloid islands off the base of the epidermis	**Dermoscopy** • Fine telangiectasias

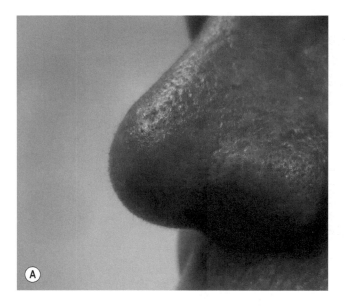

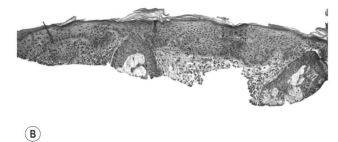

Fig. 7.6 Actinic keratosis, thin and subtle lesion that is better appreciated with palpation.

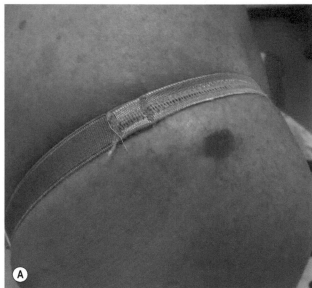

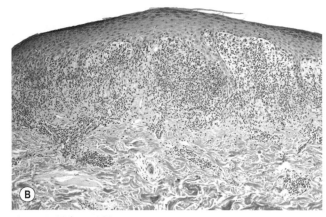

Fig. 7.7 Lichenoid keratosis.

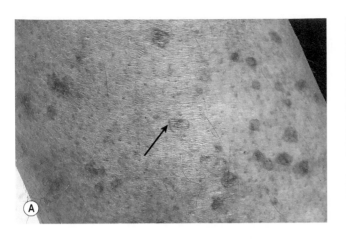

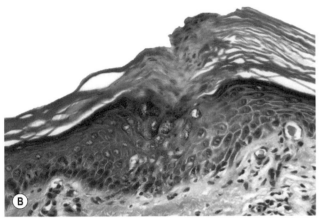

Fig. 7.8 Disseminated superficial actinic porokeratosis. *A, Courtesy, Yale Dermatology Residents' Slide Collection.*

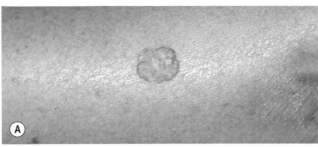

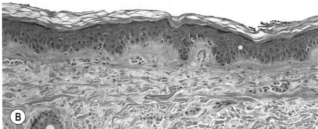

Fig. 7.9 Large cell acanthoma. *A, Courtesy, Luis Requena, MD. A, From Bolognia JL, Schaffer JV, Duncan KO, Ko CJ. Dermatology Essentials, 1e. Philadelphia: Saunders, 2014, with permission.*

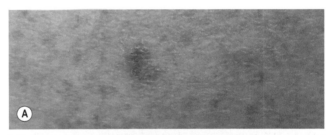

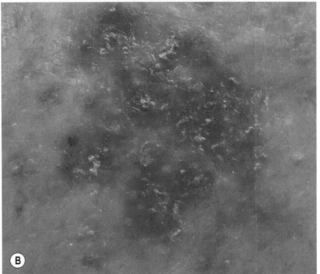

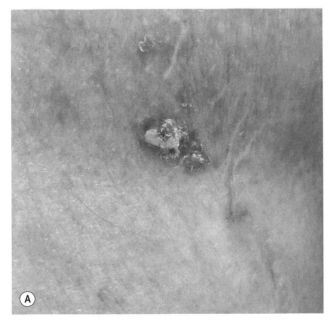

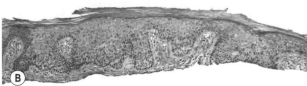

Fig. 7.10 Squamous cell carcinoma *in situ.*

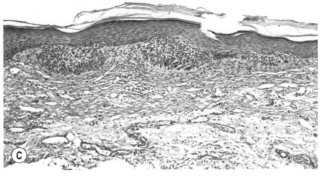

Fig. 7.11 Superficial basal cell carcinoma.

Table 7.3 Epidermal-based lesions: color – red–pink

Lesion	Appearance	Histopathology	Other clues
Clear cell acanthoma	• Well-demarcated, red, shiny papule; wafer-like collarette of scale (Fig. 7.12)	• Pale cells within the epidermis • Overlying parakeratosis	• Sharp demarcation of pale cells from adjacent normal epidermis
Poroma	• Erythematous papule (Fig. 7.13)	• Monomorphous round to oval blue cells • Vascular stroma	• Ductal structures (round spaces lined by a pink cuticle)
Paget disease (Fig. 7.14)	• Erythema, erosion, and scale	• Enlarged cells with abundant cytoplasm • Clusters of cells appear to surround a lumen	• Unilateral • Site: nipple/areola
Extramammary Paget disease (Fig. 7.15)	• Well-demarcated erythema with erosions and scale; macerated white foci		• Site: groin

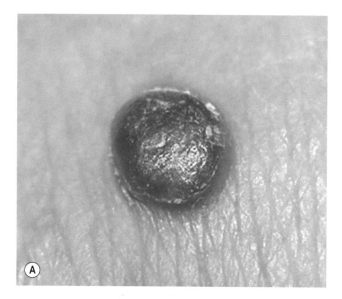

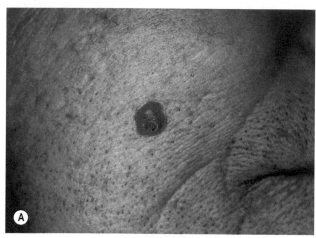

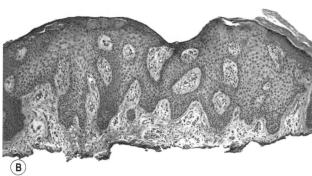

Fig. 7.12 Clear cell acanthoma. *A, Courtesy, Luis Requena, MD; B, Courtesy, Lorrenzo Cerroni, MD. A, From Bolognia JL, Schaffer JV, Duncan KO, Ko CJ. Dermatology Essentials, 1e. Philadelphia: Saunders, 2014, with permission.*

Fig. 7.13 Poroma. *A, From Bolognia JL, Jorizzo JL, Schaffer JV. Dermatology, 3e. London: Saunders, 2012, with permission.*

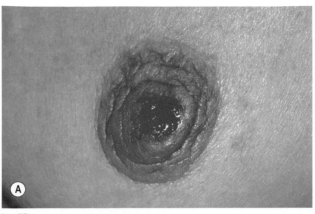

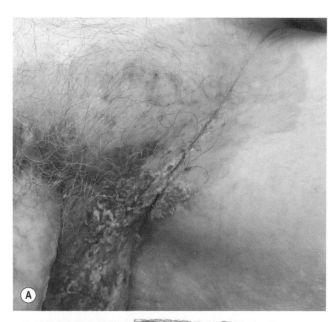

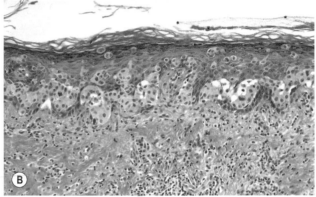

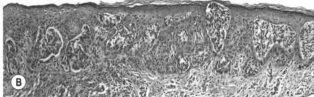

Fig. 7.14 Paget disease of the breast. *A, Courtesy, Robert Hartman, MD. A, From Bolognia JL, Jorizzo JL, Schaffer JV. Dermatology, 3e. London: Saunders, 2012, with permission.*

Fig. 7.15 Extramammary Paget disease.

Table 7.4 Epidermal-based lesions: color – white to skin-colored

Lesion	Appearance	Histopathology
Verruca vulgaris	• Finger-like projections • Punctate red–black dots	• Papillomatosis (arrows; Fig. 7.16) • Koilocytes
Molluscum (Fig. 7.17; see Fig. 6.22)	• White to light pink, pearly papules • Often with central umbilication	• Oval to round, large, pink cytoplasmic inclusions
Trichilemmoma (Fig. 7.18)	• Verrucous to smooth yellow–white papule	• Lobules of pale cells • Peripheral palisading of cells • Thickened pink basement membrane
Tumor of the follicular infundibulum (Fig. 7.19)	• White thin papules	• Anastomosing columns of pale cells
Keratoacanthoma, regressing	• Crateriform lesion consisting mostly of keratin (arrow; Fig. 7.20)	• Thinned epidermis in a cup-shape around keratin (arrow; see Fig. 7.20)

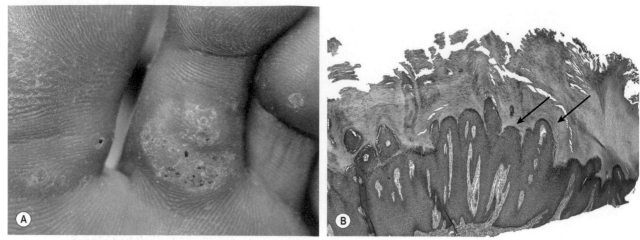

Fig. 7.16 Verruca vulgaris. *Courtesy, Yale Dermatology Residents' Slide Collection.*

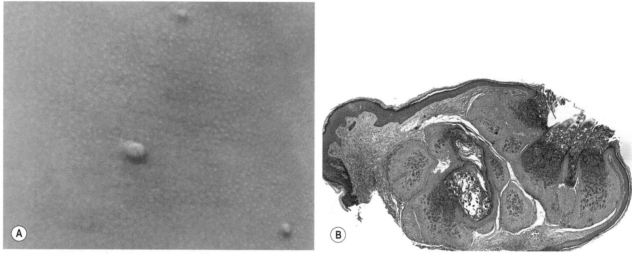

Fig. 7.17 Molluscum contagiosum.

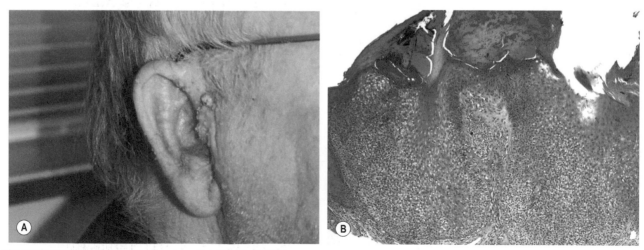

Fig. 7.18 Trichilemmoma. *A, Courtesy, Jennifer Choi, MD.*

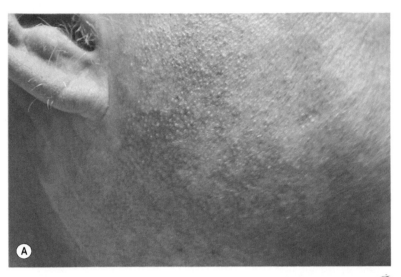

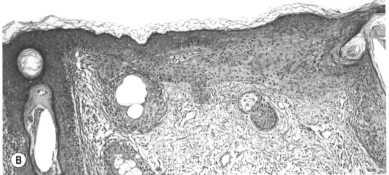

Fig. 7.19 Tumor of the follicular infundibulum.
A, Courtesy, Peter Heald, MD.

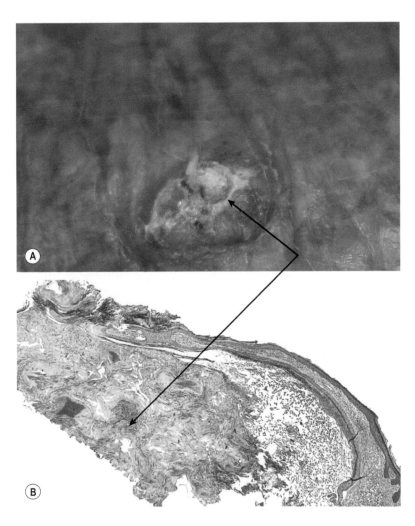

Fig. 7.20 Keratoacanthoma, regressing.
A, Courtesy, Jennifer Choi, MD.

Epidermal Injury/Necrosis | 8

Epidermal injury/necrosis may be superficial, usually manifesting as peeling or crusting of the skin (Fig. 8.1A) or may be deeper, secondary to dermal vascular injury, with early lesions presenting with a grayish hue to the skin (Fig. 8.1C; see Chapter 9). Diseases typically categorized as "interface processes" (see Fig. 1.36; erythema multiforme, lupus erythematosus, fixed drug eruption, lichen planus pigmentosus, erythema dyschromicum perstans) are also addressed in this chapter because there is damage to the epidermal–dermal junction (interface). The color of interface processes is often light pink to violaceous in lighter skin and dark gray to brown in darker skin.

The extent of epidermal injury can be important (Fig. 8.2), and this chapter organizes diseases in that vein (extensive, extensive or limited, and often limited).

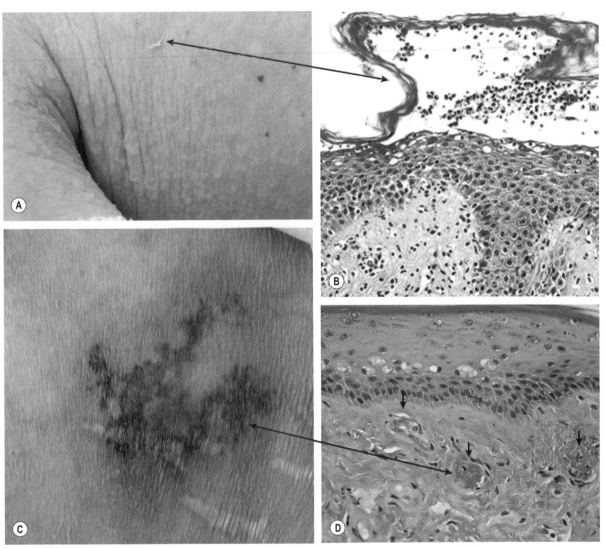

Fig. 8.1 Early epidermal necrosis. Staphylococcal scalded skin syndrome **(A,B)** and calciphylaxis **(C,D**; thrombosed dermal vessels above a deeper, calcified vessel; deeper vessel not shown). *A, Courtesy, Yale Dermatology Residents' Slide Collection. B, From Brinster NK, Liu V, McKee PH, Diwan H. Dermatopathology: High Yield Pathology. Philadelphia: Saunders, 2011. D, From Weenig RH. Pathogenesis of calciphylaxis: Hans Selye to nuclear factor kappa-B. J Am Acad Dermatol. 2008;58:458–71, © Elsevier.*

EXTENSIVE

Toxic Epidermal Necrolysis

Clinical:

Associated fever, lymphadenopathy, hepatitis
>30% of the body surface area (see Fig. 8.2; see Fig. 1.51)
Mucosal erosions
Macular atypical targets
Bullae and erosions (arrow) over the skin (Fig. 8.3)

Histopathologic:

Typically, a normal stratum corneum above epidermal
necrosis; often with detachment of the epidermis from
the dermis

Stevens–Johnson Syndrome

Clinical:

Covers <10% of the body surface area (see Fig. 8.2)
Similar lesions to toxic epidermal necrolysis, clinically
and histologically (Fig. 8.4)

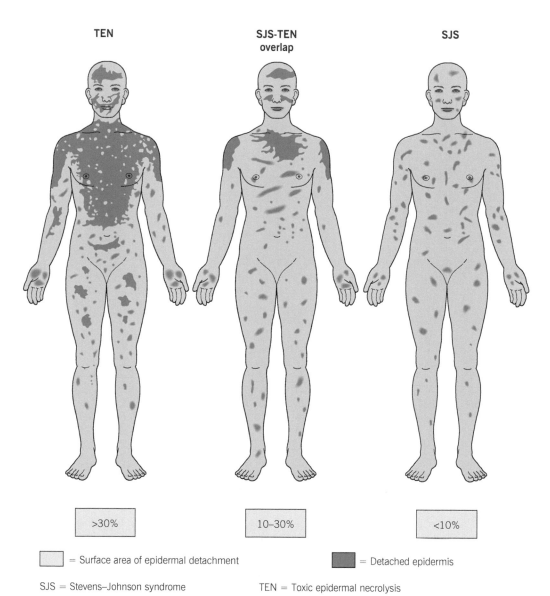

TEN

SJS-TEN
overlap

SJS

>30%   10–30%   <10%

☐ = Surface area of epidermal detachment   ▨ = Detached epidermis

SJS = Stevens–Johnson syndrome   TEN = Toxic epidermal necrolysis

Fig. 8.2 Spectrum of disease based on surface area of epidermal detachment. *Adapted from Bastuji-Garin S, Rzany B, Stern RS, et al. Clinical classification of cases of toxic epidermal necrolysis, Stevens-Johnson syndrome, and erythema multiforme. Arch Dermatol. 1993;129:92–6. From Bolognia JL, Schaffer JV, Duncan KO, Ko CJ. Dermatology Essentials, 1e. Philadelphia: Saunders, 2014, with permission.*

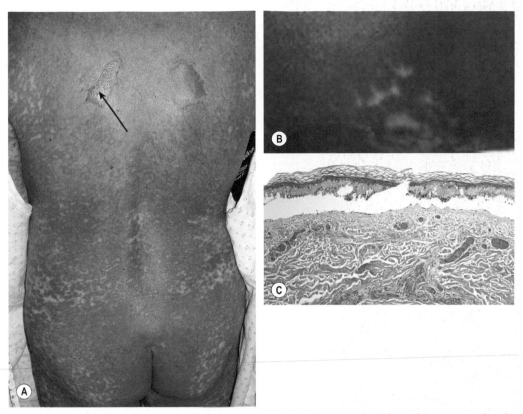

Fig. 8.3 Toxic epidermal necrolysis. **A** Sloughing of skin. **B** Macular atypical targets. **C** Epidermal necrosis with subepidermal cleft. *A,B, Courtesy, Yale Dermatology Residents' Slide Collection. B, From Bolognia JL, Schaffer JV, Duncan KO, Ko CJ. Dermatology Essentials, 1e. Philadelphia: Saunders, 2014, with permission.*

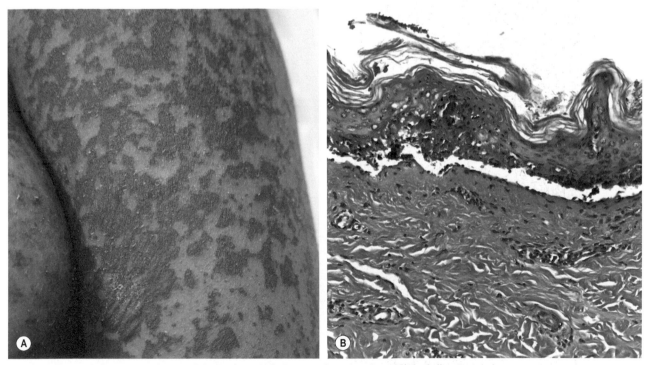

Fig. 8.4 Stevens–Johnson syndrome. *A,B, Courtesy, Yale Dermatology Residents' Slide Collection.*

EXTENSIVE OR LIMITED

Sunburn (Phototoxicity)
Clinical:
Acute erythema (Fig. 8.5)
Later stages – sloughing of skin

Thermal Burn
Clinical:
Body surface area affected can be estimated using a "rule of nines" (Fig. 8.6A)
Acute erythema; in more severe cases, sloughing, erosion, and/or ulceration (Fig. 8.6B–D)

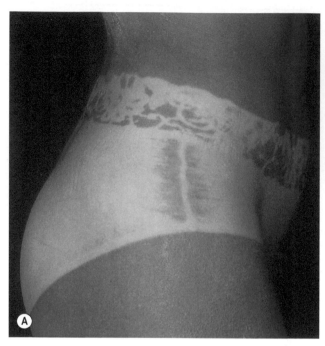

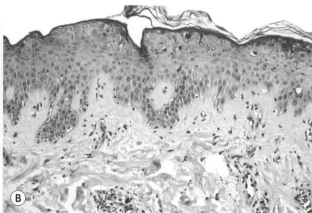

Fig. 8.5 Sunburn. **A** Twenty-four hours after an accidental 10-fold overdose of ultraviolet B (UVB) prescribed as phototherapy. **B** Scattered necrotic keratinocytes in the epidermis. *With permission, Department of Dermatology, University of Würzburg, Germany. A, From Bolognia JL, Jorizzo JL, Schaffer JV. Dermatology, 3e. London: Saunders, 2012, with permission. B, From Brinster NK, Liu V, McKee PH, Diwan H. Dermatopathology: High Yield Pathology. Philadelphia: Saunders, 2011.*

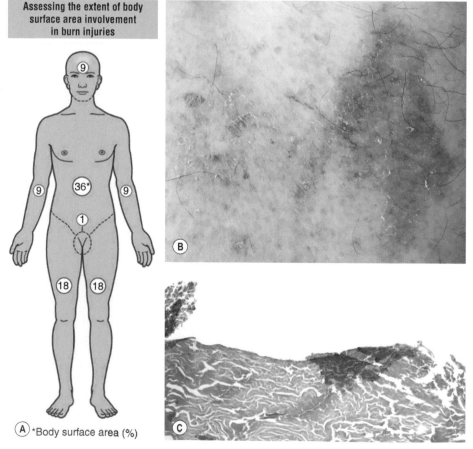

Assessing the extent of body surface area involvement in burn injuries

A *Body surface area (%)

Fig. 8.6 Thermal burn. **A** Assessing the extent of body surface area involvement: rule of nines. **B** Erythema, erosion, and scale secondary to a burn from spilling hot tea. **C** The epidermis is completely absent in this burn. *A, Courtesy, Karynne O Duncan, MD. A, From Bolognia JL, Schaffer JV, Duncan KO, Ko CJ. Dermatology Essentials, 1e. Philadelphia: Saunders, 2014, with permission.*

Erythema Multiforme

Clinical:

Favors acral sites

Classic lesion – target with central deep red erythema surrounded by a halo of lighter color and an outer red rim (Fig. 8.7A; see Figs.1.36, 1.51, 2.19A)

Papular atypical targets (only two zones; Fig. 8.7B)

Histopathologic:

Normal stratum corneum (blue arrow) above interface change (green arrow) with sparse lymphocytic inflammation (Fig. 8.7C)

Key Differences

- **Erythema multiforme** – typical targets with 3 zones of color (see Fig. 2.19A) or papular atypical targets with 2 zones of color – central deep pink to red and lighter rim (Fig. 8.8A)
- **Urticaria multiforme** – center of lesions is normal skin (Fig. 8.8B)

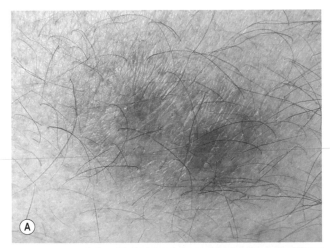

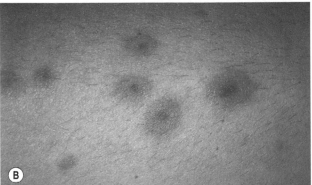

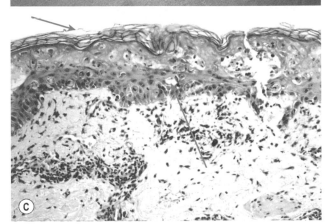

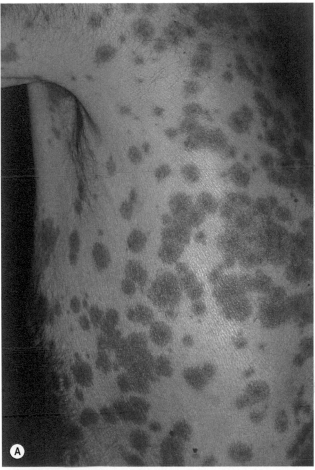

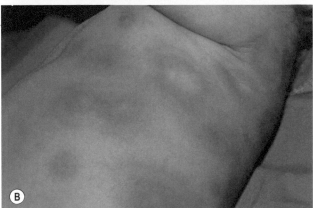

Fig. 8.7 Erythema multiforme. **A** Classic lesion. **B** Papular atypical targets. **C** Interface change and epidermal necrosis below a basket-woven stratum corneum. *A,B, Courtesy, Yale Dermatology Residents' Slide Collection. B, From Bolognia JL, Schaffer JV, Duncan KO, Ko CJ. Dermatology Essentials, 1e. Philadelphia: Saunders, 2014, with permission.*

Fig. 8.8 Lesions with two zones of color. **A** Erythema multiforme. **B** Urticaria multiforme. *A, Courtesy, Yale Dermatology Residents' Slide Collection. B, Courtesy, Julie V Schaffer, MD. A,B, From Bolognia JL, Schaffer JV, Duncan KO, Ko CJ. Dermatology Essentials, 1e. Philadelphia: Saunders, 2014, with permission.*

Paraneoplastic Pemphigus

Clinical:
Characteristic hemorrhagic crusts over the vermilion lips (Fig. 8.9)
Lesions as in erythema multiforme or pemphigus vulgaris (flaccid blisters; see Fig. 12.1)

Histopathologic:
For erythema multiforme-like lesions – interface change (Fig. 8.9B); vesicular lesions – acantholysis (Fig. 8.9C)

Direct immunofluorescence:
Linear IgG and C3 at the dermal–epidermal junction and intercellular immunoglobulin G (IgG) and C3 (Fig. 8.9D)

Lupus Erythematosus

Clinical:
In particular, subacute lupus erythematosus can lead to broad areas of epidermal damage
Papulosquamous lesions (Fig. 8.10A; see Figs. 5.31C, 6.19C), sometimes annular, over the trunk and proximal upper extremities

Histopathologic:
Interface change with scattered apoptotic cells (arrow; Fig. 8.10B)

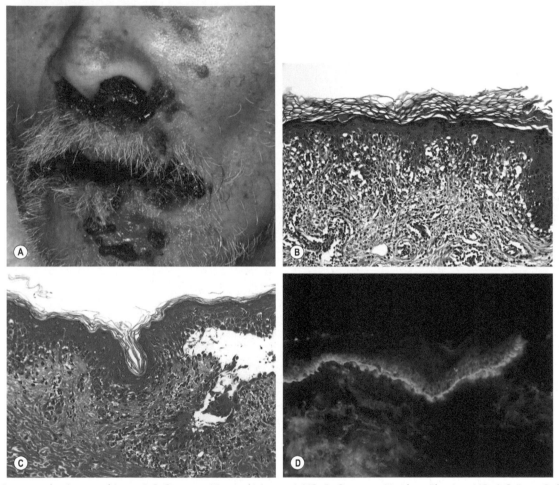

Fig. 8.9 Paraneoplastic pemphigus. *A,C, Courtesy, Masayuki Amagai, MD. D, Courtesy, Matthew Fleming, MD. A,C, From Bolognia JL, Jorizzo JL, Schaffer JV. Dermatology, 3e. London: Saunders, 2012, with permission. D, From Weidner N, Cote RJ, Suster S, Weiss LM. Modern Surgical Pathology, 2e. Philadelphia: Saunders, 2009.*

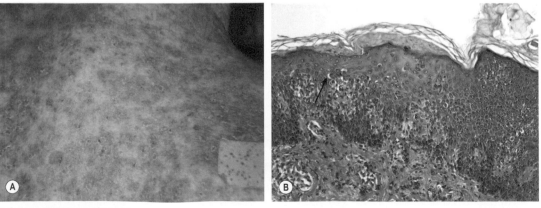

Fig. 8.10 Subacute lupus erythematosus.

Fixed Drug Eruption (Fig. 8.11)

Clinical:

Common inciting drugs include naproxen, allopurinol, antibiotics

Oval to round lesion(s), erythematous to violaceous, bullae may form

Often resolves with hyperpigmentation (see Fig. 8.11E)

Histopathologic:

Early lesions with interface change and superficial and deep mixed inflammation (see Fig. 8.11B); later lesions with pigment incontinence and variable inflammation (see Fig. 8.11F)

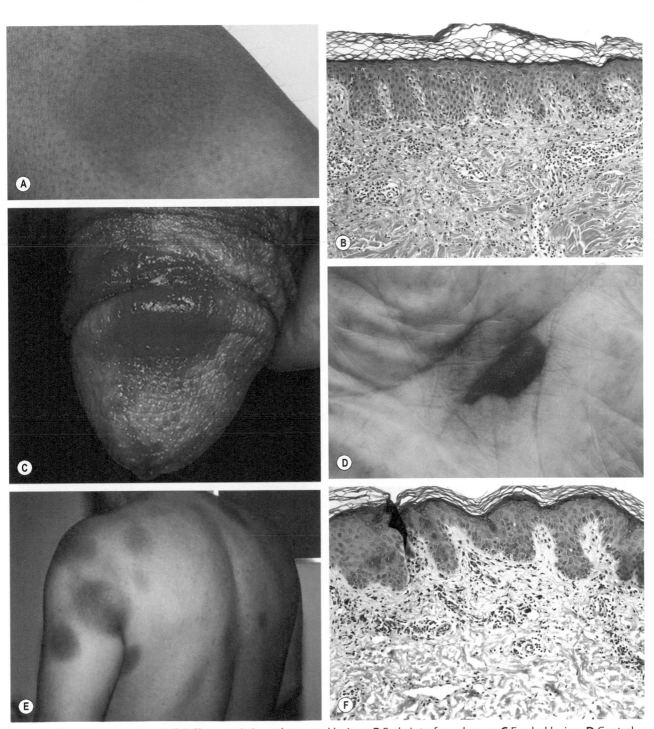

Fig. 8.11 Fixed drug eruption. **A,C,E** Characteristic oval to round lesions. **B** Early interface change. **C** Eroded lesion. **D** Central blister with detachment of the epidermis. **E** Oval areas of postinflammatory hyperpigmentation. **F** Prominent pigment incontinence in a later lesion. *A,D, Courtesy, Yale Dermatology Residents' Slide Collection; C, Courtesy, Kalman Watsky, MD; E, Courtesy, Mary Stone, MD. C,E, From Bolognia JL, Schaffer JV, Duncan KO, Ko CJ. Dermatology Essentials, 1e. Philadelphia: Saunders, 2014, with permission.*

Lichen Planus Pigmentosus

Clinical:

Brown macules or patches, may involve intertriginous sites (so-called inversus, as in this patient with inner thigh lesions; Fig. 8.12A) and/or the face and neck
May be associated with typical flat-topped, purplish lesions of lichen planus

Histopathology:

Variable lichenoid inflammation (in this example, it is moderately dense) and pigment incontinence (Fig. 8.12B)

Erythema Dyschromicum Perstans (Ashy Dermatosis)

Clinical:

There may be a thin pink border to gray–brown oval macules or patches (Fig. 8.13A)
Often on the trunk and upper arms; distribution can resemble that of pityriasis rosea

Histopathology:

Interface change, pigment incontinence, and generally mild lymphocytic inflammation

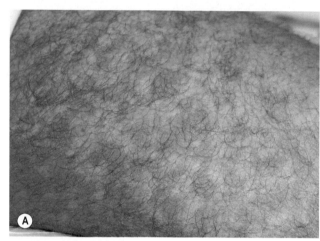
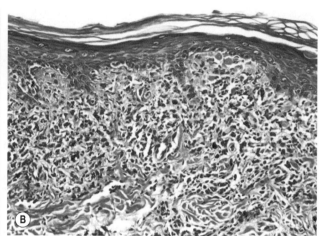

Fig. 8.12 Lichen planus pigmentosus.

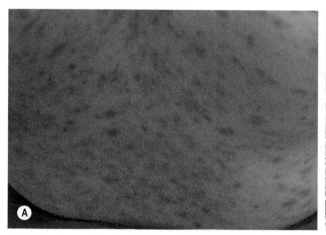
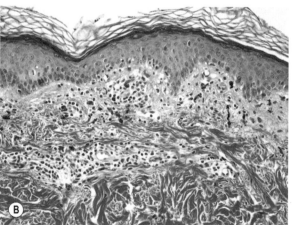

Fig. 8.13 Erythema dyschromicum perstans (ashy dermatosis).

Nutritional Deficiency

Particular nutritional deficiencies have classic associated findings (e.g. vitamin C deficiency causes bleeding gums); importantly, patients can be deficient in more than one nutrient. Several different deficiencies can produce erythema and superficial scales corresponding to superficial epidermal necrosis (Fig. 8.14); most of these present in periorificial, intertriginous, and acral areas (e.g. zinc, biotin, or essential fatty acid deficiency) except for pellagra, which favors sun-exposed sites.

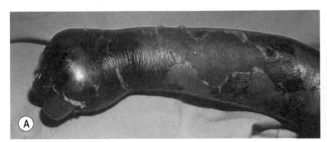

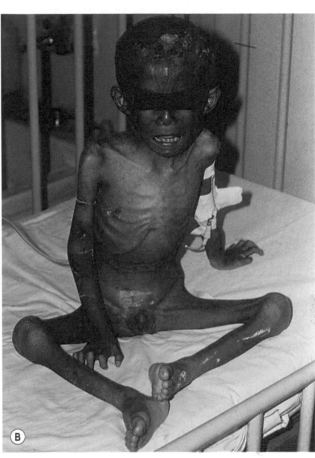

Fig. 8.14 Nutritional deficiency. **A** Marasmus. Emaciation, hyperpigmentation, and superficial necrosis of the skin. **B** Kwashiorkor. Edema and superficial epidermal necrosis with an "enamel paint" appearance. **C** Mucocutaneous clues that suggest a possible nutritional disorder. *A,B, From Bolognia JL, Jorizzo JL, Schaffer JV. Dermatology, 3e. London: Saunders, 2012, with permission. C, Courtesy, Karynne O Duncan, MD; B,C Courtesy, Ramón Ruiz-Maldonado, MD. C, From Bolognia JL, Schaffer JV, Duncan KO, Ko CJ. Dermatology Essentials, 1e. Philadelphia: Saunders, 2014, with permission.*

Mucocutaneous clues that suggest a possible nutritional disorder

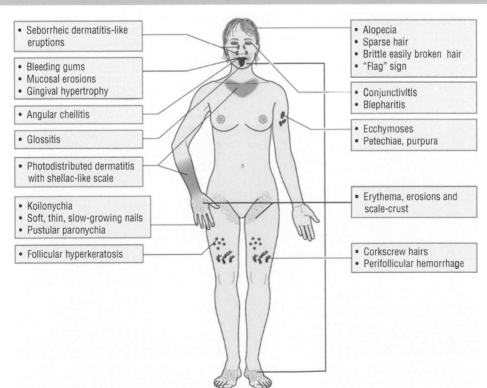

- Seborrheic dermatitis-like eruptions
- Bleeding gums
- Mucosal erosions
- Gingival hypertrophy
- Angular cheilitis
- Glossitis
- Photodistributed dermatitis with shellac-like scale
- Koilonychia
- Soft, thin, slow-growing nails
- Pustular paronychia
- Follicular hyperkeratosis
- Alopecia
- Sparse hair
- Brittle easily broken hair
- "Flag" sign
- Conjunctivitis
- Blepharitis
- Ecchymoses
- Petechiae, purpura
- Erythema, erosions and scale-crust
- Corkscrew hairs
- Perifollicular hemorrhage

Niacin/Nicotinic Acid (Vitamin B₃) Deficiency (Pellagra)

Clinical:

Classic triad – diarrhea, dementia, dermatitis
Favors sun-exposed sites (see Fig. 3.8E) and perianal areas
Erythema with subsequent hyperpigmentation, desquamation (Fig. 8.15A; see asterisk), crusting

Clinical clues – Casal's necklace (broad area of involvement around the neck)

Histopathologic:

Confluent parakeratosis and/or upper epidermal necrosis (Fig. 8.15B; see asterisk)

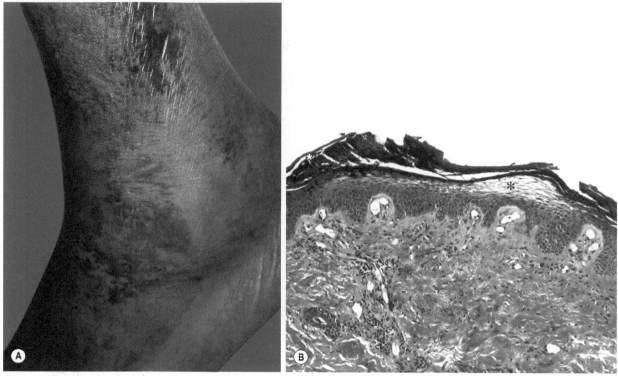

Fig. 8.15 Pellagra. *A, Courtesy, Yale Dermatology Residents' Slide Collection. A, From Bolognia JL, Jorizzo JL, Schaffer JV. Dermatology, 3e. London: Saunders, 2012, with permission.*

Zinc Deficiency (Acquired or Genetic, the Latter Is Termed *Acrodermatitis Enteropathica*)

Clinical:

Classic triad – diarrhea, dermatitis, alopecia
Favors periorificial, intertriginous, and acral sites (Fig. 8.16A–D; see Fig. 2.17F)

Erythema, erosions, crusting, and superficial desquamation
Clinical clue – pustular paronychia

Histopathologic:

Parakeratosis and/or superficial necrosis of the epidermis (Fig. 8.16E)

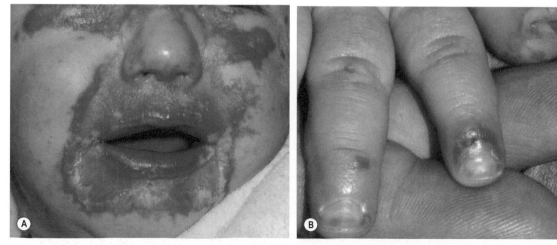

Fig. 8.16 Zinc deficiency (acrodermatitis enteropathica). *A,B, Courtesy Julie V Schaffer, MD. C, Courtesy, Jason Lott, MD; D,E Courtesy, Yale Dermatology Residents' Slide Collection. A,B, From Bolognia JL, Jorizzo JL, Schaffer JV. Dermatology, 3e. London: Saunders, 2012, with permission.*

Epidermal Injury/Necrosis

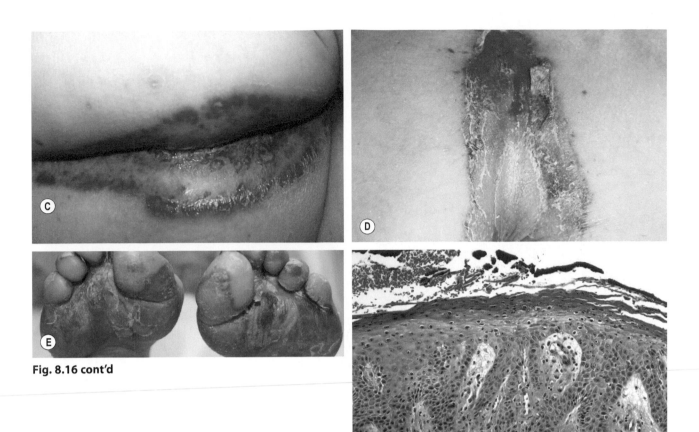

Fig. 8.16 cont'd

Necrolytic Acral Erythema

Clinical:

Associated with hepatitis C infection

Acral sites (Fig. 8.17A)

Histopathologic:

Superficial necrosis of the epidermis (Fig. 8.17B)

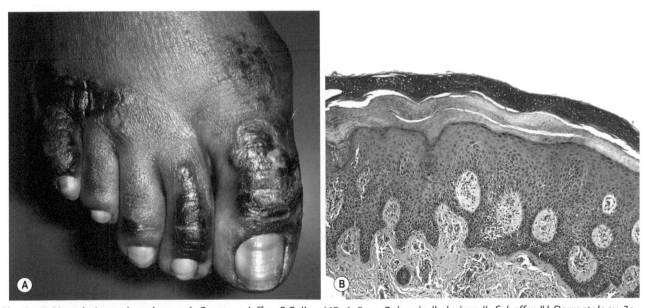

Fig. 8.17 Necrolytic acral erythema. *A, Courtesy, Jeffrey P Callen, MD. A, From Bolognia JL, Jorizzo JL, Schaffer JV. Dermatology, 3e. London: Saunders, 2012, with permission.*

Necrolytic Migratory Erythema (Fig. 8.18)

Clinical:
Associated with a glucagon-secreting pancreatic tumor
Angular cheilitis and eroded plaques with a predilection for intertriginous sites (especially the groin)

Histopathologic:
Superficial necrosis of the epidermis similar to necrolytic acral erythema

Calciphylaxis
(See Figs. 8.1C and 9.3B)

Warfarin-Induced Skin Necrosis
(See Fig. 9.3G)

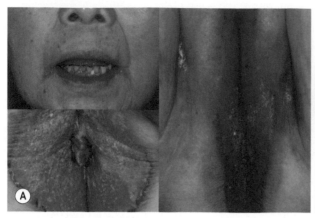
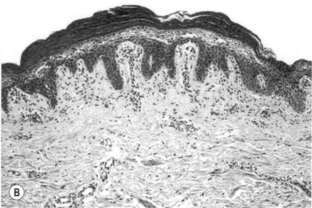

Fig. 8.18 Necrolytic migratory erythema. *A, From Tseng HC, Liu CT, Ho JC, Lin SH. Necrolytic migratory erythema and glucagonoma rising from pancreatic head. Pancreatology. 2013;13:455–7, © 2013 IAP and EPC. B, From Brinster NK, Liu V, McKee PH, Diwan H. Dermatopathology: High Yield Pathology. Philadelphia: Saunders, 2011.*

OFTEN LIMITED

Spider Bite

Clinical:
Some species of spiders will bite humans and cause epidermal and dermal necrosis (e.g. the brown recluse spider, *Loxosceles reclusa*)
Initial erythema may become dusky and eventuate in bullae and/or necrosis (Fig. 8.19)

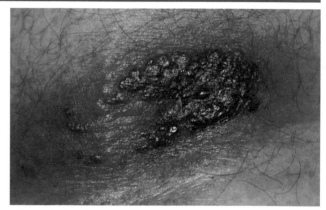

Fig. 8.19 Brown recluse spider bite. *Courtesy, Yale Dermatology Residents' Slide Collection.*

Purpura, Small Vessel Vasculitis, and Vascular Occlusion | 9

Purpura is a manifestation of extravascular erythrocytes. The morphology of purpura is important – flat vs raised and smooth/circular vs irregular/retiform/scalloped border/outline (Fig. 9.1). The irregular/retiform pattern corresponds to the cutaneous network of small vessels that produces livedo reticularis (see Figs. 1.22A,B). This chapter focuses on the distinction between palpable purpura (Fig. 9.2) and retiform purpura (Fig. 9.3). Other diseases with underlying small vessel damage include acute hemorrhagic edema of infancy (Fig. 9.4A–C), urticarial vasculitis (Fig. 9.4D,E), and erythema elevatum diutinum (Fig. 9.4H–J).

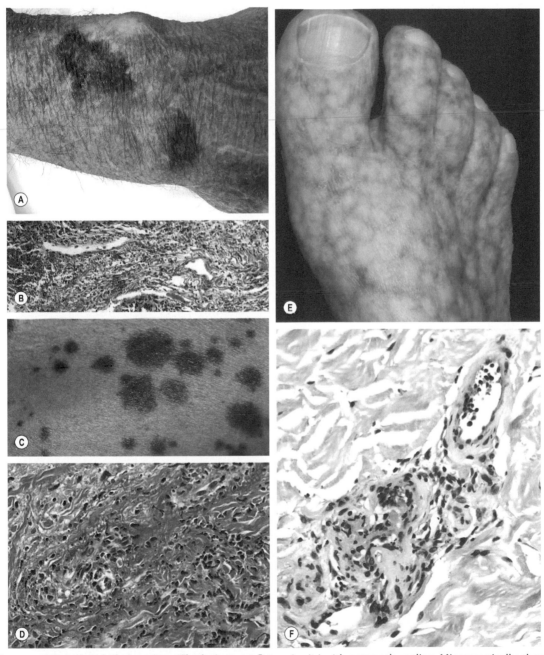

Fig. 9.1 Purpura. **A,B** Actinic (solar) purpura. The lesions are flat and solid with a smooth outline. Microscopically, there are dilated vascular spaces with extravasated erythrocytes (B). **C,D** Palpable purpura (raised with a smooth outline); leukocytoclasia and fibrin deposition microscopically (D). **E,F** Retiform purpura. The lesions are a flat network of interconnecting rings ("retiform"); vascular occlusion with sparse perivascular inflammation (F). *C, Courtesy, Yale Dermatology Residents' Slide Collection. C, From Bolognia JL, Jorizzo JL, Schaffer JV. Dermatology, 3e. London: Saunders, 2012, with permission.*

PALPABLE PURPURA

Clinical:
Palpable purpura is a common manifestation of cutaneous small vessel vasculitis. Causes are diverse and include Henoch–Schönlein purpura (see Fig. 9.2A), drug exposure, malignancies (especially hematologic; see Fig. 9.2B), systemic disease (see Fig. 9.2C–F), and infections. History, other clues on examination (see rheumatoid nodules in Fig. 9.2F), and/or laboratory studies are necessary to ascertain the ultimate cause.

The morphology is typically raised and solid circular with a smooth border (see Fig. 9.1B) and there may be surface changes, including bullae formation (see Figs. 14.2E and 14.5).

Histopathologic:
For leukocytoclastic vasculitis – classic triad of neutrophilic inflammation, leukocytoclasia, and fibrin cuffs around damaged capillaries (small vessels) (see Fig. 9.1E)

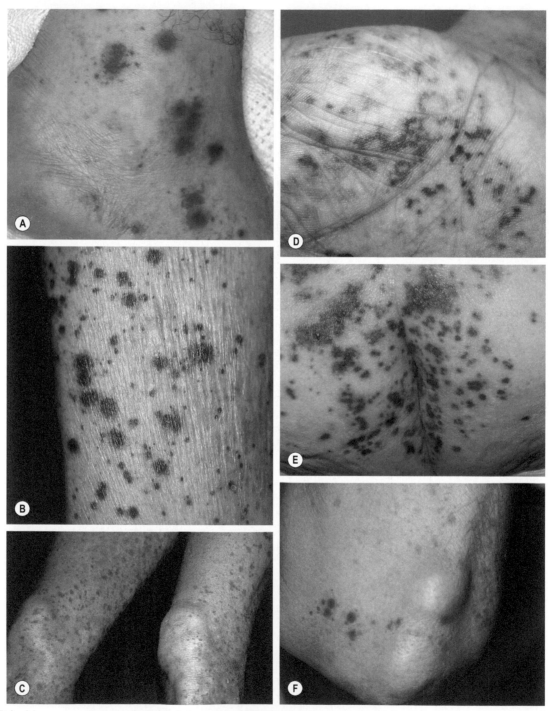

Fig. 9.2 Palpable purpura. **A** Henoch–Schönlein purpura. **B** Palpable purpura in a patient with myelodysplasia and relapsing polychondritis. **C** Mixed cryoglobulinemia. **D** Granulomatosis with polyangiitis (Wegener granulomatosis). **E** Eosinophilic granulomatosis with polyangiitis (Churg–Strauss syndrome). **F** Rheumatoid arthritis. *A,D,F, Courtesy, Yale Dermatology Residents' Slide Collection; B, Courtesy, Jean L Bolognia, MD. C, Courtesy, Lorinda Chung, MD, Bory Kea, MD and David F Fiorentino, MD. E, Courtesy, Kanade Shinkai, MD and Lindy P Fox, MD. A–C,E,F, From Bolognia JL, Jorizzo JL, Schaffer JV. Dermatology, 3e. London: Saunders, 2012, with permission.*

RETIFORM PURPURA

Clinical:

Retiform purpura is generally caused by vascular occlusion, especially when not preceded by clinical erythema. Retiform purpura that is preceded by clinical erythema may be secondary to occlusion (see Fig. 9.3A–G) or vasculitis (see Fig. 9.3H–I).

In retiform purpura, portions of the normal vascular network become fixed and visible (see Fig. 9.1E). In later stages, centers of lesions can be solid, bullous or eroded, and/or necrotic, but the borders of lesions remain scalloped/irregular, stellate, or "retiform" (see Fig. 9.3).

Histopathologic:

Inflammation may be minimal; occlusion of vessel lumina with thrombi or emboli (see Fig. 9.1F)
In some cases (e.g. levamisole-induced vasculitis, septic emboli), there can be both perivascular neutrophilic inflammation +/− leukocytoclasia and occlusion of the lumens of small vessels.

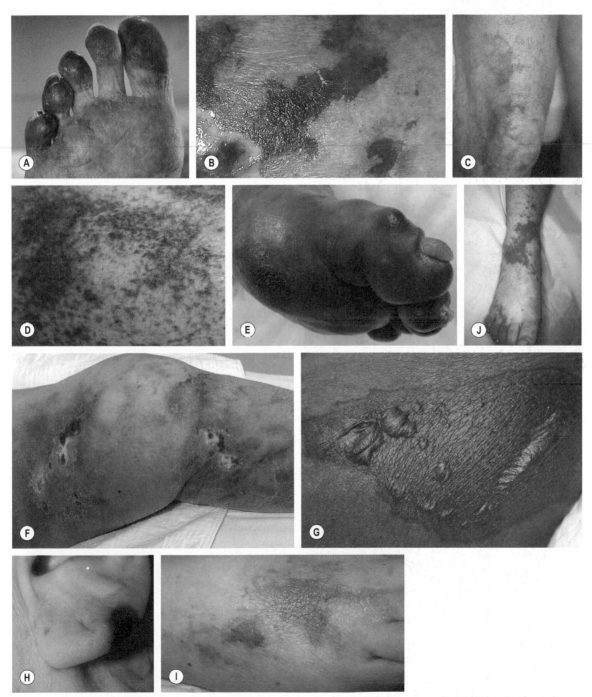

Fig. 9.3 Retiform purpura. **A** Antiphospholipid syndrome. **B** Calciphylaxis. **C** Cholesterol embolus. **D** Cryoglobulinemia, monoclonal. **E** Disseminated intravascular coagulation. **F** Intravascular lymphoma. **G** Warfarin-induced necrosis. Tendency to affect fatty areas like hips, abdomen, buttocks. **H** Levamisole-induced vasculitis. A typical site of involvement is the ear. **I** Polyarteritis nodosa. **J** Rocky Mountain spotted fever. *A,B,D,E,G–J, Courtesy, Yale Dermatology Residents' Slide Collection. C, Courtesy, Norbert Sepp, MD; F, Courtesy, Lucinda Buescher, MD. B,C,F,I,J, From Bolognia JL, Jorizzo JL, Schaffer JV. Dermatology, 3e. London: Saunders, 2012, with permission.*

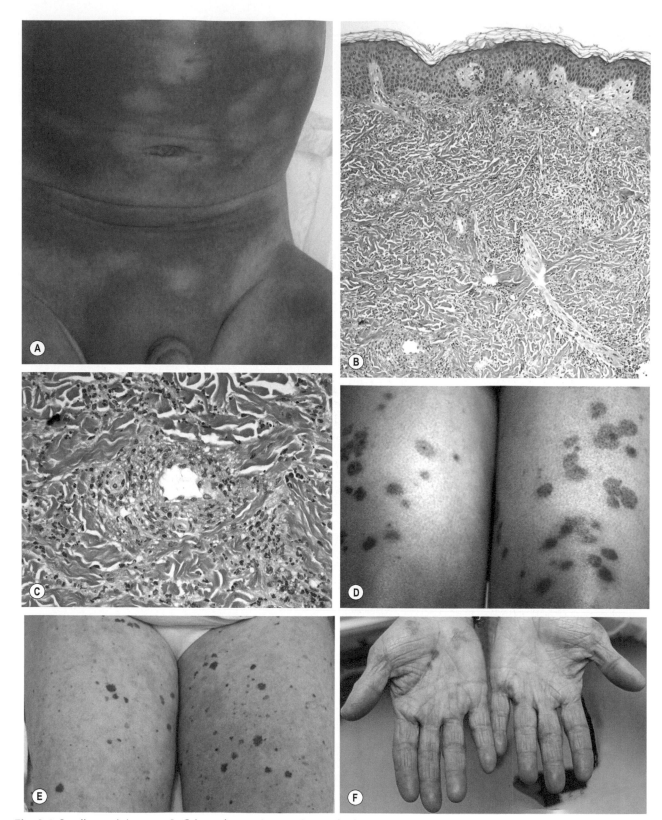

Fig. 9.4 Small vessel damage. **A–C** Acute hemorrhagic edema of infancy. **D–G** Urticarial vasculitis.

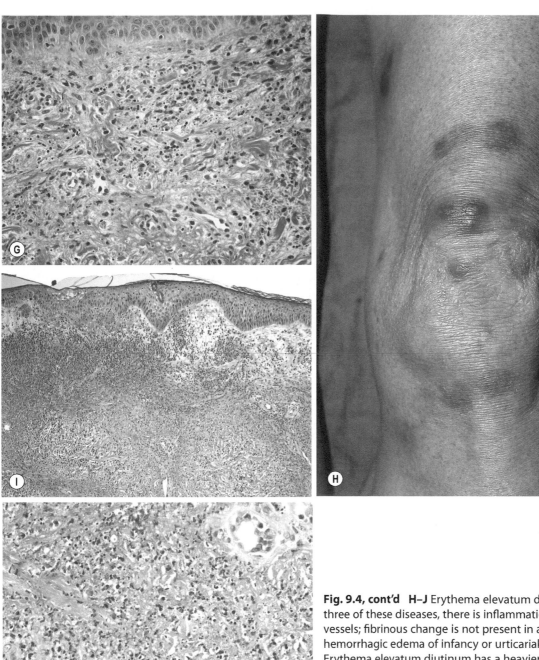

Fig. 9.4, cont'd   H–J Erythema elevatum diutinum. In all three of these diseases, there is inflammation surrounding vessels; fibrinous change is not present in acute hemorrhagic edema of infancy or urticarial vasculitis. Erythema elevatum diutinum has a heavier inflammatory infiltrate that is neutrophil-predominant. *A,D Courtesy, Yale Dermatology Residents' Slide Collection; E,F, Courtesy Ilya Lim, MD; G, Courtesy, Kenneth Greer, MD. G, From Bolognia JL, Jorizzo JL, Schaffer JV. Dermatology, 3e. London: Saunders, 2012, with permission.*

Ulcers | 10

Three major types of ulcers occur on the legs (Table 10.1), and these ulcers are often diagnosed clinically. Histopathology can be helpful in diagnosing the cause of particular ulcers, for example, pyoderma gangrenosum (Fig. 10.1), infections (Figs. 10.2–10.4), vasculitides (Figs. 10.5, 10.6), vaso-occlusive processes (Fig. 10.7), or tumors (Fig. 10.8). Selected other causes of ulcers are depicted in Figs. 10.9–10.17.

Table 10.1 Common leg ulcers – key differences

	Venous	Arterial	Neuropathic/Mal perforans*
Location	Medial malleolar region	Pressure sites (lateral malleolar region) Distal points (toes)	Pressure sites
Morphology	Irregular borders Yellow fibrinous base	Dry, necrotic base Well-demarcated ("punched out")	"Punched out"
Surrounding skin	Yellow–brown to brown discoloration caused by hemosiderin deposits Pinpoint petechiae ("stasis purpura") Lipodermatosclerosis	Shiny atrophic skin with hair loss	Thick callus
Other physical examination findings	Varicosities Leg/ankle edema ± Stasis dermatitis ± Lymphedema	Weak/absent peripheral pulses Prolonged capillary refill time (>3–4 seconds) Pallor on leg elevation (45° for 1 minute) Dependent rubor	Peripheral neuropathy with decreased sensation ± Foot deformities

*Most commonly caused by diabetes mellitus.
Images, Courtesy, David L Troutman Jr, DPM, Tammie C Ferringer, MD, Ariela Hafner, MD and Eli Sprecher, MD. Table adapted from Bolognia JL, Jorizzo JL, Schaffer JV. Dermatology, 3e. London: Saunders, 2012, with permission.

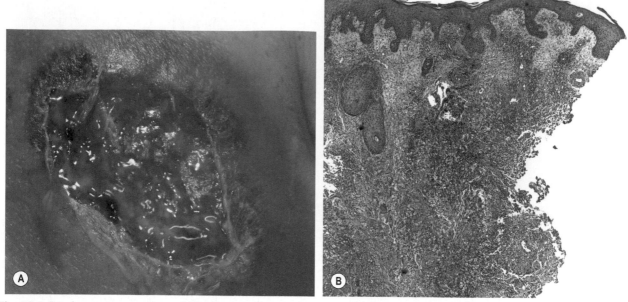

Fig. 10.1 Pyoderma gangrenosum. **A** Classic ulcerative pyoderma gangrenosum. The edge of this ulceration on the shin is undermined by violet–gray coloration and an inflammatory rim. Note the central scarring. **B** In expanding untreated lesions, a diffuse infiltrate of neutrophils is present. *A, Courtesy, Yale Dermatology Residents' Slide Collection.*

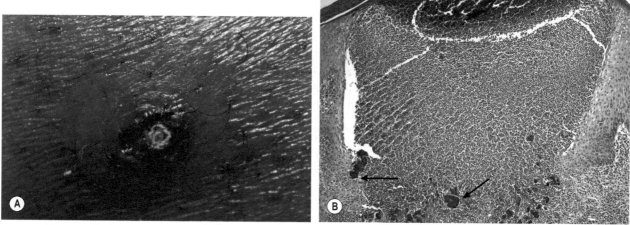

Fig. 10.2 Ecthyma. Superficial ulceration and crust on the wrist caused by infection with group A streptococci (arrows). *A, Courtesy, Yale Dermatology Residents' Slide Collection.*

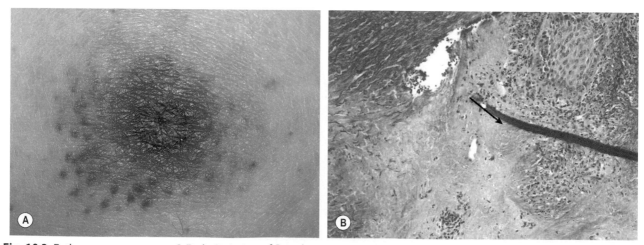

Fig. 10.3 Ecthyma gangrenosum. **A** Embolic lesion of *Pseudomonas aeruginosa* on the chest. Note the necrotic center and inflammatory border. **B** Histopathologic findings include dermal necrosis and a light blue haze of organisms (arrow). *A, Courtesy, Yale Dermatology Residents' Slide Collection.*

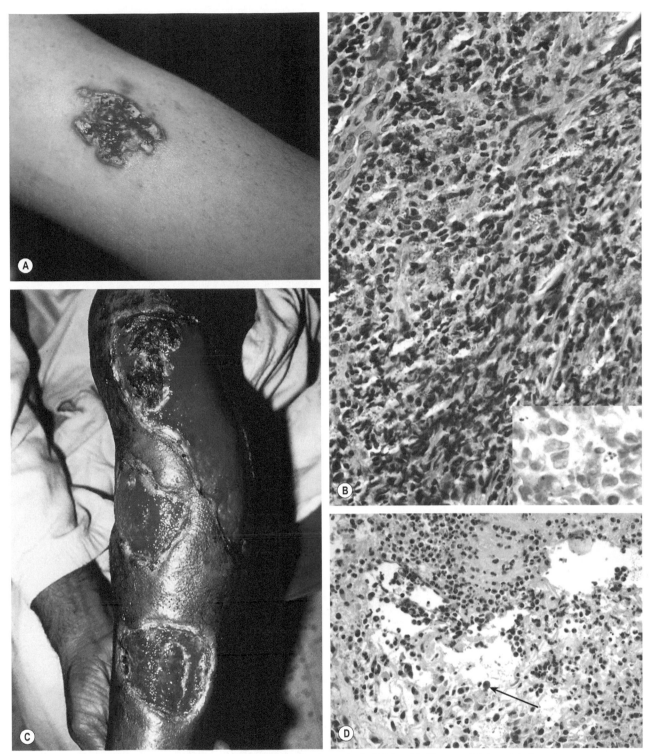

Fig. 10.4 Infectious ulcers. **A** Ulcerative form of cutaneous leishmaniasis. **B** Mixed infiltrate with intrahistiocytic organisms (round, bluish structures); inset shows staining of the organisms with CD1a. **C** Amebiasis. Multiple large, destructive ulcers. **D** Mixed inflammation and rare trophozoites (arrow). *A, Courtesy, Yale Dermatology Residents' Slide Collection; B, inset, Courtesy Shawn Cowper, MD; D, Courtesy, Omar P Sangüeza, MD. A–C, From Bolognia JL, Jorizzo JL, Schaffer JV. Dermatology, 3e. London: Saunders, 2012, with permission.*

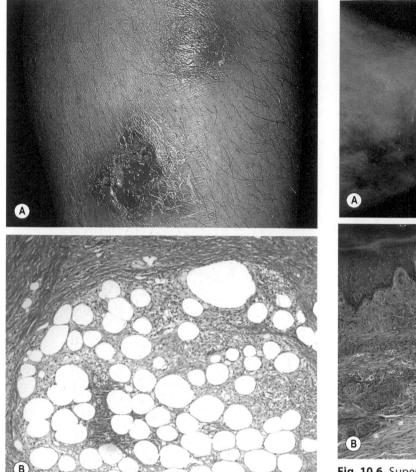

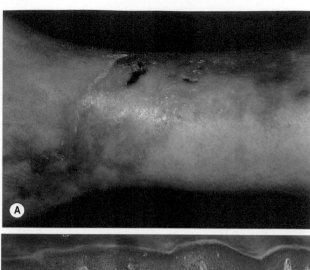

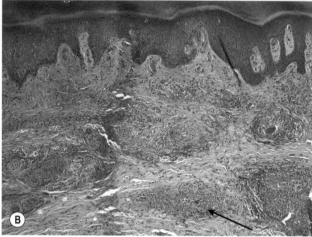

Fig. 10.5 Erythema induratum. **A** Nodular lesions on the lower leg, with evidence of ulceration. **B** Lobular panniculitis. The infiltrate is lymphocytic and granulomatous. *A, Courtesy, Kenneth E Greer, MD. A, From Bolognia JL, Jorizzo JL, Schaffer JV. Dermatology, 3e. London: Saunders, 2012, with permission.*

Fig. 10.6 Superficial ulcerating rheumatoid necrobiosis. **A** Shiny, yellow plaques with red–brown edges and areas of ulceration that clinically resemble necrobiosis lipoidica. **B** Vasculitis (fibrin and inflammation within vessel walls; arrow). *A, Courtesy, Kathryn Schwarzenberger, MD. A, From Bolognia JL, Jorizzo JL, Schaffer JV. Dermatology, 3e. London: Saunders, 2012, with permission.*

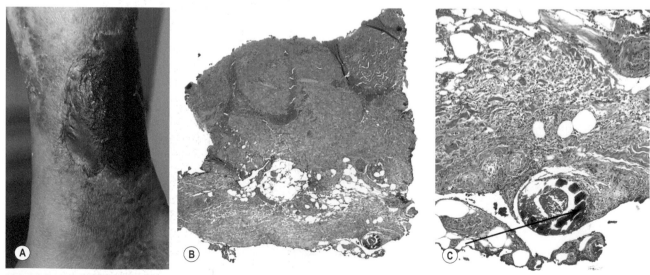

Fig. 10.7 Calciphylaxis. **A** Necrotic skin lesions in the setting of severe end-stage renal disease caused by amyloidosis of the kidney. **B,C** Calcium within a vessel (arrow). *A, Courtesy, Yale Dermatology Residents' Slide Collection.*

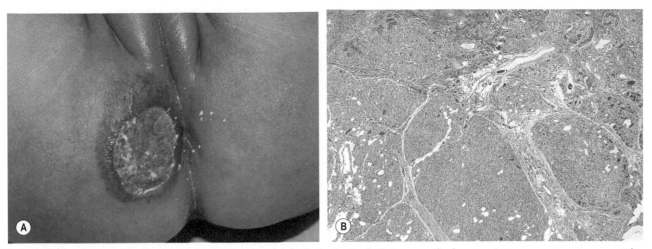

Fig. 10.8 Ulcerated minimal/arrested growth hemangioma on the buttock. **A** Because the hemangioma component may not be obvious, this diagnosis should be considered when an infant presents with an ulcer in the diaper area. **B** Lobular collections of small capillaries. *Courtesy, Julie V Schaffer, MD. From Bolognia JL, Jorizzo JL, Schaffer JV. Dermatology, 3e. London: Saunders, 2012, with permission.*

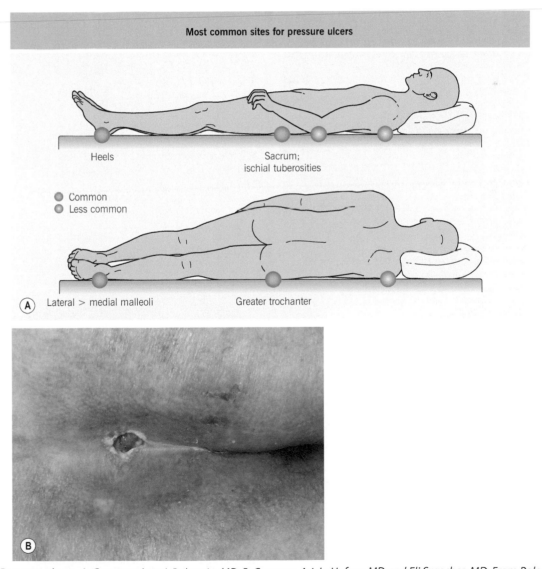

Fig. 10.9 Pressure ulcers. *A, Courtesy, Jean L Bolognia, MD. B, Courtesy, Ariela Hafner, MD and Eli Sprecher, MD. From Bolognia JL, Jorizzo JL, Schaffer JV. Dermatology, 3e. London: Saunders, 2012, with permission.*

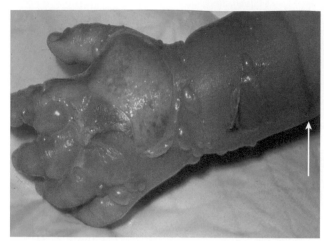

Fig. 10.10 Burn injury caused by being dunked in hot water. Note the sharp line of demarcation of the burn on the arm (arrow). *Courtesy, Sharon Ann Raimer, MD. From Bolognia JL, Jorizzo JL, Schaffer JV. Dermatology, 3e. London: Saunders, 2012, with permission.*

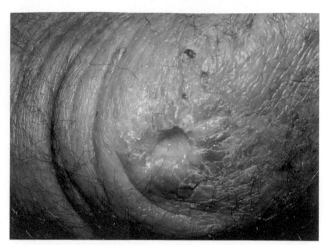

Fig. 10.11 Ulceration of the elbow in a patient with systemic sclerosis. *Courtesy, Joyce Rico, MD. From Bolognia JL, Jorizzo JL, Schaffer JV. Dermatology, 3e. London: Saunders, 2012, with permission.*

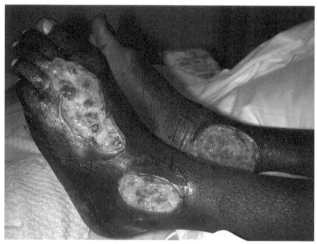

Fig. 10.12 Multiple ulcers secondary to sickle cell anemia. *Courtesy, NYU Slide Collection. From Bolognia JL, Jorizzo JL, Schaffer JV. Dermatology, 3e. London: Saunders, 2012, with permission.*

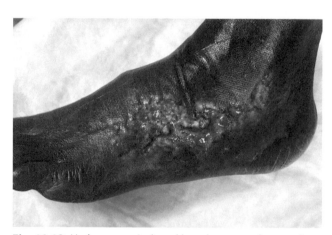

Fig. 10.13 Hydroxyurea-induced leg ulcers are often on the malleolus or tibial crest, exceedingly painful and surrounded by atrophic skin. *Courtesy, NYU Slide Collection. From Bolognia JL, Jorizzo JL, Schaffer JV. Dermatology, 3e. London: Saunders, 2012, with permission.*

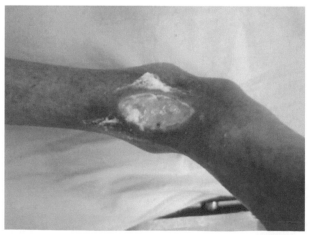

Fig. 10.14 Werner syndrome. Leg ulcerations are common in atrophic skin of the legs. *From Yeong EK, Yang CC. Chronic leg ulcers in Werner's syndrome. Br J Plast Surg 2004;57:86-88. © Elsevier.*

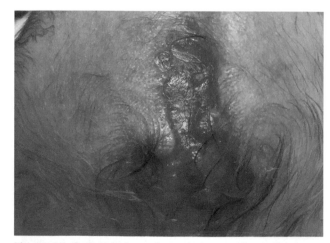

Fig. 10.15 Cutis aplasia on the scalp in a newborn. *Courtesy, Yale Dermatology Residents' Slide Collection.*

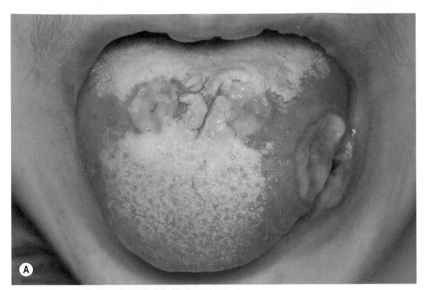

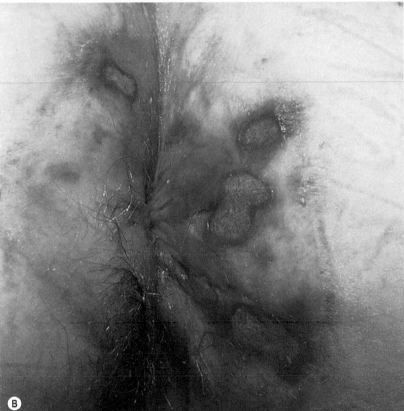

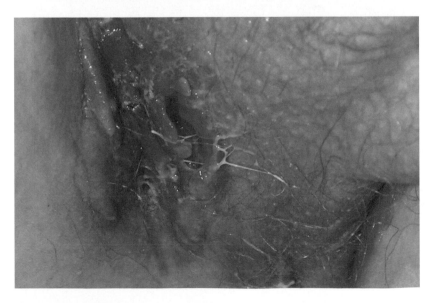

Fig. 10.16 Behçet disease. Oral **(A)** and perineal **(B)** ulcers. Acneiform and/or pustular papules are other skin manifestations of Behçet disease. *A,B Courtesy, Samuel L Moschella, MD. From Bolognia JL, Jorizzo JL, Schaffer JV. Dermatology, 3e. London: Saunders, 2012, with permission.*

Fig. 10.17 Langerhans cell histiocytosis. *Courtesy, Glen Goldman, MD.*

Epidermal Neutrophils | 11

Neutrophils within the epidermis often create pustules that may be in a background of erythema and/or erosions. This chapter mainly covers rashes that can be associated with obvious pustules, including psoriasis, acute generalized exanthematous pustulosis, subcorneal pustular dermatosis, and immunoglobulin A (IgA) pemphigus. Other disorders with more localized pustules are covered in Chapter 15.

PUSTULAR PSORIASIS, GENERALIZED

Clinical:
Widespread (Fig. 11.1) erythema and sterile pustules, many coalescing into "lakes of pus" (Fig. 11.2)

Histopathologic:
Abundant neutrophils (arrow) below the stratum corneum (Fig. 11.3); may be indistinguishable from acute generalized exanthematous pustulosis and subcorneal pustular dermatosis; other microscopic features of psoriasis (e.g. compact collections of neutrophils in the stratum corneum, hypogranulosis, regular acanthosis, prominent papillary dermal capillaries) may be present as clues

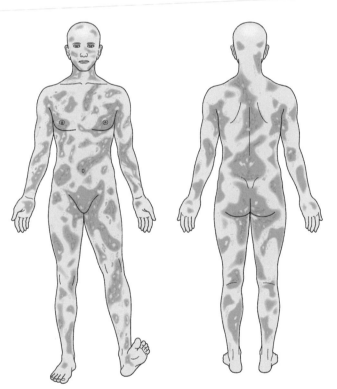

Fig. 11.1 Pustular psoriasis, generalized.

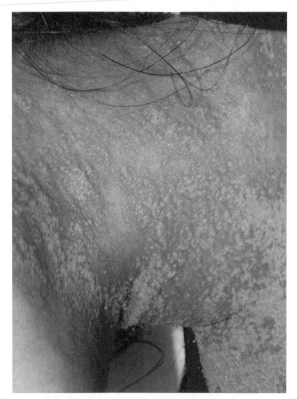

Fig. 11.2 Pustular psoriasis. *Courtesy, Julie V Schaffer, MD. From Bolognia JL, Schaffer JV, Duncan KO, Ko CJ. Dermatology Essentials, 1e. Philadelphia: Saunders, 2014, with permission.*

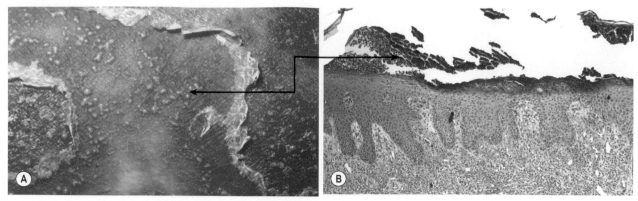

Fig. 11.3 Pustular psoriasis. Pustules correspond to subcorneal collections of neutrophils. *A, Courtesy, Kenneth Greer, MD. A, From Bolognia JL, Schaffer JV, Duncan KO, Ko CJ. Dermatology Essentials, 1e. Philadelphia: Saunders, 2014, with permission.*

PUSTULAR PSORIASIS, VARIANTS

Localized – pustules limited to plaques of psoriasis (Fig. 11.4)
Annular – rings of erythema studded with peripheral pustules (Fig. 11.5)
Palmoplantar (Fig. 11.6)
Acrodermatitis continua of Hallopeau – distal digit with erythema/scale/pustules (see Fig. 5.11B)

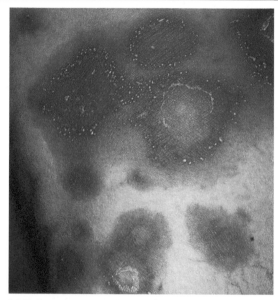

Fig. 11.5 Pustular psoriasis, annular. *Courtesy, Yale Dermatology Residents' Slide Collection. From Bolognia JL, Schaffer JV, Duncan KO, Ko CJ. Dermatology Essentials, 1e. Philadelphia: Saunders, 2014, with permission.*

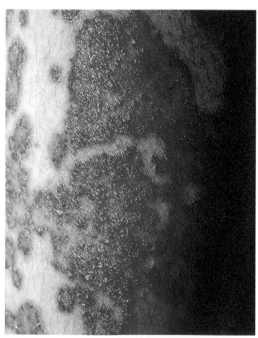

Fig. 11.4 Pustular psoriasis, localized. Well-demarcated, mostly solid red plaques studded with tiny pustules. *Courtesy, Yale Dermatology Residents' Slide Collection. From Bolognia JL, Schaffer JV, Duncan KO, Ko CJ. Dermatology Essentials, 1e. Philadelphia: Saunders, 2014, with permission.*

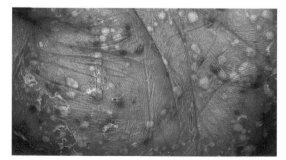

Fig. 11.6 Pustulosis of the palm. *Courtesy, Yale Dermatology Residents' Slide Collection. From Bolognia JL, Schaffer JV, Duncan KO, Ko CJ. Dermatology Essentials, 1e. Philadelphia: Saunders, 2014, with permission.*

ACUTE GENERALIZED EXANTHEMATOUS PUSTULOSIS

Clinical:
Commonly induced by antibiotics (penicillins, macrolides)

Begins on the face/body folds and becomes generalized (Fig. 11.7)

Small, sterile pustules over edema and erythema (Figs. 11.8, 11.9)

Histopathologic:
Subcorneal collections of neutrophils; eosinophils may be prominent in the dermis (Fig. 11.9B)

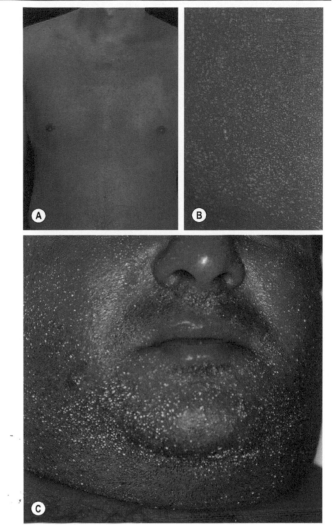

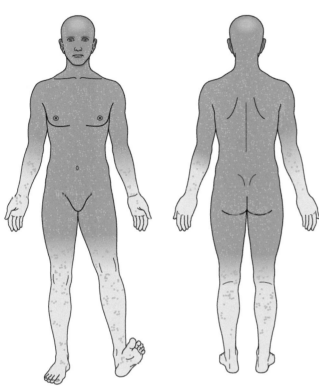

Fig. 11.7 Acute generalized exanthematous pustulosis, distribution.

Fig. 11.8 Acute generalized exanthematous pustulosis. *C, Courtesy, Kalman Watsky, MD. A,B, From Min JA, Park HJ, Cho BK, Lee JY. Acute generalized exanthematous pustulosis induced by Rhus (lacquer). J Am Acad Dermatol. 2010;63:166–8, © Elsevier. C, From Bolognia JL, Jorizzo JL, Schaffer JV. Dermatology, 3e. London: Saunders, 2012, with permission.*

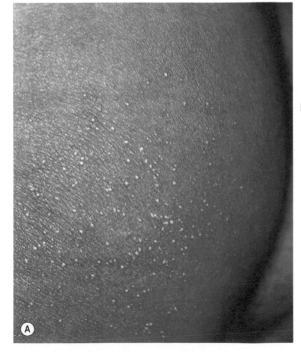

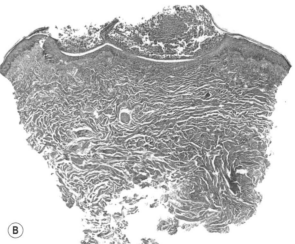

Fig. 11.9 Acute generalized exanthematous pustulosis. *Courtesy, Yale Dermatology Residents' Slide Collection. From Bolognia JL, Schaffer JV, Duncan KO, Ko CJ. Dermatology Essentials, 1e. Philadelphia: Saunders, 2014, with permission.*

SUBCORNEAL PUSTULAR DERMATOSIS (SNEDDON–WILKINSON DISEASE)

Clinical:
Considered by some to be a variant of psoriasis
Tends to affect body folds (Fig. 11.10)
Annular lesions studded with pustules (Fig. 11.11)
Pustules may be "half and half" with clear fluid above pus
(Fig. 11.12)

Histopathologic:
Findings can be identical to pustular psoriasis, acute
generalized exanthematous pustulosis, and IgA
pemphigus (subcorneal pustular dermatosis type)

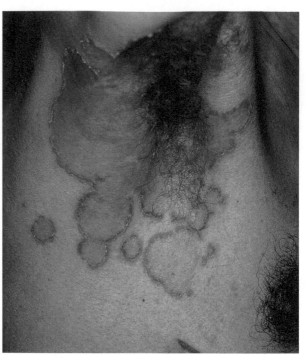

Fig. 11.11 Subcorneal pustular dermatosis. *Courtesy, Yale Dermatology Residents' Slide Collection. From Bolognia JL, Schaffer JV, Duncan KO, Ko CJ. Dermatology Essentials, 1e. Philadelphia: Saunders, 2014, with permission.*

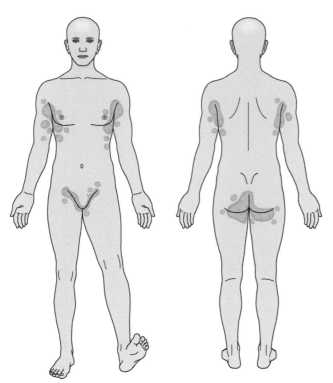

Fig. 11.10 Subcorneal pustular dermatosis, distribution.

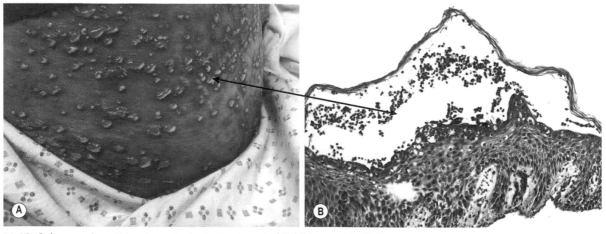

Fig. 11.12 Subcorneal pustular dermatosis. *A, Courtesy, Jeff Gehlhausen, MD, PhD.*

OTHER CAUSES OF PUSTULES

Pustules can be seen in a variety of other settings. Sterile pustules are seen in acne (Fig. 11.13) and other acneiform processes and in neutrophil-rich processes, such as early pyoderma gangrenosum (Fig. 11.14; see Chapter 16 and Figs. 16.1–16.4) or acropustulosis of infancy (Fig. 11.15). Scabies infestation may also present with pustules (Fig. 11.16). Other organisms can also present with nonsterile pustules (Fig. 11.17); special stains and/or culture studies may be helpful.

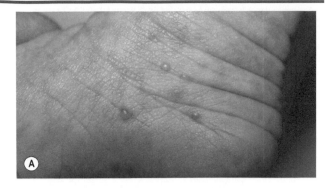

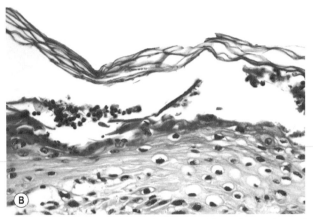

Fig. 11.15 Acropustulosis of infancy. Vesicles and pustules with absent burrows. *Courtesy, Deborah S Goddard, MD, Amy E Gilliam, MD, and Ilona J Frieden, MD. From Bolognia JL, Jorizzo JL, Schaffer JV. Dermatology, 3e. London: Saunders, 2012, with permission.*

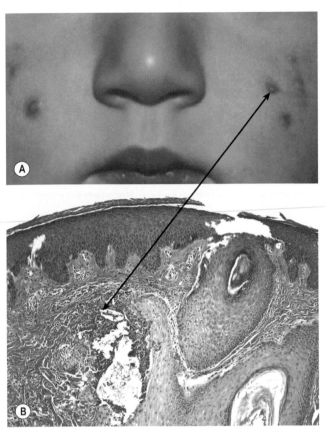

Fig. 11.13 Acne. *Courtesy, Kalman Watsky, MD. From Bolognia JL, Schaffer JV, Duncan KO, Ko CJ. Dermatology Essentials, 1e. Philadelphia: Saunders, 2014, with permission.*

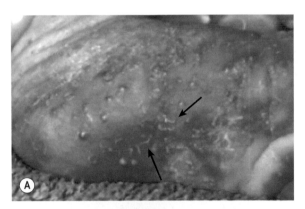

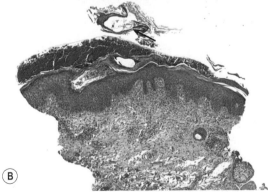

Fig. 11.16 Scabies infestation. **A** Multiple burrows (arrows) and small pustules. **B** Egg casings (arrow) are evident. *Courtesy, Anne Lucky, MD. From Schachner LA, Hansen RE. Pediatric Dermatology, 4e. London: Mosby, 2011.*

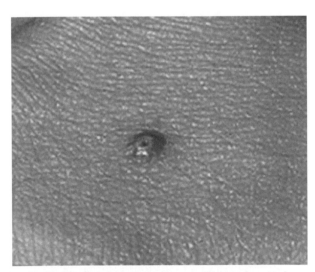

Fig. 11.14 Pyoderma gangrenosum, early papulopustule. *Courtesy, Yale Dermatology Residents' Slide Collection. From Bolognia JL, Schaffer JV, Duncan KO, Ko CJ. Dermatology Essentials, 1e. Philadelphia: Saunders, 2014, with permission.*

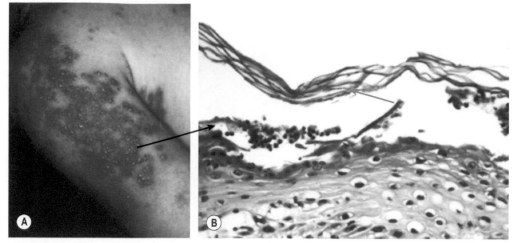

Fig. 11.17 Tinea corporis. Pustules within figurate plaques. Dermatophytes are evident (green arrow). *Courtesy, Yale Dermatology Residents' Slide Collection. From Bolognia JL, Schaffer JV, Duncan KO, Ko CJ. Dermatology Essentials, 1e. Philadelphia: Saunders, 2014, with permission.*

IgA PEMPHIGUS

Clinical:

Two types, both with intercellular IgA deposition on immunofluorescence (Fig. 11.18A)

1. Subcorneal pustular dermatosis type (Fig. 11.18B; histologically indistinguishable from Sneddon–Wilkinson disease; see Fig. 11.12B)
2. Intraepidermal neutrophilic type (Fig. 11.18C)

Typically affects the axillae/groin (Fig. 11.19)

Central crusts surrounded by flaccid vesicles or pustules (Fig. 11.20)

Histopathologic:

Subcorneal pustular dermatosis type – subcorneal collections of neutrophils; acantholysis generally not prominent

Intraepidermal neutrophilic type – surface often abnormal without an intact stratum corneum; neutrophils pepper the epidermis

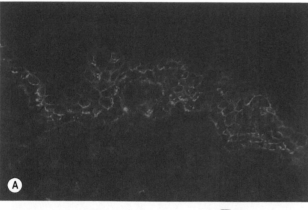

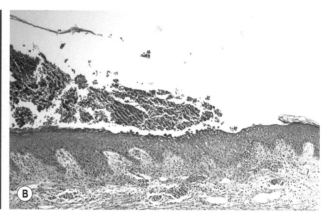

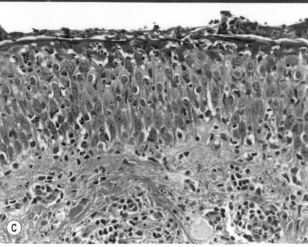

Fig. 11.18 Immunoglobulin A (IgA) pemphigus. **A** Direct immunofluorescence – intercellular IgA deposition. **B** Subcorneal neutrophils in the subcorneal pustular dermatosis type. **C** Superficial erosion and intraepidermal neutrophils in the intraepidermal neutrophilic type. *C, Courtesy, Lorenzo Cerroni, MD. From Bolognia JL, Jorizzo JL, Schaffer JV. Dermatology, 3e. London: Saunders, 2012, with permission.*

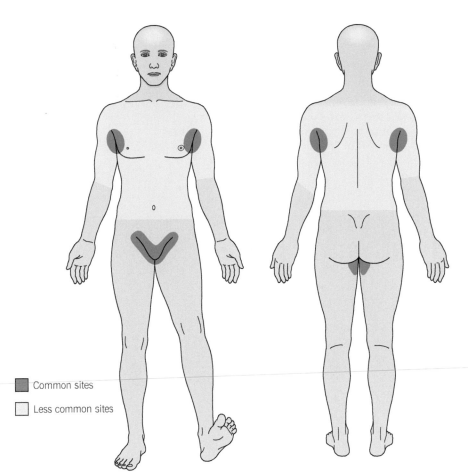

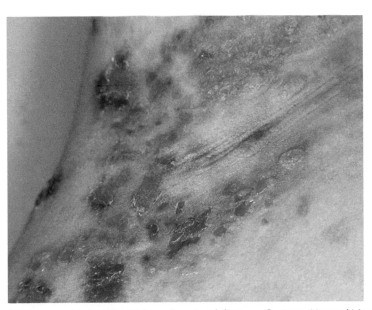

Fig. 11.19 Immunoglobulin A (IgA) pemphigus, distribution.

Common sites

Less common sites

Fig. 11.20 Immunoglobulin A (IgA) pemphigus, intraepidermal neutrophilic type. *Courtesy, Masayuki Amagai, MD. From Bolognia JL, Jorizzo JL, Schaffer JV. Dermatology, 3e. London: Saunders, 2012, with permission.*

RASHES WITH PUSTULES

Key Differences (Fig. 11.21)

- **Pustular psoriasis** – lakes of pus (arrow)
- **Acute generalized exanthematous pustulosis** – edema may be present, small monomorphous pustules
- **Subcorneal pustular dermatosis of Sneddon and Wilkinson** – annular lesions with relatively normal center

- **IgA pemphigus, subcorneal pustular dermatosis type** – central crusts (arrows) surrounded by vesicles/pustules

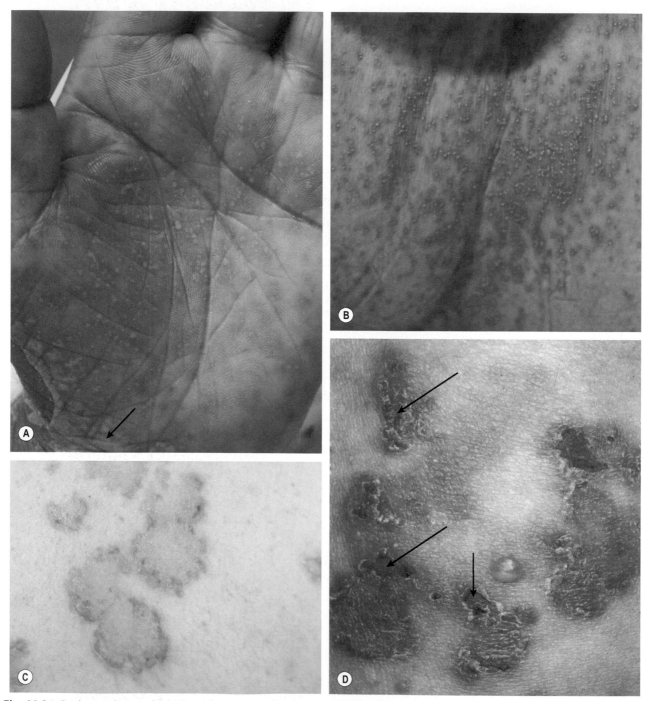

Fig. 11.21 Rashes with pustules. **A** Pustular psoriasis. **B** Acute generalized exanthematous pustulosis. **C** Subcorneal pustular dermatosis of Sneddon and Wilkinson. **D** Immunoglobulin A (IgA) pemphigus, subcorneal pustular dermatosis type. *A, Courtesy, Yale Dermatology Residents' Slide Collection; B, Courtesy, Yale Dermatology Residents' Slide Collection; C, Courtesy, Dirk Elston, MD. D, Courtesy, Masayuki Amagai, MD. C, From Elston D. Clinical image collection. Dermatopathology, 2e. London: Saunders, 2014. D, From Bolognia JL, Jorizzo JL, Schaffer JV. Dermatology, 3e. London: Saunders, 2012, with permission.*

Vesiculobullous, Numerous Lesions | 12

Many different factors are clues to the diagnosis of blistering disorders. Some diseases have particular sites of predilection (Table 12.1). The morphology and arrangement of the individual lesions are important (i.e. tense vs flaccid, erythematous vs nonerythematous base [Fig. 12.1], clustered [Fig. 12.2]). The location of the split is also a key factor to consider (Table 12.2). For many blistering disorders, there are particular direct immunofluorescence patterns (Table 12.3) and characteristic circulating antibodies (Table 12.4). This chapter focuses on bullous pemphigoid, pemphigoid gestationis, mucous membrane pemphigoid, epidermolysis bullosa acquisita, porphyria cutanea tarda, linear immunoglobulin A (IgA) disease, dermatitis herpetiformis, bullous lupus erythematosus, bullous lichen planus, pemphigus, herpesvirus infection, and coxsackievirus infection.

Table 12.1 Blistering disorders – characteristic distribution

Blistering disorder	Site(s)
Bullous pemphigoid Pemphigus vulgaris Pemphigus foliaceus Linear immunoglobulin A (IgA) disease	Trunk and extremities
Pemphigoid gestationis	Abdomen
Mucous membrane pemphigoid (Brunsting-Perry variant)	Scalp
Epidermolysis bullosa acquisita* Porphyria cutanea tarda Hand-foot-and-mouth disease	Acral
Dermatitis herpetiformis	Elbows/knees Buttocks Scalp
Pemphigus vegetans	Body folds

*May also be generalized.

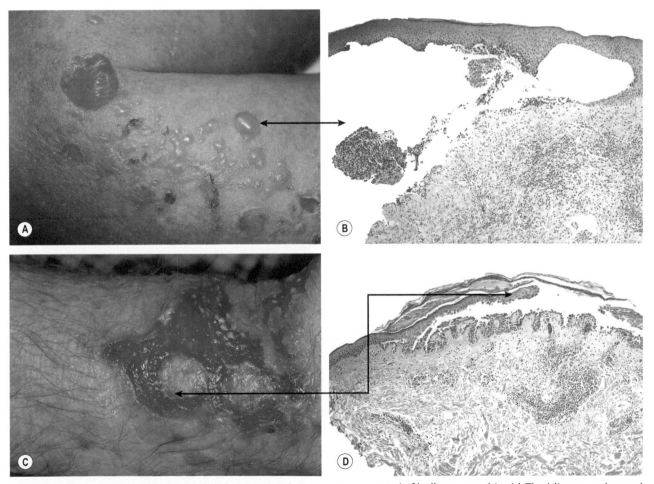

Fig. 12.1 Bullous pemphigoid vs pemphigus vulgaris. **A,B** Tense blisters typical of bullous pemphigoid. The blisters are located within pink, urticarial plaques. **C,D** Flaccid blister break easily into typical erosions of pemphigus vulgaris. Skin surrounding the blisters is nonerythematous. *A, Courtesy, Yale Dermatology Residents' Slide Collection. C, From Schwarzenberger K et al., Requisites in Dermatology: General Dermatology, with permission.*

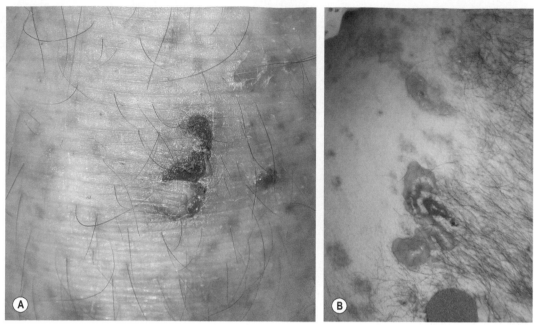

Fig. 12.2 Clustered vesicles/bullae. **A** Dermatitis herpetiformis. Clustered small vesicles ("herpetiform") and erosions. **B** Linear immunoglobulin A (IgA) disease. Clusters of larger vesicles/bullae in annular arrangements. *Courtesy, Yale Dermatology Residents' Slide Collection.*

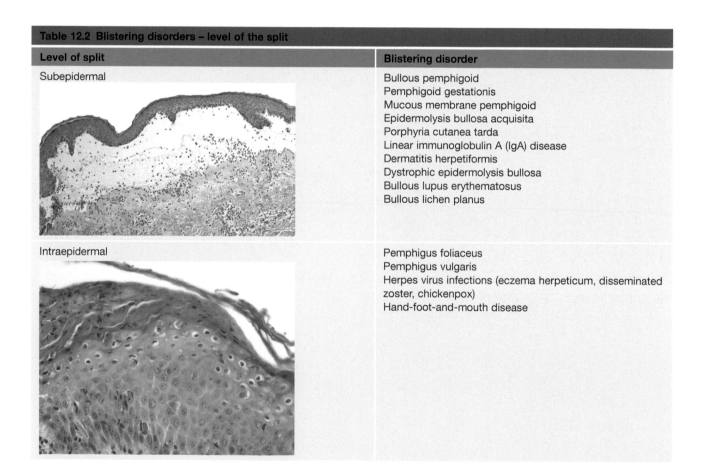

Table 12.2 Blistering disorders – level of the split	
Level of split	**Blistering disorder**
Subepidermal	Bullous pemphigoid Pemphigoid gestationis Mucous membrane pemphigoid Epidermolysis bullosa acquisita Porphyria cutanea tarda Linear immunoglobulin A (IgA) disease Dermatitis herpetiformis Dystrophic epidermolysis bullosa Bullous lupus erythematosus Bullous lichen planus
Intraepidermal	Pemphigus foliaceus Pemphigus vulgaris Herpes virus infections (eczema herpeticum, disseminated zoster, chickenpox) Hand-foot-and-mouth disease

Table 12.3 Blistering disorders – usual direct immunofluorescence patterns

Direct immunofluorescence pattern	Blistering disorder
Linear C3 and IgG at the dermal–epidermal junction 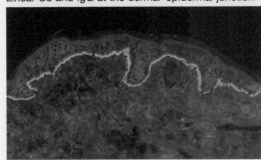	Bullous pemphigoid Pemphigoid gestationis Mucous membrane pemphigoid Epidermolysis bullosa acquisita Bullous lupus erythematosus*
Intercellular IgG and C3 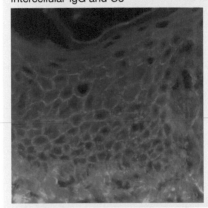	Pemphigus vulgaris Pemphigus foliaceus
Linear IgA at the dermal–epidermal junction 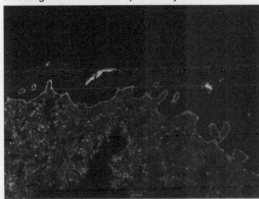	Linear IgA disease Mucous membrane pemphigoid
Granular IgA in the papillary dermis 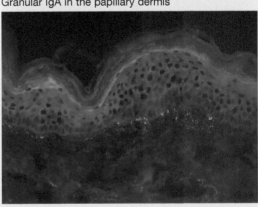	Dermatitis herpetiformis

*Often has IgA and IgM as well.
IgA, Immunoglobulin A; *IgG*, immunoglobulin G.

Table 12.4 Blistering disorders – antibody profiles

Blistering disorder	Antibodies directed against
Bullous pemphigoid	BPAg1, BPAg2
Pemphigus vulgaris	Desmoglein 3
Pemphigus foliaceus	Desmoglein 1
Dermatitis herpetiformis	Epidermal transglutaminase
Linear IgA	BPAg2
Mucous membrane pemphigoid	BPAg2
Pemphigoid gestationis	BPAg2
Epidermolysis bullosa acquisita	Type VII collagen
Bullous lupus erythematosus	

BPAg1, Bullous pemphigoid antigen 1; *BPAg2*, bullous pemphigoid antigen 2; *IgA*, immunoglobulin A.

BULLOUS PEMPHIGOID

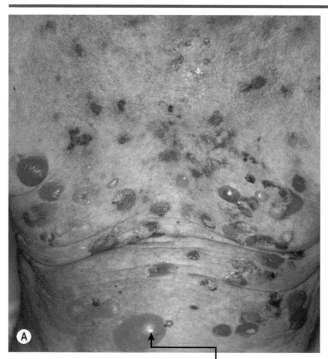

Clinical:
Generalized or localized tense blisters (Fig. 12.3A)
Blister base erythematous or skin-colored

Histopathologic:
Subepidermal split with numerous eosinophils
(Fig. 12.3B,C)

Direct Immunofluorescence:
Linear C3 and immunoglobulin G (IgG) at the
dermal–epidermal junction

Salt-Split Skin:
Localization of immunoreactants to the blister roof (most
common pattern), base, or both

Bullous Pemphigoid, Variants
(Fig. 12.4; see Fig. 4.15)

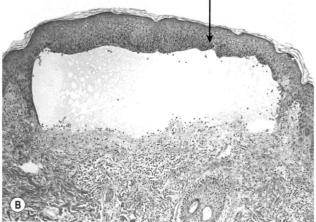

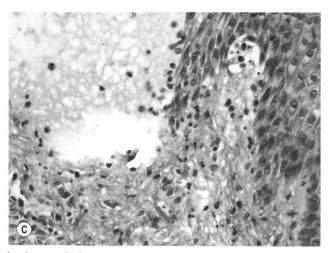

Fig. 12.3 Bullous pemphigoid. **A** Tense blisters and erosions on a background of erythematous skin. **B** Tense blister with separation between the epidermis and dermis. **C** Eosinophils are present at the blister base. *A, Courtesy, Yale Dermatology Residents' Slide Collection. A, From Bolognia JL, Jorizzo JL, Schaffer JV. Dermatology, 3e. London: Saunders, 2012, with permission.*

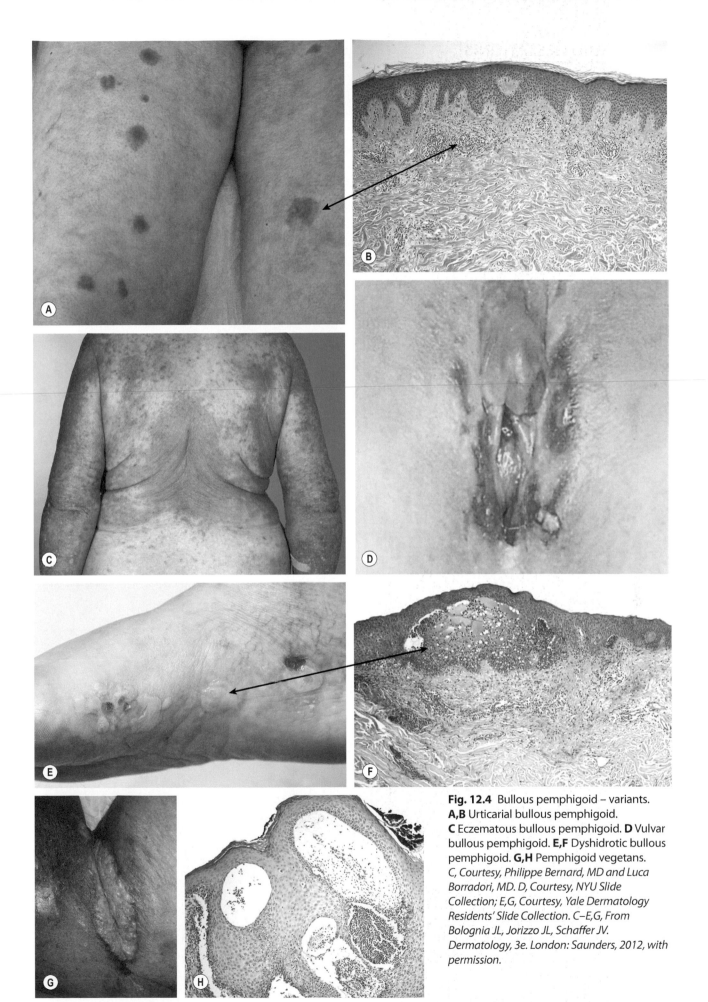

Fig. 12.4 Bullous pemphigoid – variants.
A,B Urticarial bullous pemphigoid.
C Eczematous bullous pemphigoid. **D** Vulvar
bullous pemphigoid. **E,F** Dyshidrotic bullous
pemphigoid. **G,H** Pemphigoid vegetans.
*C, Courtesy, Philippe Bernard, MD and Luca
Borradori, MD. D, Courtesy, NYU Slide
Collection; E,G, Courtesy, Yale Dermatology
Residents' Slide Collection. C–E,G, From
Bolognia JL, Jorizzo JL, Schaffer JV.
Dermatology, 3e. London: Saunders, 2012, with
permission.*

PEMPHIGOID GESTATIONIS

Clinical:
Affects pregnant women
Tense blisters, initially on the abdomen (Fig. 12.5)

Direct immunofluorescence:
Linear C3 at the dermal–epidermal junction
(Fig. 12.5C)

Histopathologic:
Similar to bullous pemphigoid
Biopsy of an urticarial lesion may only show mixed
perivascular inflammation (Fig. 12.5B)

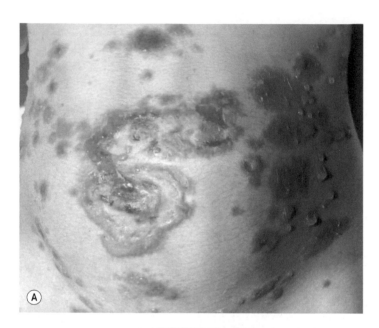

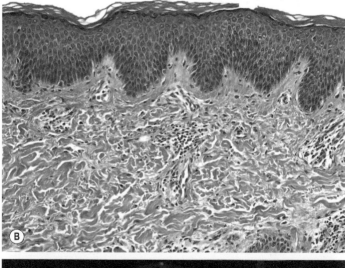

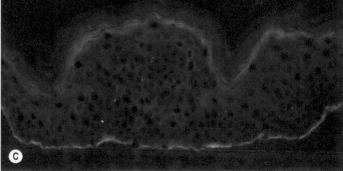

Fig. 12.5 Pemphigoid gestationis. Tense blisters on the abdomen of a pregnant woman. *A, Courtesy, Christina M Ambros-Rudolph, MD. From Bolognia JL, Jorizzo JL, Schaffer JV. Dermatology, 3e. London: Saunders, 2012, with permission.*

MUCOUS MEMBRANE PEMPHIGOID

Clinical:
Brunsting-Perry variant – blisters/ulcerations localized to the scalp (Fig. 12.6A)
Blisters may reform in scars from previous blisters (Fig. 12.6B)
Desquamative gingivitis, ocular lesions (Fig. 12.7)

Histopathologic:
Features may resemble bullous pemphigoid (dermal scarring may be a clue)

Direct immunofluorescence:
Like bullous pemphigoid (linear IgG and C3 at the dermal–epidermal junction)

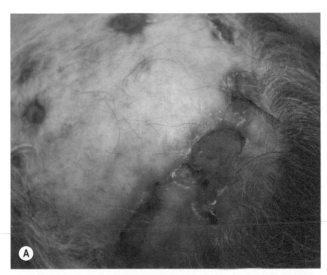

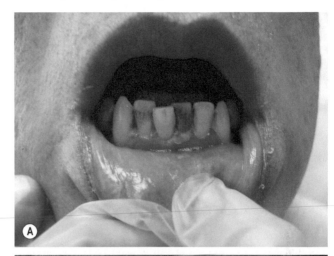

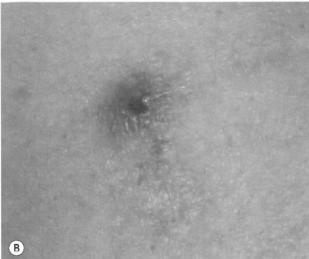

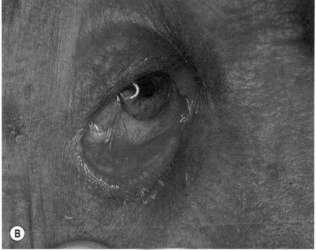

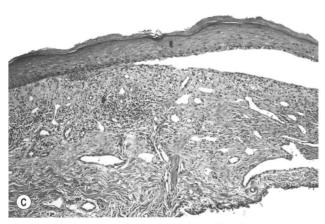

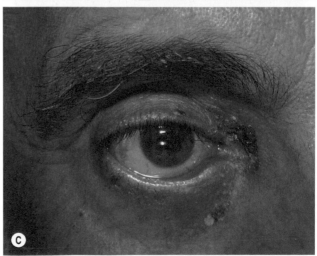

Fig. 12.6 Mucous membrane pemphigoid. **A** Scarring alopecia and ulcerated lesions on the scalp. **B** Recurrent lesion at the site of a scar from a prior lesion. **C** Dermal fibrosis is a clue.

Fig. 12.7 Mucous membrane pemphigoid. **A** Desquamative gingivitis. **B,C** Ocular lesions. *B, Courtesy, Yale Dermatology Residents' Slide Collection; C, Courtesy, Louis A Fragola, MD. B,C, From Bolognia JL, Jorizzo JL, Schaffer JV. Dermatology, 3e. London: Saunders, 2012, with permission.*

EPIDERMOLYSIS BULLOSA ACQUISITA

Clinical:
Classically, localized to areas of frequent trauma (hands/elbows; Fig. 12.8)
May be generalized

Histopathologic:
Subepidermal split with variable inflammation

Direct Immunofluorescence:
Linear C3 and IgG, sometimes with immunoglobulin M (IgM) and/or IgA

Salt-Split Skin:
Localization of immunoreactants to the blister base

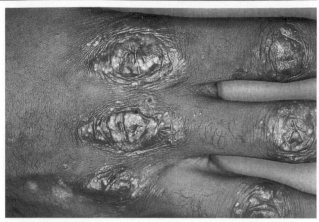

Fig. 12.8 Epidermolysis bullosa acquisita. *Courtesy, Yale Dermatology Residents' Slide Collection. From Bolognia JL, Jorizzo JL, Schaffer JV. Dermatology, 3e. London: Saunders, 2012, with permission.*

PORPHYRIA CUTANEA TARDA

Clinical:
Tense blisters or crusted lesions on dorsal hands (Fig. 12.9A)
Hypertrichosis of lateral face

Histopathologic:
Noninflamed subepidermal split with thickened basement membrane (Fig. 12.9B)

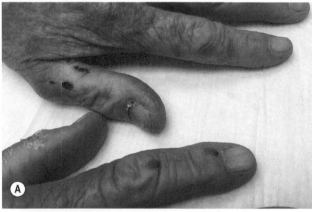

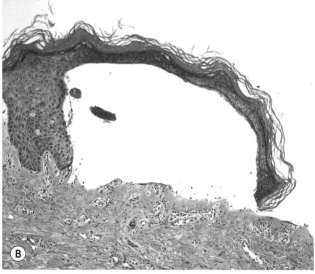

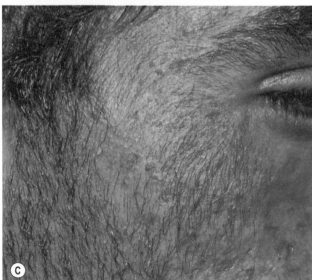

Fig. 12.9 Porphyria cutanea tarda. **A** Crusted erosions on dorsal fingers. **B** Subepidermal split with minimal inflammation. **C** Hypertrichosis. *A, Yale Dermatology Residents' Slide Collection; C, Courtesy, Kurt Stenn, MD. C, From Bolognia JL, Jorizzo JL, Schaffer JV. Dermatology, 3e. London: Saunders, 2012, with permission.*

LINEAR IgA DISEASE

Clinical:
Predilection for body folds but may be generalized
Clusters of tense vesicles or bullae that may form annular rings (Fig. 12.10A,B)

Histopathologic:
Subepidermal split with neutrophils (Fig. 12.10C)

Direct Immunofluorescence:
Linear IgA at the dermal–epidermal junction

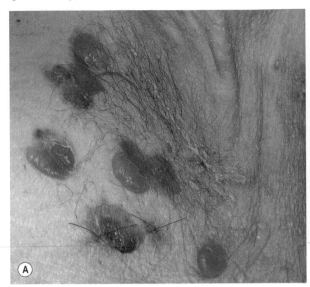

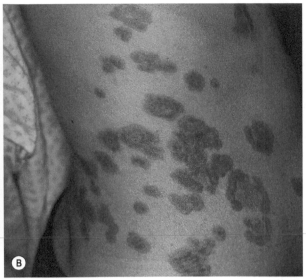

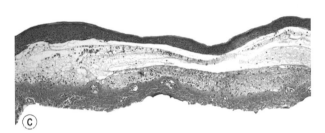

Fig. 12.10 Linear immunoglobulin A (IgA) disease. Tense blisters at the edges of pink–red plaques. *A, Courtesy, Yale Dermatology Residents' Slide Collection. B, Courtesy, John J Zone, MD. B, From Bolognia JL, Jorizzo JL, Schaffer JV. Dermatology, 3e. London: Saunders, 2012, with permission.*

DERMATITIS HERPETIFORMIS

Clinical:
Favors the elbows/knees, scalp, lower back
Excoriated vesicles; intact blisters rare because of intense pruritus and scratching (Fig. 12.11A)

Histopathologic:
Neutrophils in dermal papillae +/− subepidermal split (Fig. 12.11B)

Direct Immunofluorescence:
Granular (rarely fibrillar) IgA in the dermal papillae

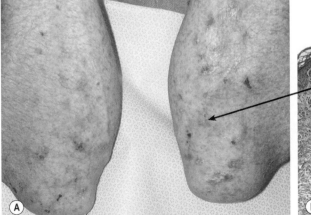

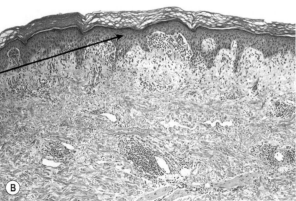

Fig. 12.11 Dermatitis herpetiformis. Crusted erosions on the elbows, a typical site. *Courtesy, Yale Dermatology Residents' Slide Collection.*

BULLOUS LUPUS ERYTHEMATOSUS

Clinical:
Bullae in a patient with underlying systemic lupus erythematosus (Fig. 12.12A)

Histopathologic:
Subepidermal split with neutrophils (Fig. 12.12B)

Direct Immunofluorescence:
Linear IgG, IgM, IgA; intranuclear labeling of antinuclear antibodies may be seen (Fig. 12.12C)

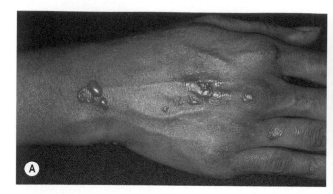

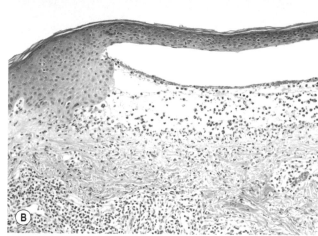

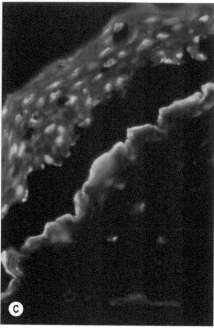

Fig. 12.12 Bullous lupus erythematosus. Tense blisters on the hand of a patient with systemic lupus erythematosus. *A, Courtesy, Yale Dermatology Residents' Slide Collection. A, From Bolognia JL, Jorizzo JL, Schaffer JV. Dermatology, 3e. London: Saunders, 2012, with permission. C, From Patterson JW. Practical Skin Pathology: A Diagnostic Approach. Philadelphia: Saunders, 2013.*

BULLOUS LICHEN PLANUS

Clinical:
Violaceous papule/plaque that blisters (Fig. 12.13A)

Histopathologic:
Subepidermal cleft with lymphocytes, pigment incontinence (Fig. 12.13B)

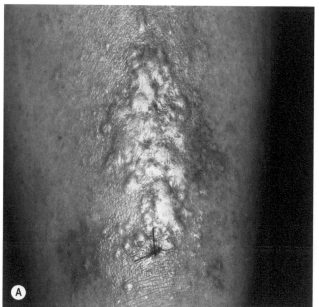

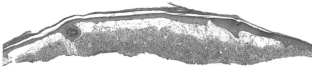

Fig. 12.13 Bullous lichen planus. Blisters forming within polygonal, purple plaques. *A, Courtesy, Yale Dermatology Residents' Slide Collection. A, From Bolognia JL, Jorizzo JL, Schaffer JV. Dermatology, 3e. London: Saunders, 2012, with permission.*

PEMPHIGUS VULGARIS

Clinical:
Often generalized, may be localized
Flaccid bullae and erosions (Fig. 12.14A)

Histopathologic:
Suprabasilar acantholysis (see Fig. 12.1D)

Direct Immunofluorescence:
Intercellular IgG and C3 (see Table 12.3)

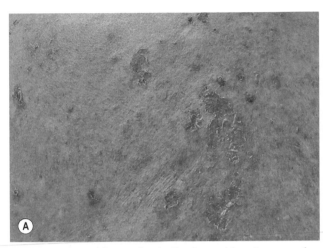
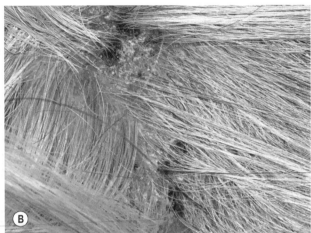

Fig. 12.14 A Pemphigus vulgaris. Erosions with collarettes of scale on the back. **B** Pemphigus foliaceus. Crusted, eroded papules on the scalp, a typical location. *B, Courtesy, Karynne O. Duncan, MD.*

PEMPHIGUS, VARIANTS

Pemphigus Foliaceus
Clinical:
Scalp, face, and upper body are typically affected (Fig. 12.14B; see Chapter 5)
Lesions may be crusted, eroded, or have cornflakes-like scales (see Fig. 1.55H)

Histopathologic:
Subcorneal acantholysis

IgA Pemphigus
(See Chapter 11)

Pemphigus Vegetans
Clinical:
Favors body folds
Thick, vegetative, eroded plaques (Fig. 12.15A)

Histopathologic:
Acanthosis with eosinophilic abscesses (Fig. 12.15B)
Acantholysis may not be evident

Paraneoplastic Pemphigus
(see Chapter 8)

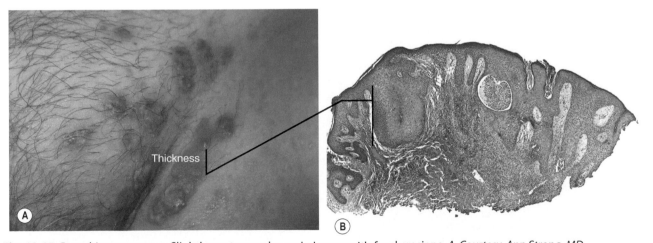

Thickness

Fig. 12.15 Pemphigus vegetans. Slightly warty papules and plaques with focal erosions. *A, Courtesy, Ann Strong, MD.*

HERPES VIRUS INFECTIONS (ECZEMA HERPETICUM, DISSEMINATED ZOSTER, CHICKENPOX)

Histopathologic features of herpes simplex virus and varicella zoster virus infections are similar, with acantholysis within the epidermis, multinucleate cells, and rimmed chromatin in nuclei of acantholytic cells

Eczema Herpeticum
Clinical:
Background of atopic dermatitis
Punched out 3- to 5-mm monomorphous ulcerations (Fig. 12.16A)

Disseminated Zoster
Clinical:
Individual lesions similar to chickenpox or eczema herpeticum (Fig. 12.16B)

Varicella (Chickenpox)
Clinical:
2- to 4-mm papule on an erythematous base (Fig. 12.16C; see Fig. 6.22)

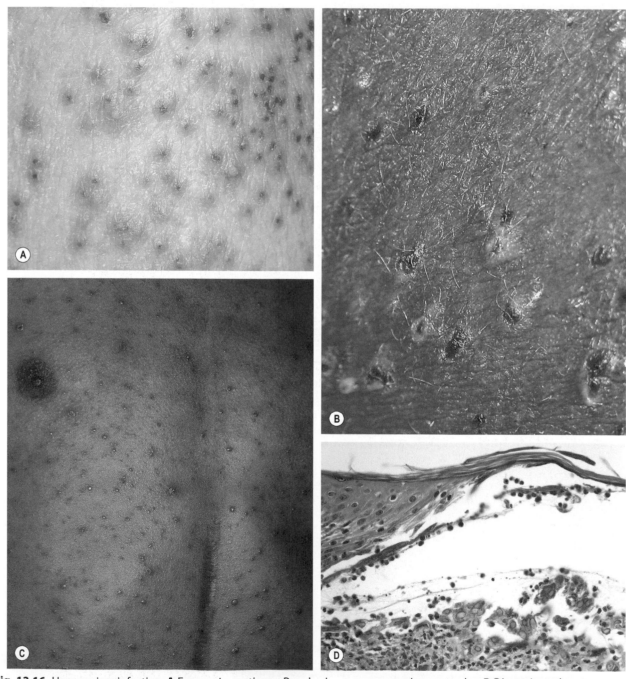

Fig. 12.16 Herpes virus infection. **A** Eczema herpeticum. Punched out, monomorphous papules. **B** Disseminated zoster. Monomorphous, eroded papules. **C** Varicella. **D** Histologic findings in herpes virus infections. Acantholytic cells and multinucleate cells with rimming of chromatin. *A,B, Courtesy, Yale Dermatology Residents' Slide Collection; C, Courtesy, Robert Hartman, MD. C, From Bolognia JL, Jorizzo JL, Schaffer JV. Dermatology, 3e. London: Saunders, 2012, with permission.*

HAND-FOOT-AND-MOUTH DISEASE

Clinical:
Caused by enteroviruses, particularly coxsackievirus
Typical acral distribution (hands, feet, intraoral)
Atypical variants can involve the skin more extensively
(Fig. 12.17A; see Fig. 6.22) and/or affect sites of atopic
dermatitis (eczema coxsackium; Fig. 12.17B)
Oval vesicles, may be crusted or eroded

Histopathologic:
Superficial necrotic keratinocytes (arrow), papillary
dermal edema, lymphocytic infiltrate (Fig. 12.17C)

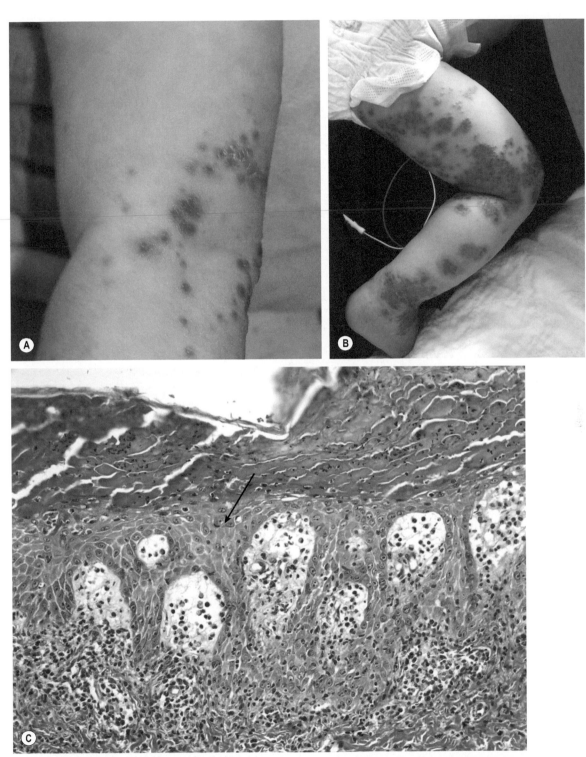

Fig. 12.17 Hand-foot-and-mouth disease. Eroded vesicles, in some areas becoming confluent. *A,B, Courtesy, Robert Stavert, MD.*

ADDITIONAL DIRECT IMMUNOFLUORESCENCE IMAGES

(Figs. 12.18–12.20)

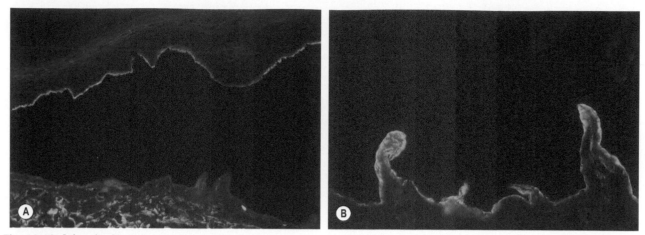

Fig. 12.18 Salt-split skin patterns. **A** Deposition of immunoreactant on the base of the roof, a typical pattern of bullous pemphigoid. **B** Deposition of immunoreactant on the floor (dermis), a typical pattern of epidermolysis bullosa acquisita that can also be associated with bullous pemphigoid.

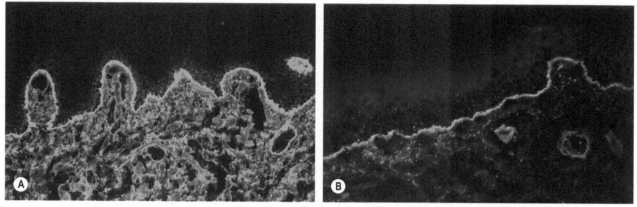

Fig. 12.19 Serrated patterns on direct immunofluorescence testing. **A** n-serrated (bullous pemphigoid). **B** u-serrated (epidermolysis bullosa acquisita or bullous lupus erythematosus).

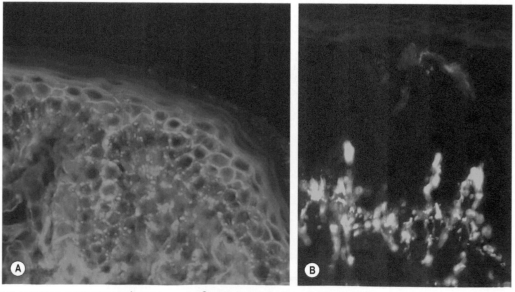

Fig. 12.20 Less common patterns on direct immunofluorescence testing. **A** Punctate intercellular pattern of immunoglobulin G (IgG) deposition in pemphigus. **B** Fibrillar immunoglobulin A (IgA) deposition in the papillary dermis in dermatitis herpetiformis.

Vesicles, Blisters, and Papulopustules in Infants | 13

Vesiculobullous and papular disorders in infants often have a characteristic distribution (i.e. head, body folds, acral).

HEAD

Neonatal Cephalic Pustulosis (Fig. 13.1)
Clinical:
Papulopustules on the face of infants from about 2 to 3 weeks of age to 2 to 3 months of age
Absent comedones

Eosinophilic Folliculitis
(See Chapter 15)

Benign Cephalic Histiocytosis (Fig. 13.2)
Clinical:
Typically on the face or neck
Small (<5 mm) brown–red papules
Spontaneous resolution over time (months to years)

Histopathologic:
Histiocytes (CD1a-negative) within the dermis

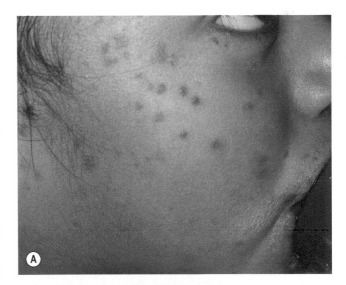

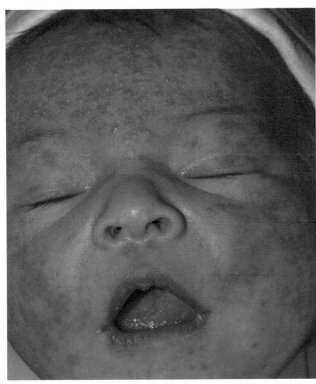

Fig. 13.1 Neonatal cephalic pustulosis. *Courtesy, Julie V Schaffer, MD. From Bolognia JL, Schaffer JV, Duncan KO, Ko CJ. Dermatology Essentials, 1e. Philadelphia: Saunders, 2014, with permission.*

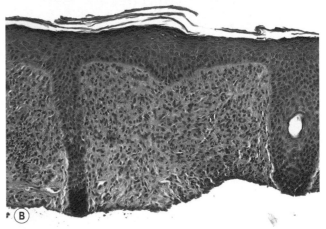

Fig. 13.2 Benign cephalic histiocytosis. *A, Courtesy, Yale Dermatology Residents' Slide Collection. A, From Bolognia JL, Schaffer JV, Duncan KO, Ko CJ. Dermatology Essentials, 1e. Philadelphia: Saunders, 2014, with permission.*

BODY FOLDS

Langerhans Cell Histiocytosis (Fig. 13.3)

Clinical:

Favors the scalp and body folds (see Figs. 2.14, 6.22, 20.2, 20.3 and Table 20.1)

Pink to red–brown papules, often with petechiae, sometimes eroded/ulcerated

Histopathologic:

Histiocytes with reniform (kidney-shaped) nuclei that are langerin, CD1a, and S100 positive

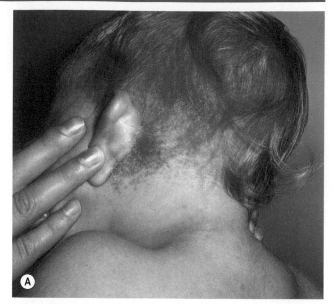

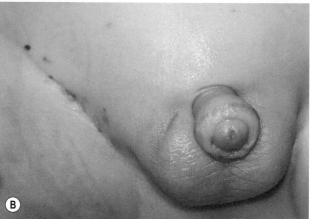

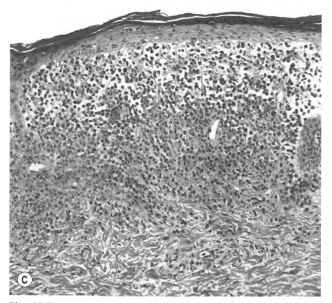

Fig. 13.3 Langerhans cell histiocytosis. *A, Courtesy, Irwin Braverman, MD; B, Courtesy, Jonathan Leventhal, MD.*

ACRAL

Acropustulosis of Infancy (Fig. 13.4)
Clinical:
Cyclic, typical age is 3 to 6 months up to 2 to 3 years
Pruritic vesicles

Histopathologic:
Intraepidermal pustules

Scabies (Fig. 13.5; see Fig. 11.16A,B)
Clinical:
Can present like acropustulosis of infancy (see Fig. 11.15)
Presence of burrows (see Figs. 2.20, 23.5–23.8) may be helpful

Histopathologic:
Evidence of scabies (mite; arrow) infestation on scraping or biopsy

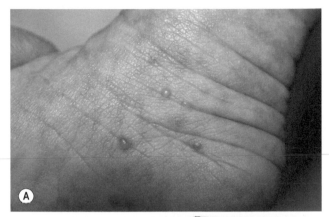

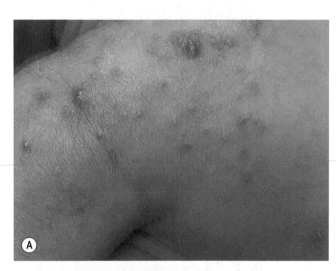

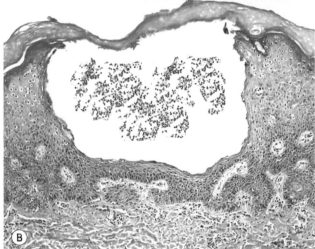

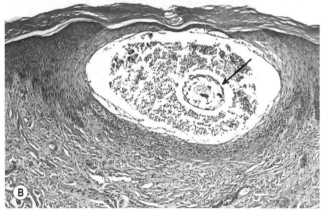

Fig. 13.4 Acropustulosis of infancy. *A, Courtesy, Deborah S Goddard, MD, Amy E Gilliam, MD, and Ilona J Frieden, MD. A, From Bolognia JL, Schaffer JV, Duncan KO, Ko CJ. Dermatology Essentials, 1e. Philadelphia: Saunders, 2014, with permission.*

Fig. 13.5 Scabies. *A, Courtesy, Yale Dermatology Residents' Slide Collection.*

OTHER DISORDERS

Erythema Toxicum Neonatorum (Fig. 13.6)

Clinical:

Typically develops on day 1 or 2 of life and resolves within a week

Progresses from the face to the body

Erythematous papules and vesicles and pustules that may be surrounded by a pink flare

Histopathologic:

Eosinophilic pustules within the epidermis

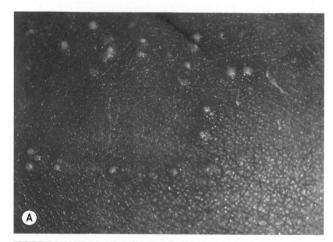

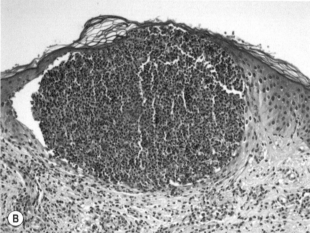

Fig. 13.6 Erythema toxicum neonatorum. *A, Courtesy, Yale Dermatology Residents' Slide Collection. B, From Patterson JW. Practical Skin Pathology: A Diagnostic Approach. Philadelphia: Saunders, 2013.*

Transient Neonatal Pustular Melanosis (Fig. 13.7)

Clinical:

Favors the face, neck, back, and shins

Superficial small vesiculopustules that rupture and leave collarettes of scale, resulting in brown macules

Histopathologic:

Neutrophils below the stratum corneum

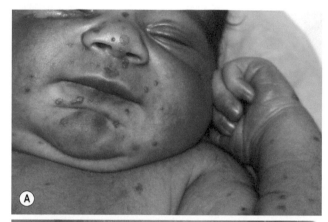

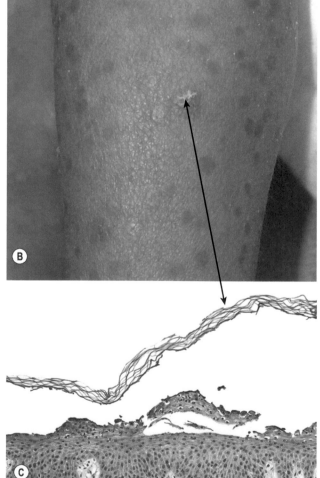

Fig. 13.7 Transient neonatal pustular melanosis. *A,B, Courtesy, Yale Dermatology Residents' Slide Collection. B, From Bolognia JL, Schaffer JV, Duncan KO, Ko CJ. Dermatology Essentials, 1e. Philadelphia: Saunders, 2014, with permission.*

Miliaria Crystallina (Fig. 13.8)

Clinical:
Often secondary to increased perspiration
Favors the face, trunk, and arms
Clear, short-lived vesicles, noninflamed

Miliaria Rubra (Fig. 13.9)

Clinical:
Favors occluded areas, such as the neck and the trunk
Clear vesicles surrounded by a pink–red border

Histopathologic:
Spongiosis and inflammation of the eccrine duct where it enters the epidermis

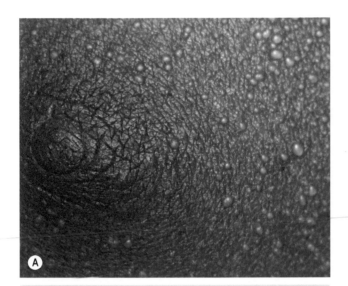

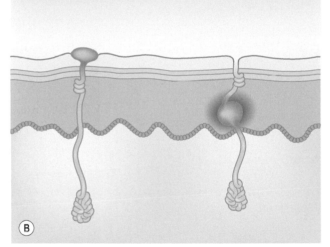

Fig. 13.8 Miliaria crystallina. **A** Miliaria crystallina. **B** Miliaria crystallina affects the surface of the acrosyringium; miliaria rubra affects the acrosyringium as it crosses the stratum spinosum. *A, Courtesy, Yale Dermatology Residents' Slide Collection. B, From Weston WL, Lane AT, Morelli JG. Color Textbook of Pediatric Dermatology, 4e. St Louis: Mosby, 2007.*

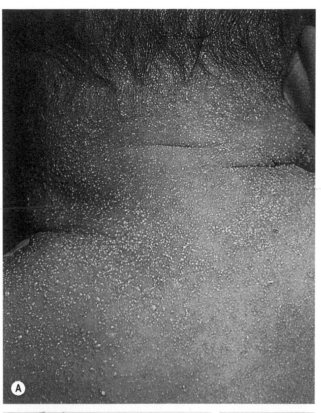

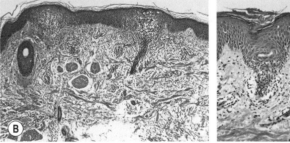

Fig. 13.9 Miliaria rubra. *A, Courtesy, Lawrence Eichenfeld, MD. A, From Bolognia JL, Schaffer JV, Duncan KO, Ko CJ. Dermatology Essentials, 1e. Philadelphia: Saunders, 2014, with permission. B, From Patterson JW. Weedon's Skin Pathology, 4e. London: Churchill Livingstone, 2015.*

Candidiasis (Fig. 13.10)

Clinical:

Acquired in utero

Often evident at birth

Erythematous papules and/or pustules with fine scale; in premature infants, diffuse erythema and erosions

Histopathologic:

Yeast and pseudohyphae in the stratum corneum

Herpes Virus Infection (Fig. 13.11)

Clinical:

Grouped vesicles on an erythematous base, scalloped borders

Histopathologic:

Acantholysis, rimmed chromatin, multinucleate cells

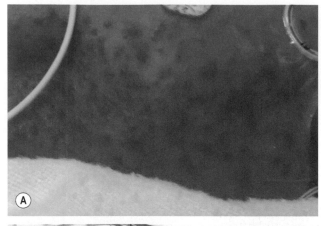

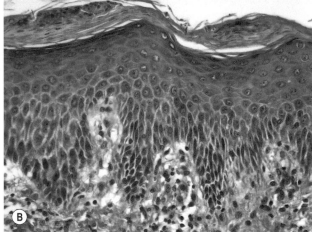

Fig. 13.10 Candidiasis. *A, Courtesy, Yale Dermatology Residents' Slide Collection.*

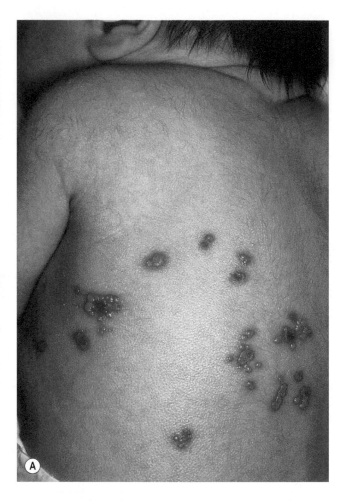

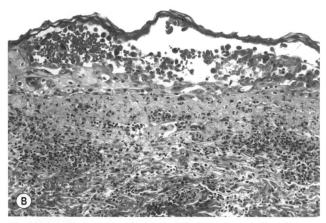

Fig. 13.11 Herpes simplex virus infection. *A, Courtesy, Yale Dermatology Residents' Slide Collection. A, From Bolognia JL, Schaffer JV, Duncan KO, Ko CJ. Dermatology Essentials, 1e. Philadelphia: Saunders, 2014, with permission.*

Epidermolysis Bullosa

Clinical:
Group of inherited disorders that often present with vesicles/bullae in infancy

Histopathologic:
Blistering within or below the epidermis (Figs. 13.12, 13.13)

Incontinentia Pigmenti
(See Table 13.1; Fig. 1.28A)

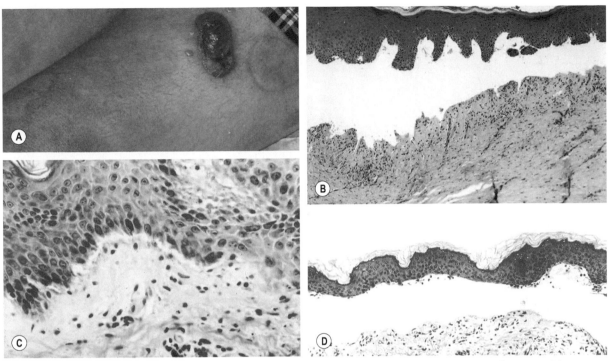

Fig. 13.12 Epidermolysis bullosa. **A** Dystrophic epidermolysis bullosa. Blistering and scarring at sites of previous blisters. **B** Location of the split in dystrophic epidermolysis bullosa (in the papillary dermis, with scarring). **C** The split is higher in epidermolysis bullosa simplex (within the basal cell). **D** Also in junctional epidermolysis bullosa (below the basal cell). *A, Courtesy, Yale Dermatology Residents' Slide Collection. B–D, From Patterson JW. Practical Skin Pathology: A Diagnostic Approach. Philadelphia: Saunders, 2013.*

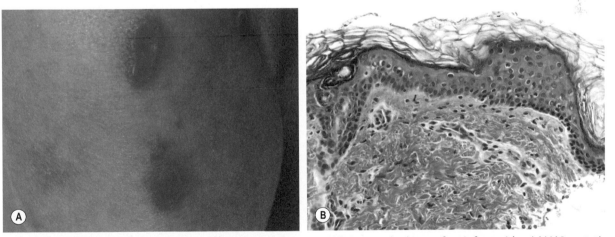

Fig. 13.13 Junctional epidermolysis bullosa. **A** Flaccid, erythematous blisters on the knee of an infant with a *LAMA3* mutation. **B** Noninflammatory split between the epidermis and dermis on the right side of the photomicrograph. *A,B, Courtesy, Yale Dermatology Residents Slide Collection.*

Table 13.1 Four stages of incontinentia pigmenti (see Fig. 1.29)

Stage	Typical age of presentation	Typical resolution
1 – Vesicular (see Fig. 3.12G)	Rarely congenital; birth to 2–3 weeks	In weeks to months
2 – Verrucous	2–6 weeks	In weeks to months
3 – Hyperpigmented	2–6 months	Fades during childhood
4 – Hypopigmented	Puberty	None

Blistering, Localized | 14

In addition to morphology, body site affected, and clues from history, the microscopic findings (i.e. subcorneal, intraepidermal, or subepidermal split) in localized blistering conditions can aid in making the correct diagnosis (Fig. 14.1).

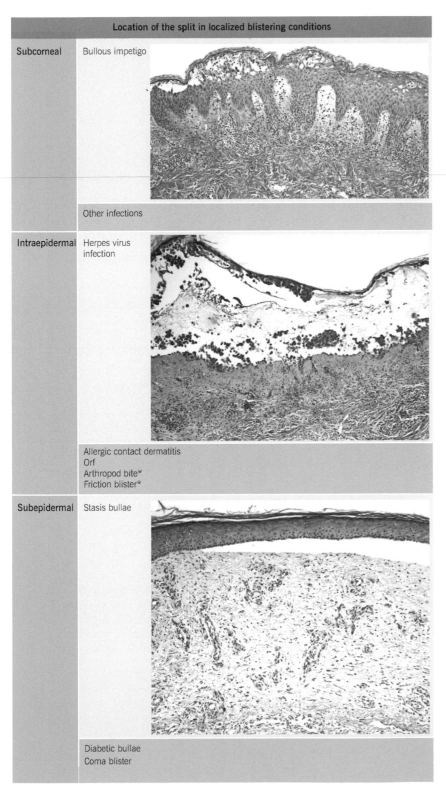

Location of the split in localized blistering conditions	
Subcorneal	Bullous impetigo
	Other infections
Intraepidermal	Herpes virus infection
	Allergic contact dermatitis Orf Arthropod bite* Friction blister*
Subepidermal	Stasis bullae
	Diabetic bullae Coma blister

Fig. 14.1 Microscopy of selected localized blistering conditions. *Can also be subepidermal.

DISORDERS WITH A CHARACTERISTIC MORPHOLOGY (FIG. 14.2)

Key Differences

- **Bullous impetigo** – Somewhat tense vesicles/bullae or superficial erosions with collarettes of scale, solitary or multiple lesions
- **Herpes virus infection** – Clustered vesicles and crusts (borders of coalescing lesions may be scalloped), often

on an erythematous base; older lesions may be eroded/ulcerated; typical locations include the lips and genitalia/buttocks
- **Leukocytoclastic vasculitis** – Palpable purpura, sometimes with focal blisters, often acral

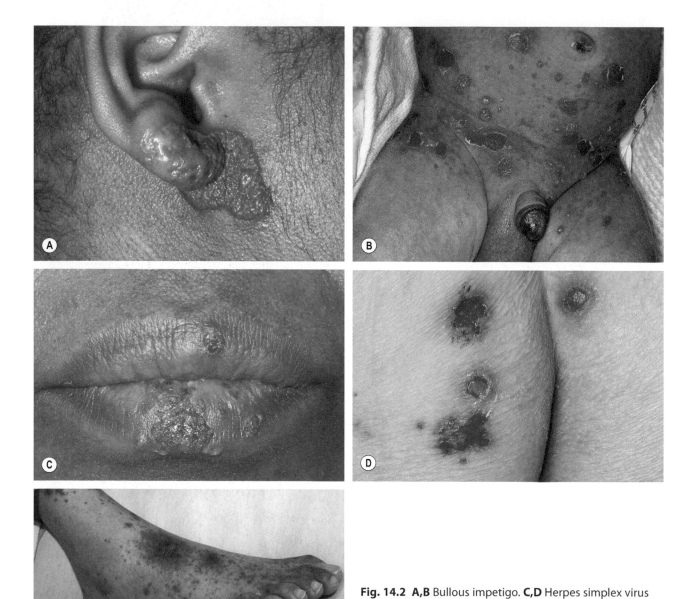

Fig. 14.2 A,B Bullous impetigo. **C,D** Herpes simplex virus infection. **E** Leukocytoclastic vasculitis. *A–D, Courtesy, Yale Dermatology Residents' Slide Collection. E, Courtesy, William Damsky, MD. B, From Bolognia JL, Jorizzo JL, Schaffer JV. Dermatology, 3e. London: Saunders, 2012, with permission.*

DISORDERS THAT ARE OFTEN ACRAL

Dyshidrotic Eczema

Clinical:
Deep-seated vesicles, often on the margins of the fingers/hand (see Figs. 2.18B, 2.20A)
Occasionally larger bullae
May be pruritic

Histopathologic:
Vesicles within acral skin

Orf (Fig. 14.3)

Clinical:
Generally on the hand; varying morphology depending on stage

Histopathologic:
Necrosis (reticular degeneration) of the epidermis with cytoplasmic pink inclusions, variable inflammation

Diabetic Bullae (Fig. 14.4)

Clinical:
Predilection for the legs; often tense, noninflamed blisters; occurs in patient with a history of diabetes mellitus

Stasis Bullae

Clinical:
Predilection for the legs; other signs of venous insufficiency (i.e. venulectasia, brown discoloration secondary to hemosiderin deposition)

Histopathologic:
Clustered, thick-walled capillaries in the dermis below the split

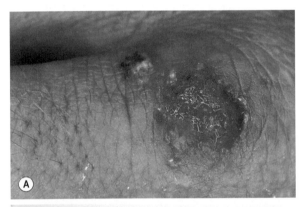

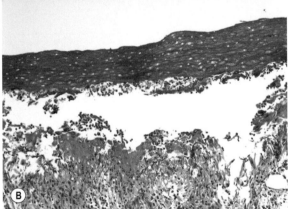

Fig. 14.3 Orf. Reticular degeneration is shown in **(B)**. *A, Courtesy, Anthony Mancini, MD. From Bolognia JL, Jorizzo JL, Schaffer JV. Dermatology, 3e. London: Saunders, 2012, with permission.*

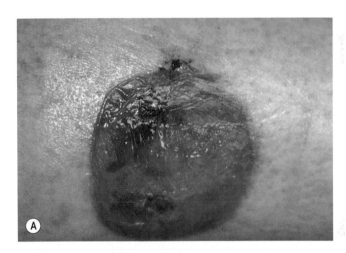

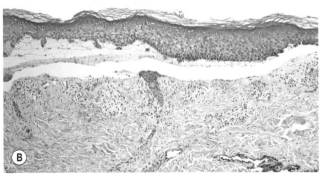

Fig. 14.4 Diabetic bullae, noninflamed subepidermal split.

Leukocytoclastic Vasculitis, Bullous

Clinical:
Palpable purpura, typically on the lower extremities (Fig. 14.5A)

Histopathologic:
Subepidermal split above neutrophils and leukocytoclasia around vessels that have fibrin cuffs (Fig. 14.5B)

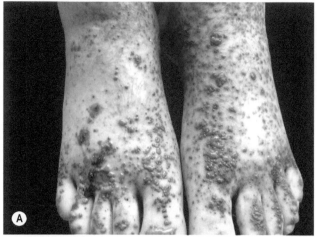

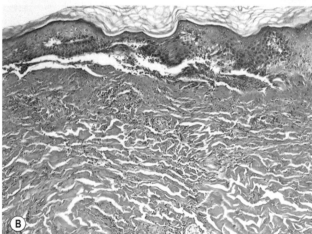

Fig. 14.5 Leukocytoclastic vasculitis, bullous. *A, Courtesy, Karynne O. Duncan, MD.*

Localized Epidermolysis Bullosa (Fig. 14.6)

Clinical:
Favors feet or other areas prone to trauma

Histopathologic:
Separation of the epidermis from dermis; basal cells may appear disrupted (see Fig. 13.12)

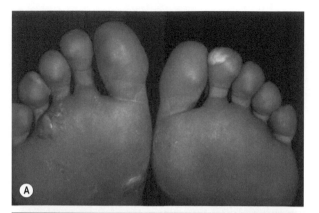

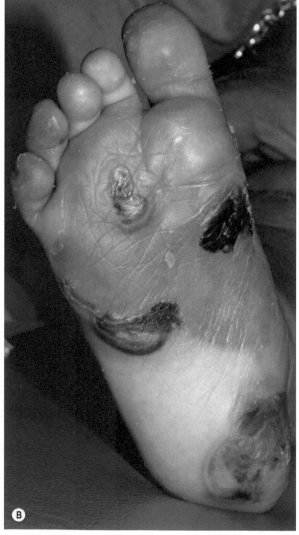

Fig. 14.6 Localized epidermolysis bullosa. *A, Courtesy, Yale Dermatology Residents' Slide Collection; B, Courtesy, Julie V Schaffer, MD. A,B, From Bolognia JL, Jorizzo JL, Schaffer JV. Dermatology, 3e. London: Saunders, 2012, with permission.*

TYPICAL HISTORY

Bullous Arthropod Bite (Fig. 14.7)
Clinical:
History of outdoor activity and contact with arthropods

Histopathologic:
Characteristic intraepidermal split with serum and mixed dermal inflammation

Friction Blister
Clinical:
History of friction

Histopathologic:
Typically an intraepidermal split with minimal inflammation

Coma Bulla (Fig. 14.8)
Clinical:
History of pressure on the affected area during a coma

Histopathologic:
Necrosis of eccrine glands +/− epidermal and dermal necrosis, minimal inflammation

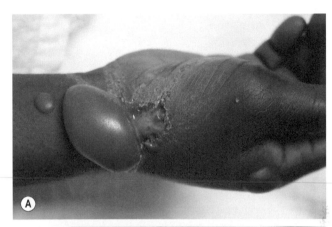

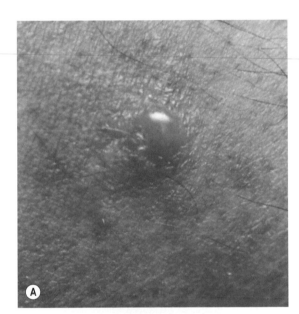

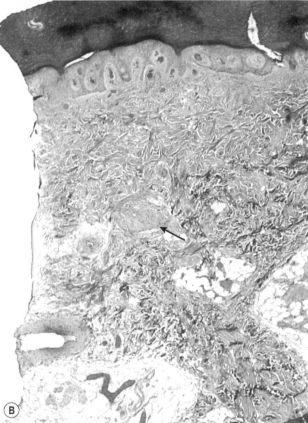

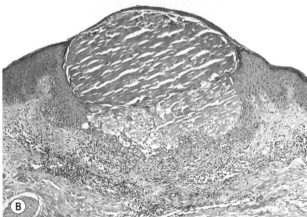

Fig. 14.7 Bullous arthropod bites. Intraepidermal serum and mixed inflammation **(B)**. *A, Courtesy, Yale Dermatology Residents' Slide Collection.*

Fig. 14.8 Coma bullae. Eccrine gland necrosis (arrow) is shown in **(B)**. *A, Courtesy, Yale Dermatology Residents' Slide Collection.*

Burn (Fig. 14.9)

Clinical:

History of exposure of affected skin to high temperatures

Histopathologic:

Partial to full-thickness necrosis/loss of epidermis +/− dermal necrosis

Artifactual Split Secondary to Topical Anesthetic Use Before Biopsy

Clinical:

History of use of topical anesthetic to numb the skin prior to biopsy

Usually, no blister is visible clinically at the time of biopsy

Histopathologic:

Separation of the epidermis from the dermis (Fig. 14.10); on biopsy, other features of the particular disease/process can be present

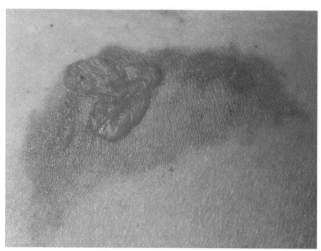

Fig. 14.9 Burn. There is blistering of the skin overlying erythema. The patient splashed boiling water onto her skin when pouring it out from a pot.

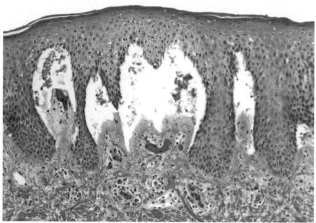

Fig. 14.10 Artifactual split below the epidermis secondary to use of a topical anesthetic before biopsy. There are also changes of a papulosquamous dermatitis, with parakeratosis and acanthosis.

Follicular Processes │ 15

Follicular processes have lesions that are either pierced by a hair shaft or are distributed in a pattern corresponding to hair follicles. This chapter covers acne vulgaris, acne rosacea, folliculitis, keratosis pilaris, pityriasis rubra pilaris, discoid lupus erythematosus, lichen planopilaris, follicular mucinosis, scurvy, vitamin A deficiency, and trichodysplasia spinulosa.

ACNE VULGARIS

Clinical:
Typically affects the face, chest, and back
Lesions include comedones, papules, pustules, and nodules (Figs. 15.1, 15.2; see Figs. 2.2A, 2.3A, 2.4)
Sequelae include scarring and postinflammatory pigmentary changes (see Fig. 15.2)

Histopathologic:
Inflamed lesions often correspond to rupture of a follicle with acute inflammation

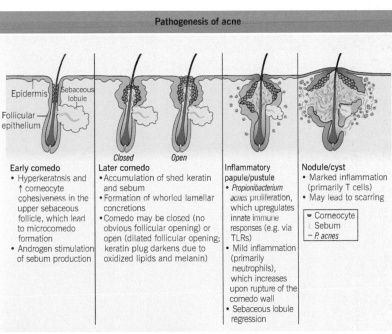

Pathogenesis of acne

Epidermis / Sebaceous lobule
Follicular epithelium

Closed   *Open*

Early comedo
- Hyperkeratosis and ↑ corneocyte cohesiveness in the upper sebaceous follicle, which lead to microcomedo formation
- Androgen stimulation of sebum production

Later comedo
- Accumulation of shed keratin and sebum
- Formation of whorled lamellar concretions
- Comedo may be closed (no obvious follicular opening) or open (dilated follicular opening; keratin plug darkens due to oxidized lipids and melanin)

Inflammatory papule/pustule
- *Propionibacterium acnes* proliferation, which upregulates innate immune responses (e.g. via TLRs)
- Mild inflammation (primarily neutrophils), which increases upon rupture of the comedo wall
- Sebaceous lobule regression

Nodule/cyst
- Marked inflammation (primarily T cells)
- May lead to scarring

Corneocyte
Sebum
P. acnes

Fig. 15.1 Pathogenesis of acne. *From Bolognia JL, Schaffer JV, Duncan KO, Ko CJ. Dermatology Essentials, 1e. Philadelphia: Saunders, 2014, with permission.*

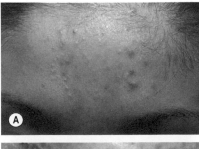

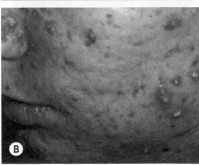

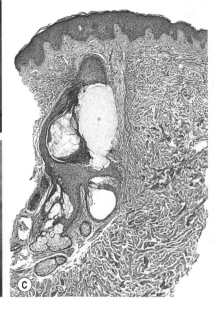

Fig. 15.2 Acne. **A** Open and closed comedones and several inflammatory papules. **B** Papulopustules and scarring. **C** Follicular rupture and inflammation. *A, Courtesy Kalman Watsky, MD; B, Courtesy, Andrew Zaenglein, MD and Diane Thiboutot, MD. A,B, From Bolognia JL, Schaffer JV, Duncan KO, Ko CJ. Dermatology Essentials, 1e. Philadelphia: Saunders, 2014, with permission.*

ACNE ROSACEA

Clinical:
Most commonly affects the face (Fig. 15.3; see Figs. 2.2B,C, 2.4, 2.6A); rarely scalp, chest
Papulopustular form and granulomatous variant are folliculocentric

Histopathologic:
Perifollicular and perivascular lymphocytes +/− histiocytes
Dilated vessels

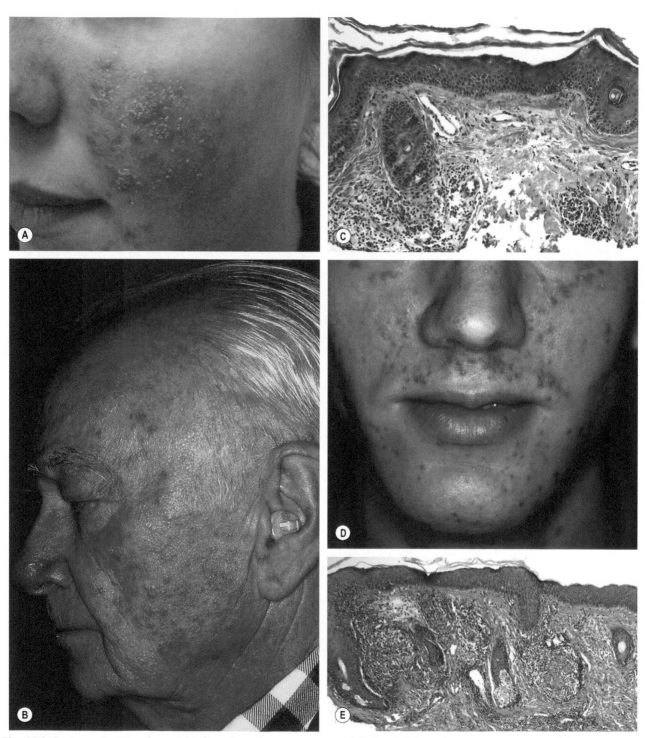

Fig. 15.3 Rosacea. **A–C** Papulopustular form. Lymphocytes surround follicles. **D,E** Granulomatous rosacea (perifollicular granulomas). *A, Courtesy, Kalman Watsky, MD; B,D, Courtesy, Yale Dermatology Residents' Slide Collection. B,D, From Bolognia JB, Jorizzo JL, Rapini RP. Dermatology, 2e. London: Saunders, 2008, with permission.*

FOLLICULITIS

Folliculitis is inflammation of hair follicles and can be superficial or deep, infectious (Fig. 15.4) or noninfectious (Figs. 15.5, 15.6; see Figs. 2.25C, 6.22)

Papules and/or pustules, sometimes crusted, affect various sites

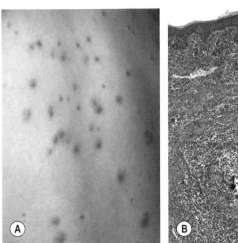

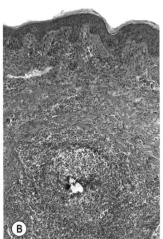

Fig. 15.4 Infectious folliculitis. **A,B** Bacterial (*Staphylococcus aureus*) folliculitis. Clumps of bacteria are present in an inflamed follicle. **C,D** Fungal folliculitis. Around the hair shaft, there are hyphae cut in cross-section (arrow). In addition to erythematous papules, there are plaques with annular scale. **E,F** Viral (herpes simplex virus) folliculitis. There is acantholysis with multinucleate cells. **G,H** *Demodex* folliculitis. *Demodex* mites (arrow) are located in the dermis with surrounding inflammation. *A, Courtesy, Julie V Schaffer, MD; E, Courtesy, Yale Dermatology Residents' Slide Collection; G, Courtesy, Peter Heald, MD. A, From Bolognia JL, Schaffer JV, Duncan KO, Ko CJ. Dermatology Essentials, 1e. Philadelphia: Saunders, 2014, with permission.*

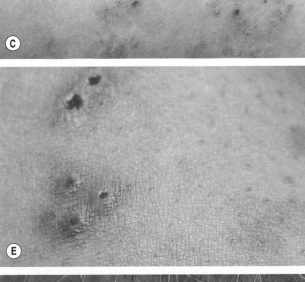

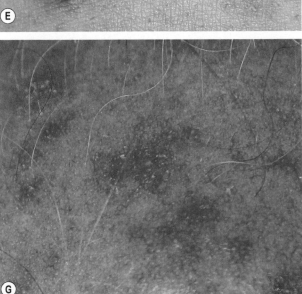

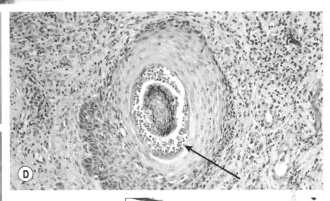

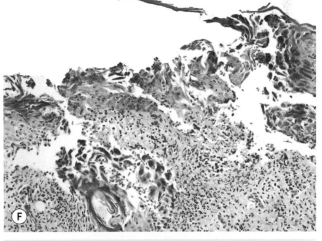

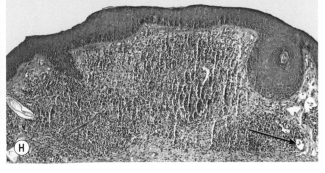

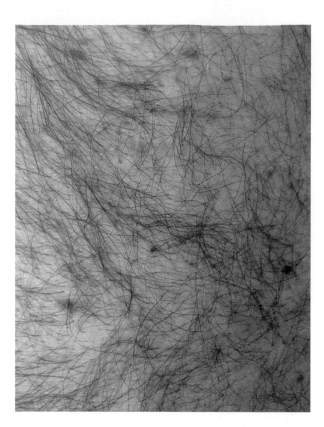

Fig. 15.5 Sterile (culture-negative) folliculitis. Note the pustule pierced by a hair shaft.

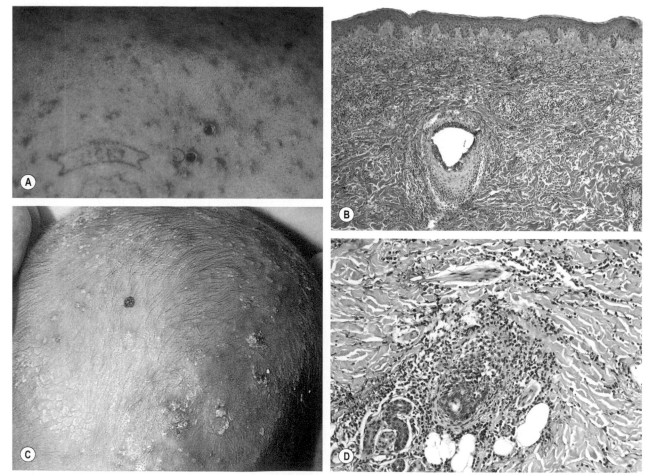

Fig. 15.6 Eosinophilic folliculitis. **A,B** Acquired immunodeficiency syndrome (AIDS)–associated. **C,D** In infancy, typical scalp involvement. *A, Courtesy, Yale Dermatology Residents' Slide Collection. A, From Bolognia JL, Schaffer JV, Duncan KO, Ko CJ. Dermatology Essentials, 1e. Philadelphia: Saunders, 2014, with permission. C, From Schachner LA, Hansen RE. Pediatric Dermatology, 4e. London: Mosby, 2011.*

KERATOSIS PILARIS

Clinical:
Favors the upper arms (Fig. 15.7) and thighs and the lateral cheeks in children
Keratotic follicular papules, +/− erythema

Histopathologic:
Keratin-plugged hair follicle, sometimes with surrounding inflammation

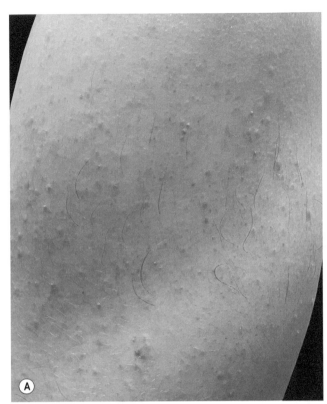
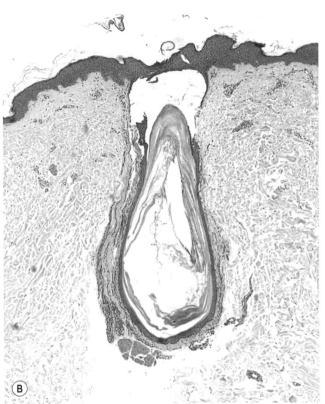

Fig. 15.7 Keratosis pilaris. *A, Courtesy, Karynne O. Duncan, MD.*

PITYRIASIS RUBRA PILARIS (SEE ALSO CHAPTER 5)

Clinical:
Nutmeg grater–like follicular papules (Fig. 15.8)

Histopathologic:
Follicular plugging; there may be hyperkeratosis with alternating parakeratosis in the stratum corneum

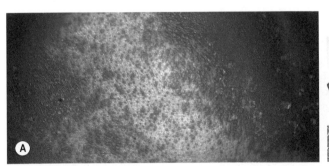
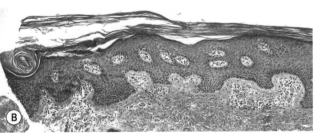

Fig. 15.8 Pityriasis rubra pilaris. **A,B** Follicular papules and confluent erythema with follicular plugging and alternating orthokeratosis and parakeratosis. *A, Courtesy, Yale Dermatology Residents' Slide Collection. A, From Bolognia JL, Schaffer JV, Duncan KO, Ko CJ. Dermatology Essentials, 1e. Philadelphia: Saunders, 2014, with permission.*

DISCOID LUPUS ERYTHEMATOSUS

Clinical:
Follicular plugging, often easily appreciated in the conchal bowl (Fig. 15.9)
Associated scarring, dyspigmentation, and/or atrophy

Histopathologic:
Follicular plugging, interface change (variable inflammation at the dermal–epidermal junction), superficial and deep perivascular and periadnexal lymphocytic inflammation (Fig. 15.9B,C); there may be clusters of CD123-positive lymphocytes

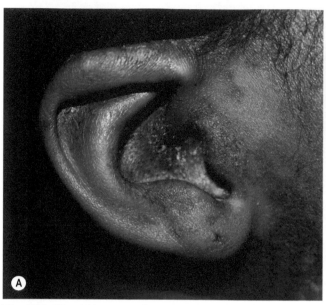

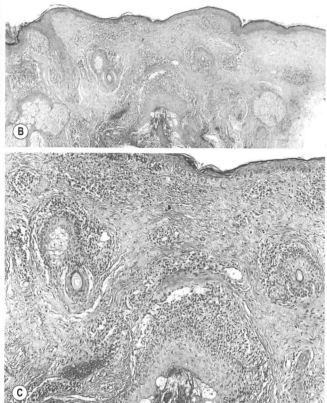

Fig. 15.9 Discoid lupus erythematosus. *Courtesy, Yale Dermatology Residents' Slide Collection.*

LICHEN PLANOPILARIS

Clinical:
Scalp with areas of hair loss (Fig. 15.10) sometimes with plugged, erythematous follicles
Skin, mucosa, or nails may show signs of lichen planus

Histopathologic:
Lymphocytes surrounding the upper part of the follicle, with destruction of the follicular epithelium

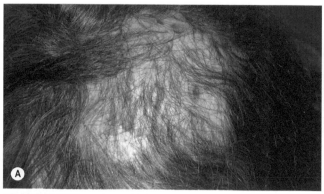

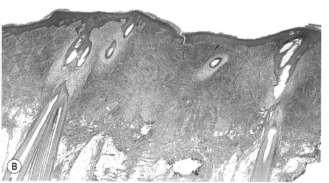

Fig. 15.10 Lichen planopilaris.

FOLLICULAR MUCINOSIS

Clinical:
Grouped follicular papules with alopecia (Fig. 15.11; see also Fig. 2.7A)

Violet–brown plaques may be present

Histopathologic:
Mucin within follicles creating white–blue space between keratinocytes

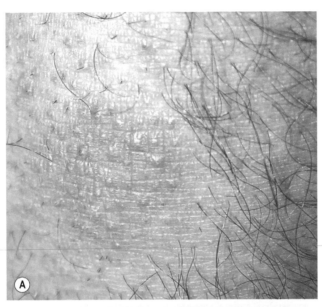

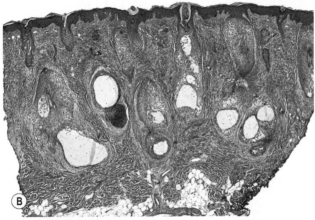

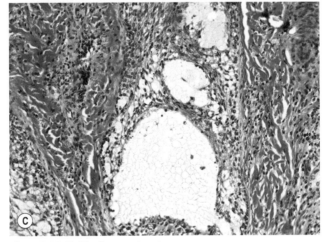

Fig. 15.11 Follicular mucinosis.

SCURVY

Clinical:
Perifollicular hemorrhage and corkscrew hairs (Fig. 15.12)
Other clues – gingival bleeding, purpura

Histopathologic:
Keratin-plugged follicles surrounded by inflammation and erythrocytes

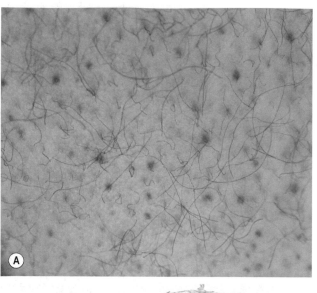

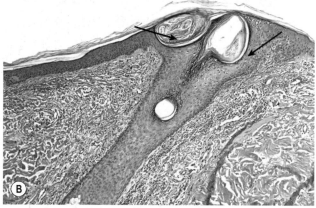

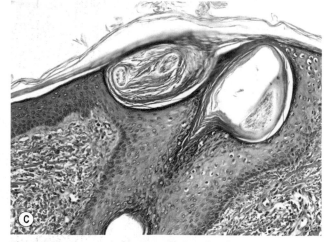

Fig. 15.12 Scurvy. *A, Courtesy, Christopher Stamey, MD.*

VITAMIN A DEFICIENCY

Clinical:
Phrynoderma (clusters of hyperkeratotic follicular papules) over extensor surfaces (Fig. 15.13)
Xerosis
Night blindness

Histopathologic:
Keratin-plugged follicle

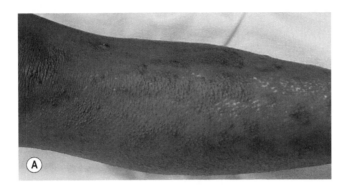

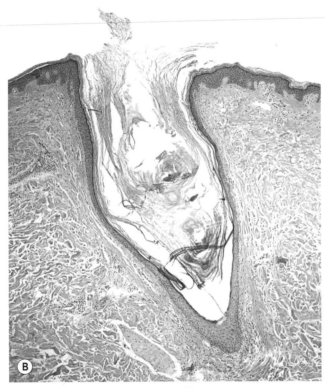

Fig. 15.13 Phrynoderma. *A, Courtesy, Chad M Hivnor, MD. A, From Bolognia JL, Schaffer JV, Duncan KO, Ko CJ. Dermatology Essentials, 1e. Philadelphia: Saunders, 2014, with permission.*

TRICHODYSPLASIA SPINULOSA

Clinical:
Follicular papules (Fig. 15.14), sometimes with prominent protruding spines

Histopathologic:
Expanded follicles with abnormal outer root sheath and absent hair shaft

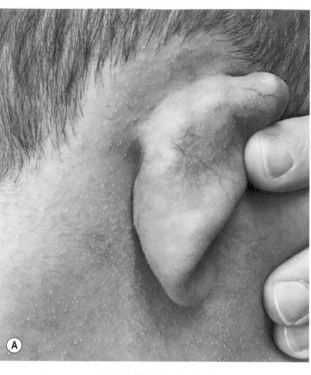

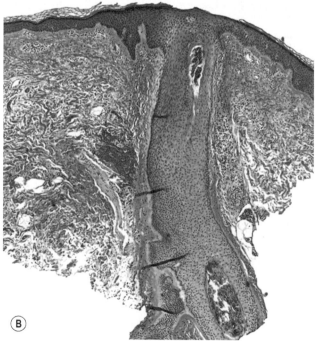

Fig. 15.14 Viral-associated trichodysplasia. **A** Follicular papules on the face. **B** Dilated follicle with abnormal parakeratosis. *A, Courtesy, Richard Antaya, MD.*

Dermal Inflammation | 16

Neutrophilic infiltrates may have a characteristic acute, nontreated appearance that is red and "hot" as a result of inflammation (see Fig. 1.48). Mixed inflammatory infiltrates (lymphocytes and histiocytes with neutrophils or eosinophils) are often a lighter pink–red. Granulomatous disorders typically have a red–brown to pink color (see Chapter 20 and Fig. 2.7G). This chapter covers neutrophilic, mixed, and lymphocytic infiltrates.

NEUTROPHILIC ("HOT")

Sweet Syndrome
Clinical:
Any site, but predilection for facial and acral locations Edematous/pseudovesicular to crusted papules and plaques, sometimes targetoid (Fig. 16.1A,B; see Fig. 2.7F)

Histopathologic:
Dense dermal infiltrate of neutrophils (Fig. 16.1C,D); sometimes with papillary dermal edema

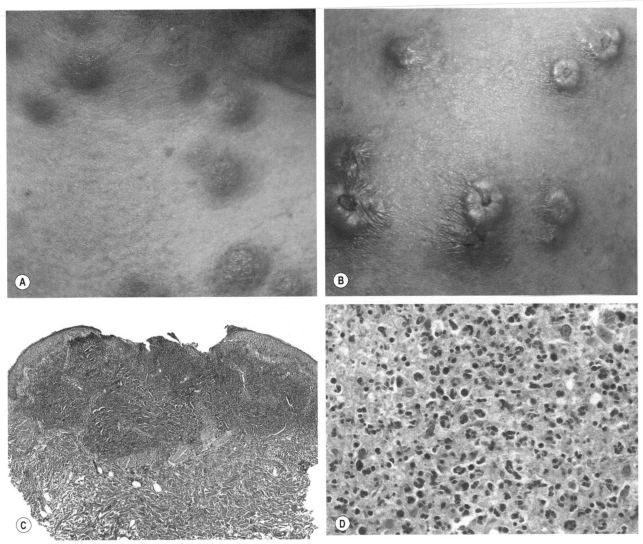

Fig. 16.1 Sweet syndrome. *A,B, Courtesy, Yale Dermatology Residents' Slide Collection.*

Pyoderma Gangrenosum (Fig. 16.2)

Clinical:
Any site, but commonly on the legs
Early lesion is an inflamed pustule (see Fig. 11.14)
Well-developed lesions often ulcerated with a violet–gray undermined border

Histopathologic:
Acute, inflamed lesions have a dense dermal infiltrate of neutrophils

Erythema Elevatum Diutinum, Acute Stage (Fig. 16.3)

Clinical:
Symmetric, often acral (extensor surfaces of elbows/hands), red–violet to pink–brown papules and plaques

Histopathologic:
Infiltrate of neutrophils with vascular damage
Late stage becomes clinically indurated and histologically fibrotic (see Fig. 21.16)

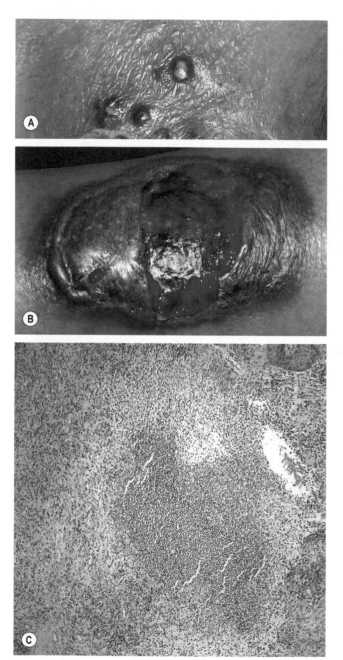

Fig. 16.2 Pyoderma gangrenosum. *A, B, Courtesy, Yale Dermatology Residents' Slide Collection.*

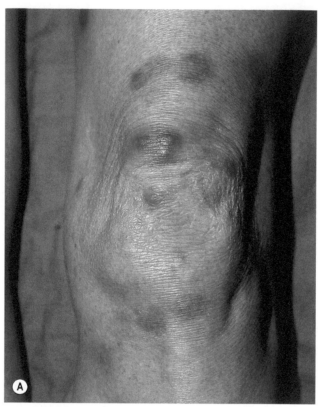

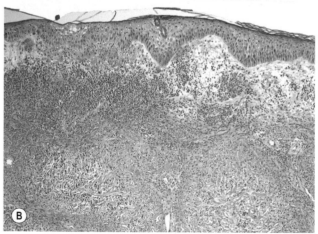

Fig. 16.3 Erythema elevatum diutinum. *A, Courtesy, Kenneth Greer, MD. A, From Bolognia JL, Jorizzo JL, Schaffer JV. Dermatology, 3e. London: Saunders, 2012, with permission.*

Cellulitis (Fig. 16.4)

Clinical:
Any site, but commonly affects the lower legs
Warm, tender, bright red plaque
Often associated fever and elevated white cell count

Histopathologic:
Interstitial infiltrate of neutrophils

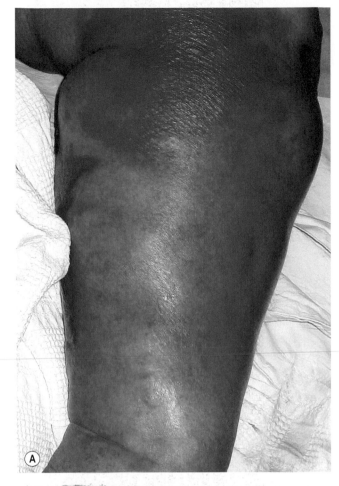

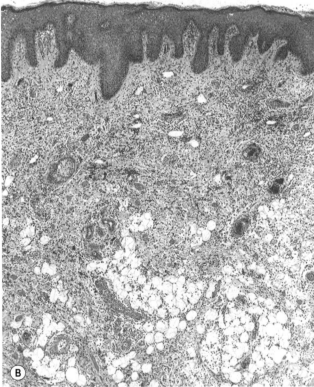

Fig. 16.4 Cellulitis (group A streptococci). *A, Courtesy, Yale Dermatology Residents' Slide Collection. A, From Bolognia JL, Jorizzo JL, Schaffer JV. Dermatology, 3e. London: Saunders, 2012, with permission. B, From Guarner J. Skin and soft tissue infections. In: Procop GW, Pritt BS (eds). Pathology of Infectious Diseases. London: Saunders, 2015.*

MIXED WITH NEUTROPHILS AND EOSINOPHILS OR PREDOMINANT EOSINOPHILS (PINK–RED)

Wells Syndrome (Eosinophilic Cellulitis; Fig. 16.5)

Clinical:
Pink edematous plaques that may resemble cellulitis

Histopathologic:
Interstitial infiltrate of eosinophils and neutrophils, often with flame figures (collagen encrusted with granular red–purple material) (Fig. 16.5C)

Arthropod Bite Reaction (Fig. 16.6)

Clinical:
Various arthropods can assault or bite humans
Lesions are pink–red papules, sometimes crusted or vesicular

Histopathologic:
Superficial and deep perivascular and interstitial mixed infiltrate; there may be epidermal changes

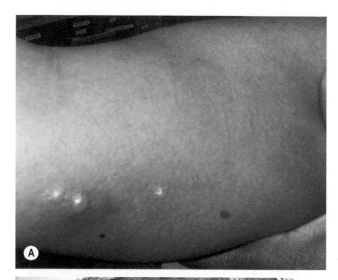

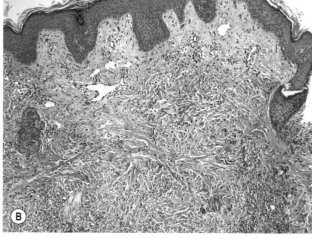

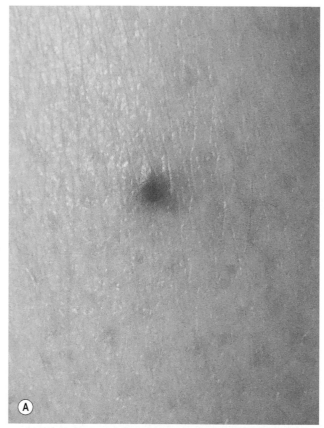

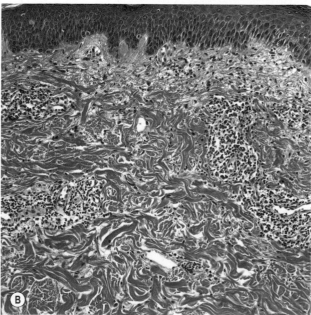

Fig. 16.5 Wells syndrome. *A, Courtesy, Yale Dermatology Residents' Slide Collection.*

Fig. 16.6 Arthropod bite reaction.

Palisaded Neutrophilic and Granulomatous Disorder (Fig. 16.7)

Clinical:

Associated with connective tissue disorders, such as rheumatoid arthritis, lupus erythematosus, and granulomatosis with polyangiitis

Erythematous papules, sometimes with central "punched out" ulceration

Favors the elbows and extensor digits

Histopathologic:

Neutrophilic infiltrates with vasculitis and/or palisading granulomas

Granuloma Faciale (Fig. 16.8; see Fig. 2.7E)

Clinical:

Typically on the face but may affect other sites

Red–brown papule or plaque, often with prominent follicular openings

Histopathologic:

Mixed infiltrate below a grenz zone (rim of spared papillary dermis)

Dilated, plugged follicles may be present

Fixed Drug Eruption

(See Chapter 8)

Urticaria (see Fig. 1.48M,N)

Clinical:

Transient (duration <24 hours), edematous pink papules/ plaques

Histopathologic:

Perivascular and interstitial neutrophils, lymphocytes, and/or eosinophils

Urticarial Bullous Pemphigoid

(See Chapter 12)

Eosinophilic Folliculitis

(See Chapter 15)

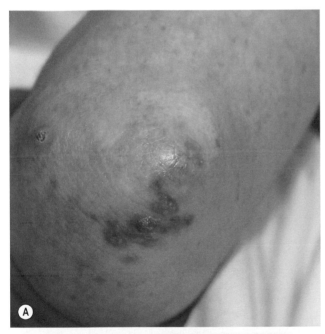

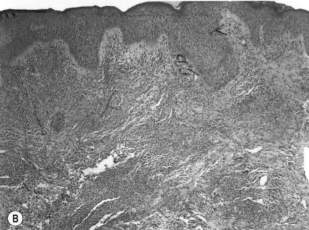

Fig. 16.7 Palisaded neutrophilic and granulomatous disorder.

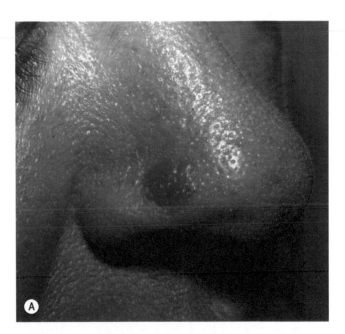

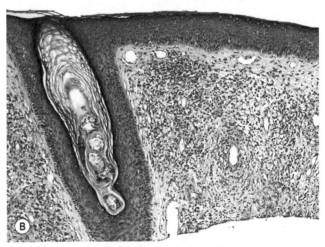

Fig. 16.8 Granuloma faciale. *A, Courtesy, Cloyce L Stetson, MD; B, Courtesy, Anjela Galan, MD. A, From Bolognia JL, Schaffer JV, Duncan KO, Ko CJ. Dermatology Essentials, 1e. Philadelphia: Saunders, 2014, with permission.*

PREDOMINANTLY LYMPHOCYTIC

Polymorphic Eruption of Pregnancy (Pruritic Urticarial Papules and Plaques of Pregnancy) (Fig. 16.9)

Clinical:

Abdomen and upper thighs, sparing the umbilicus
Pink to pink–brown (the latter in darker skin types)
papules and plaques; can be urticarial, targetoid, vesicular,
or eczematous

Histopathologic:

Perivascular lymphocytic infiltrate, +/− eosinophils;
epidermal changes may be present, depending on the type
of lesion sampled for biopsy

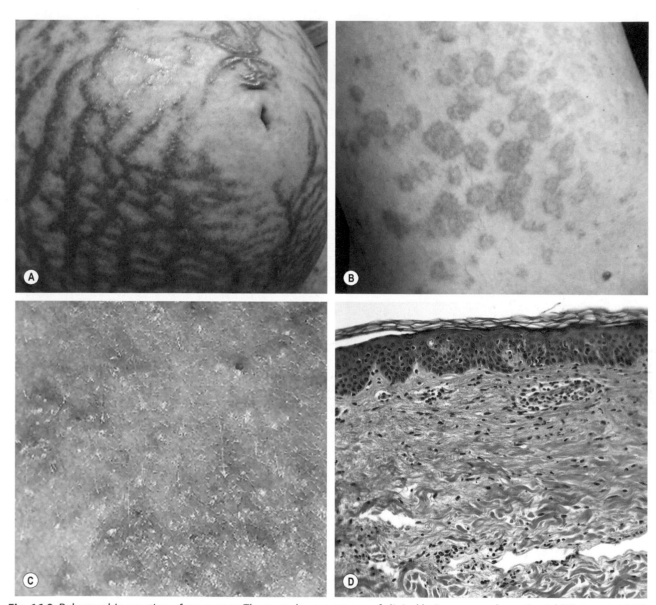

Fig. 16.9 Polymorphic eruption of pregnancy. There can be a spectrum of clinical lesions – macular, urticarial **(A)**, targetoid **(B)**, vesicular, and eczematous **(C)**. *A, Courtesy, Yale Dermatology Residents' Slide Collection; B,C, Courtesy, Christina M Ambros-Rudolph, MD. B,C, From Bolognia JL, Schaffer JV, Duncan KO, Ko CJ. Dermatology Essentials, 1e. Philadelphia: Saunders, 2014, with permission.*

Lyme Disease (Fig. 16.10)

Clinical:

Classic lesion is targetoid with darker center and 1- to 2-cm-wide pink rim

Lesions may be multiple

Histopathologic:

Nonspecific perivascular inflammation, plasma cells may or may not be present

Perniosis (Fig. 16.11)

Clinical:

Pink to purple macules and/or papules, sometimes with petechiae, typically on the digits (acral sites)

Histopathologic:

Superficial and deep perivascular and perieccrine lymphocytic inflammation, often with papillary dermal edema

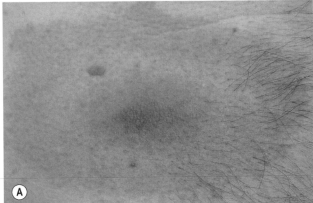

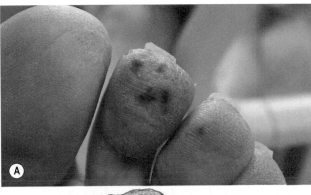

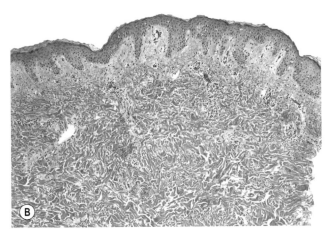

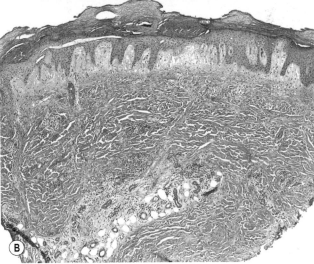

Fig. 16.10 Lyme disease. *A, Courtesy, Yale Dermatology Residents' Slide Collection.*

Fig. 16.11 Perniosis. *A, Courtesy, Jean L Bolognia, MD. A, From Bolognia JL, Jorizzo JL, Schaffer JV. Dermatology, 3e. London: Saunders, 2012, with permission.*

Lupus Tumidus

Clinical:
Typically affects the face/upper trunk (see Fig. 2.7B)
Edematous, pink papules and plaques (Fig. 16.12A)

Histopathologic:
Perivascular lymphocytic inflammation, classically with
increased dermal mucin (Fig. 16.12C)

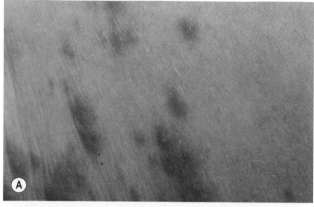

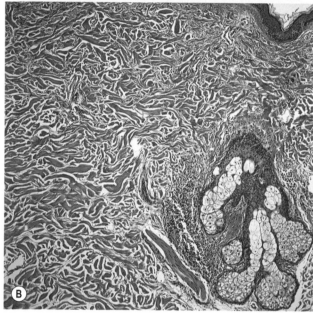

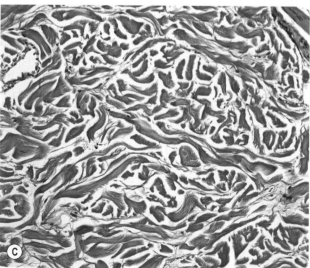

Fig. 16.12 Lupus tumidus. Increased mucin is shown in **(C)**.
A, Courtesy, Yale Dermatology Residents' Slide Collection.

Lymphocytic Infiltrate of Jessner

Clinical:
Typically affects the upper trunk or face (Fig. 16.13; see
Fig. 2.7C)
Juicy pink papules or plaques, sometimes annular

Histopathologic:
Perivascular lymphocytic inflammation, classically
without increased dermal mucin

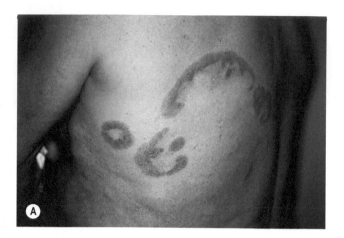

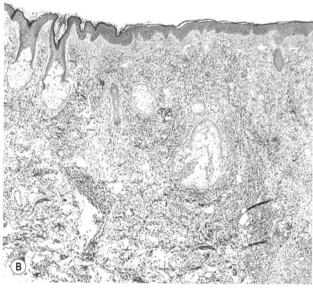

Fig. 16.13 Lymphocytic infiltrate of Jessner. Typical arciform
plaques on the back. *A, From Rémy-Leroux V, Léonard F,
Lambert D, et al. Comparison of histopathologic-clinical
characteristics of Jessner's lymphocytic infiltration of the skin
and lupus erythematosus tumidus: Multicenter study of 46 cases.
J Am Acad Dermatol. 2008;58:217–23, © Elsevier.*

Deep Soft Tissue Disorders: Panniculitis and Deep Soft Tissue Inflammation

17

This chapter addresses inflammatory disorders that primarily affect the tissues below the dermis in fat and/or fascia (Table 17.1; Figs. 17.1–17.4).

Table 17.1 Common panniculitides

Entity	Clinical		Histopathologic
	Site (Fig. 17.1)	**Morphology**	
Erythema nodosum	• Especially on shins • Also thighs, forearms	• Bilateral, tender erythematous nodules (Fig. 17.2A)	• Septal fibrosis and inflammation (Fig. 17.2B)
Erythema induratum	• Posterior lower legs	• Erythematous nodules • May ulcerate (Fig. 17.2C)	• Lobular panniculitis with mixed inflammation, sometimes granulomatous, +/− vasculitis (Fig. 17.2D)
Lipodermatosclerosis	• Favors the lower medial legs	• Indurated pink to red–brown plaques (Fig. 17.2E,F)	• Lipomembranous change within fat lobules (Fig. 17.2G)
Lupus panniculitis	• Proximal extremities/hips • Upper trunk/face	• May have overlying changes of discoid lupus and/or skin may be tethered down (Fig. 17.2H)	• Hyaline necrosis of fat with lymphoid follicles (Fig. 17.2I)

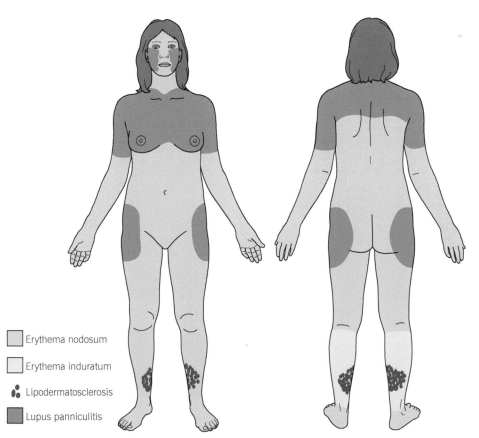

☐ Erythema nodosum

☐ Erythema induratum

⚬ Lipodermatosclerosis

▓ Lupus panniculitis

Fig. 17.1 Most common locations for several forms of panniculitis. *Adapted from Bolognia JL, Jorizzo JL, Schaffer JV. Dermatology, 3e. London: Saunders, 2012, with permission.*

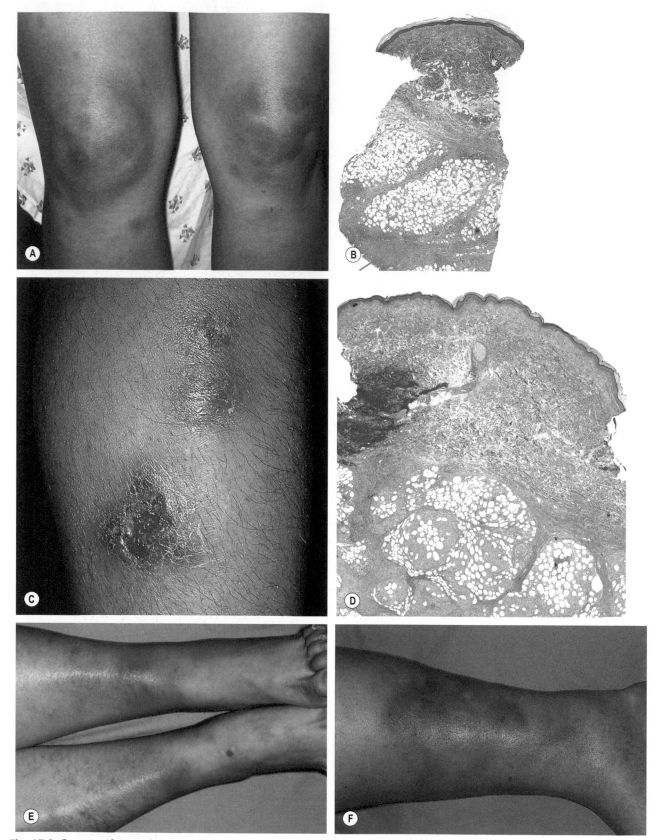

Fig. 17.2 Common forms of panniculitis. **A,B** Erythema nodosum. Septal fibrosis, thickening (blue arrow), and inflammation (orange arrow). The septae, rather than the lobules of fat, are affected primarily. **C,D** Erythema induratum. Unlike erythema nodosum (A), lesions tend to affect the calf and may be ulcerated. Inflammation is primarily centered within the lobules of fat. **E–G** Lipodermatosclerosis. Inflammation within the lobules of fat with some septal fibrosis.

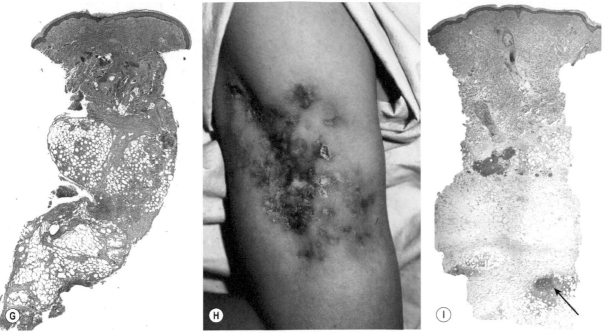

Fig. 17.2, cont'd   H,I Lupus panniculitis. Hyaline fat necrosis with a lymphoid follicle (black arrow). *A, Courtesy, Yale Dermatology Residents' Slide Collection. C,F,H, Courtesy, Kenneth E Greer, MD. E, Courtesy, James Patterson, MD. C,E,F,H, From Bolognia JL, Jorizzo JL, Schaffer JV. Dermatology, 3e. London: Saunders, 2012, with permission.*

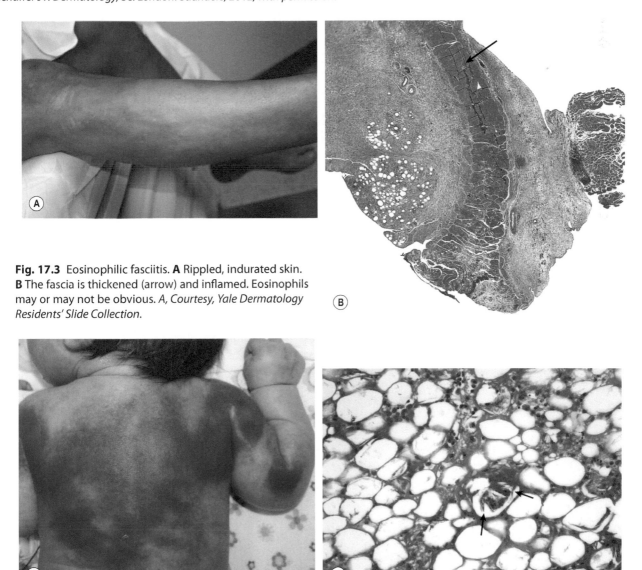

Fig. 17.3 Eosinophilic fasciitis. **A** Rippled, indurated skin. **B** The fascia is thickened (arrow) and inflamed. Eosinophils may or may not be obvious. *A, Courtesy, Yale Dermatology Residents' Slide Collection.*

Fig. 17.4 Subcutaneous fat necrosis of the newborn. Erythematous, indurated plaques with inflammation and crystals (arrows) in the fat. *A, Courtesy, Yale Dermatology Residents' Slide Collection.*

Dermal-Based Lesions | 18

Dermal tumors of different origins can have similar appearances, so history and biopsy are important for determining the correct diagnosis (Fig. 18.1). This chapter focuses on the characteristic presentations of dermal-based tumors (Tables 18.1, 18.2).

CONGENITAL/INFANTILE NODULES

Causes of congenital nodules include vascular tumors (see Fig. 18.1; Figs. 18.2, 18.3) and malformations; solid tumors (e.g. myofibroma [Fig. 18.4]; rhabdomyosarcoma [see Fig. 18.1B]); hematologic processes (e.g. mastocytoma, leukemia cutis, dermal erythropoiesis); and developmental anomalies (see Chapter 19).

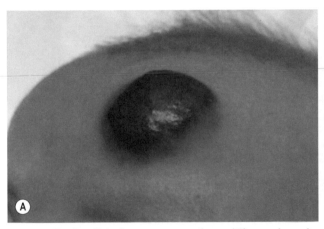
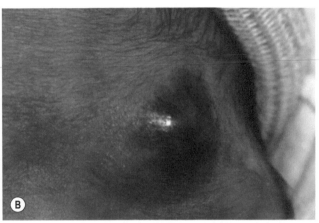

Fig. 18.1 Similar clinical appearances of two different dermal tumors. **A** Infantile hemangioma. Bright red color like that of a ripe strawberry. **B** Rhabdomyosarcoma. *From Eichenfield LF, Frieden IJ, Zaenglein AL, Mathes E. Neonatal and Infant Dermatology, 3e. London: Saunders, 2014.*

Table 18.1 Dermal-based lesions

Entity	Classic morphologic clues*	Histopathology
Vascular tumors		
Infantile hemangioma	• **History:** Not present at birth, grows rapidly over first couple of months • Bright red nodule (Fig. 18.1A); a white halo caused by vascular steal is sometimes present	• Lobules of small capillaries (glucose transporter 1 [GLUT1]-positive) • Often extends into the subcutaneous
Congenital hemangioma	• **History:** Present at birth • **Site:** Predilection for pressure points • Oval shape • Blue–red nodule with white–green halo (Fig. 18.2)	• Lobules of small capillaries (GLUT1-negative)
Tufted angioma	• Mottled to solid red patches and red papules (Fig. 18.3A,B)	• Small lobules (tufts) of small capillaries • Dilated lymphatic spaces
Glomuvenous malformation (glomangioma)	• May be autosomal dominant inheritance, particularly if multiple lesions • Clustered blue papules (Fig. 18.3C,D)	• Dilated spaces lined by one to two layers of monomorphous cells with round blue nuclei
Fibrous tumors		
Myofibroma	• **Site:** Often on the head/neck or trunk • Firm or rubbery nodule or infiltrative plaque • Skin-colored to red–purple • May be multiple (Fig. 18.4)	• Biphasic with increased vascularity and spindle cells (myofibroblasts)
Infantile digital fibroma	• **Site:** Typically on the 2nd toe • Firm, pink nodule (Fig. 18.5)	• Elongated spindle cells with cytoplasmic pink inclusions

205

Continued

Table 18.1 Dermal-based lesions—cont'd

Entity	Classic morphologic clues*	Histopathology
Hematologic processes		
Mastocytoma	• **History:** Intermittent blistering • Brown–pink to red papulonodule • Leathery surface (Fig. 18.6)	• Fried egg–shaped cells with granular cytoplasm

*Not every case will have these features.

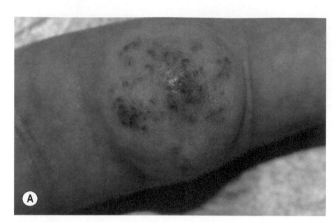
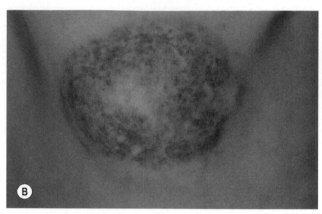

Fig. 18.2 Congenital hemangioma. **A** Rapidly involuting congenital hemangioma. As hemangiomas involute, any red coloration generally progressively lightens/disappears. **B** Noninvoluting congenital hemangioma. These lesions are distinguished by clinical course. *From Eichenfield LF, Frieden IJ, Zaenglein AL, Mathes E. Neonatal and Infant Dermatology, 3e. London: Saunders, 2014.*

NONCONGENITAL LESIONS

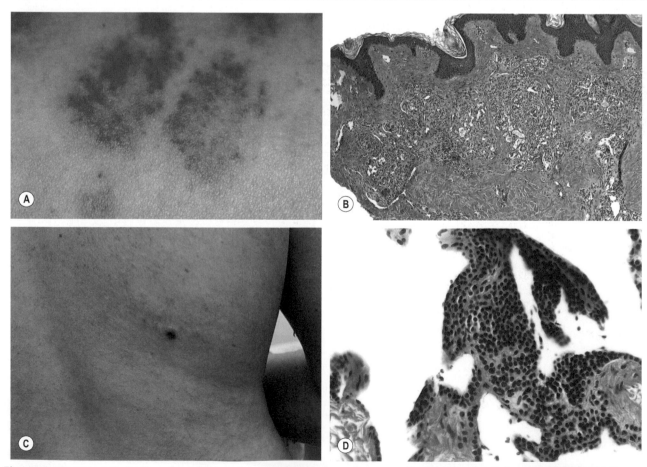

Fig. 18.3 Characteristic findings for tufted angioma **(A,B)** and glomuvenous malformation **(C,D).** Tufted angiomas typically have darker red, minimally raised papules in a mottled, irregular distribution over a lighter pink background. Glomuvenous malformations often are on the trunk and are clustered blue–purple papules. *A,C, Courtesy, Yale Dermatology Residents' Slide Collection; D, Courtesy, Nemanja Rodic, MD, PhD.*

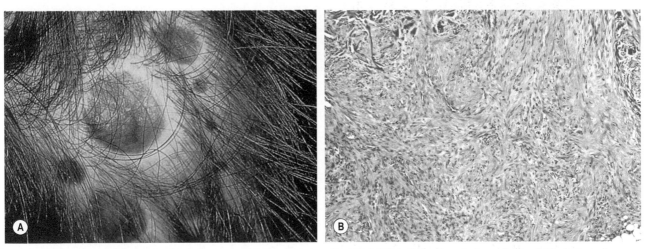

Fig. 18.4 Infantile myofibromatosis. *A, Courtesy, Yale Dermatology Residents' Slide Collection. A, From Bolognia JL, Jorizzo JL, Schaffer JV. Dermatology, 3e. London: Saunders, 2012, with permission.*

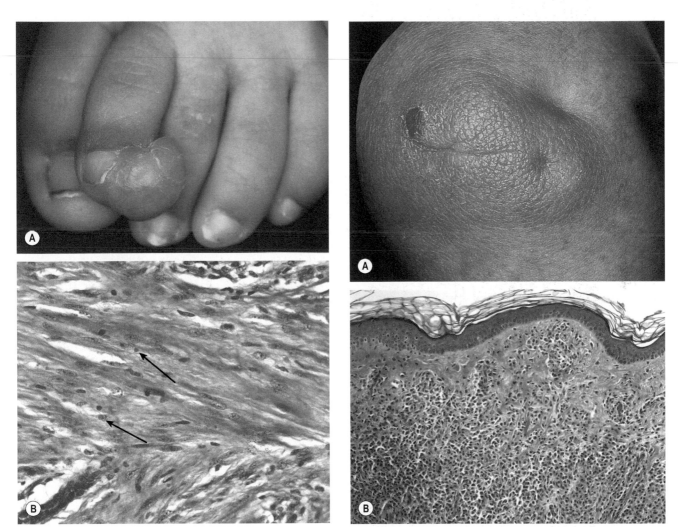

Fig. 18.5 Infantile digital fibroma. The second toe is characteristically involved. *A, Courtesy, Yale Dermatology Residents' Slide Collection. A, From Bolognia JL, Schaffer JV, Duncan KO, Ko CJ. Dermatology Essentials, 1e. Philadelphia: Saunders, 2014, with permission.*

Fig. 18.6 Mastocytoma. The surface appears leathery. *Courtesy, Michael Tharp, MD. A, From Bolognia JL, Schaffer JV, Duncan KO, Ko CJ. Dermatology Essentials, 1e. Philadelphia: Saunders, 2014, with permission.*

Table 18.2 Characteristic papulonodules in children/adults

Entity	Classic morphologic clues*	Histopathology
Adnexal tumors		
Apocrine hidrocystoma (see Fig. 19.4)	• **Site:** Eyelid • Bluish, translucent papule	• Cuboidal cells lining a lumen
Pilomatricoma (Fig. 18.7)	• Bluish tinge • Firm to hard plate-like papulonodule • Lesion will "teeter totter" with pressure on one side or another	• Shadow cells within butterscotch-colored keratin
Sebaceous hyperplasia (see Fig. 2.1E)	• **Site:** Face • Yellow papule with central dell	• Dilated follicular infundibulum surrounded by sebaceous glands
Syringoma (see Fig. 2.1D)	• **Site:** Eyelids • Flesh-colored papules	• Tadpole-shaped epithelium with clear cells and ductal differentiation
Vascular tumors		
Cherry angioma (Fig. 18.8)	• Bright red papule	• Clusters of dilated spaces lined by endothelial cells
Pyogenic granuloma (Fig. 18.9)	• **Site:** Predilection for head/neck, fingers • History of rapid growth • Eroded red papule, often pedunculated	• Polypoid • Lobules of small vessels
Superficial hemosiderotic lymphatic malformation (hobnail hemangioma; targetoid hemosiderotic hemangioma; Fig. 18.10)	• Three-colored zones	• Dilated vessels superficially and centrally • Slit-like vessels deeper • Hemosiderin at periphery
Neural tumor		
Neurofibroma (Fig. 18.11; see Fig. 2.24E)	• Soft, compressible pink papule	• Delicate spindle cells with pink stroma
Plexiform neurofibroma (Fig. 18.12)	• On palpation, the lesion feels like a "bag of worms"	• Multiple separate cords of spindle cells with pink stroma
Fibrous tumors		
Fibrous papule (Fig. 18.13)	• **Site:** Commonly on the nose • Firm, skin-colored to pink papule	• Dense pink collagen • Dilated vessels • Stellate fibroblasts
Dermatofibroma (Fig. 18.14)	• **Site:** Often on the lower legs • Various colors • Firm papule • Becomes slightly depressed with lateral pressure • **Dermoscopy:** delicate peripheral pseudo-network	• Busy dermis filled with spindle cells • Collagen entrapment
Keloid (Fig. 18.15)	• **Site:** Favors the upper trunk/proximal arms • Firm dark pink papulonodule • May be in linear configurations	• Thickened "bubble gum" collagen
Malignant tumors of epidermal origin		
Basal cell carcinoma, pigmented (Fig. 18.16)	• Translucent papule with globules of dark pigment	• Basaloid islands with brown pigment
Basal cell carcinoma, nodular (Fig. 18.17)	• Light pink translucent nodule • Telangiectasias	• Large basaloid islands with peripheral palisading
Squamous cell carcinoma (Fig. 18.18)	• Indurated pink nodule +/− overlying keratin	• Keratin within atypical islands of keratinocytes
Melanocytic tumors		
Blue nevus	• **Site:** Predilection for the hands/feet, but also the face, scalp and other sites • Blue–black papule • **Dermoscopy:** uniform blue–gray color	• Dendritic pigmented cells with associated melanophages
Malignant melanoma, nodular (Fig. 18.19)	• Rapidly growing black nodule	• Large melanocytes in irregular nests
Lymphoma		
Patch/plaque-stage mycosis fungoides (Fig. 18.20)	• **Site:** Double-covered skin (see Fig. 1.16B) • Annular to solid deeply pink plaques • Wrinkled surface and dry scale	• Atypical lymphocytes within the epidermis and in a dermal band

*Not every case will have these features.

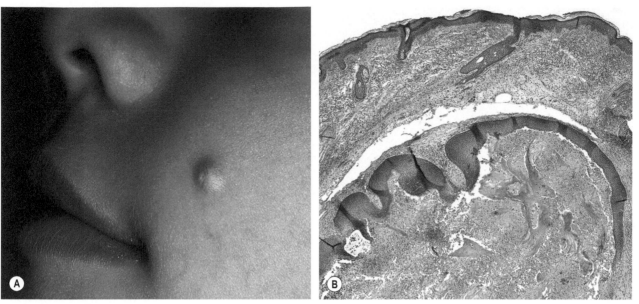

Fig. 18.7 Pilomatricoma. Palpation will often help with the diagnosis, as the lesion is typically very firm and may feel somewhat plate-like. *A, Courtesy, Yale Dermatology Residents' Slide Collection. A, From Bolognia JL, Schaffer JV, Duncan KO, Ko CJ. Dermatology Essentials, 1e. Philadelphia: Saunders, 2014, with permission.*

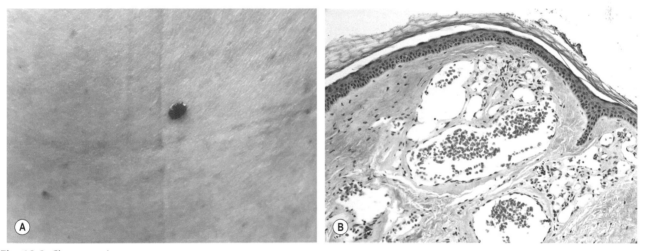

Fig. 18.8 Cherry angioma.

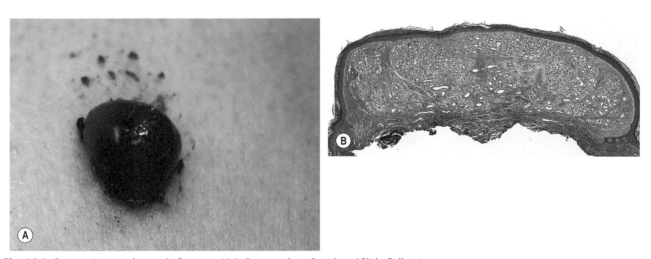

Fig. 18.9 Pyogenic granuloma. *A, Courtesy, Yale Dermatology Residents' Slide Collection.*

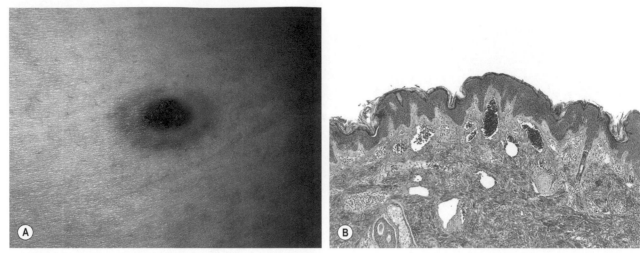

Fig. 18.10 Superficial hemosiderotic lymphatic malformation (hobnail hemangioma; targetoid hemosiderotic hemangioma). Not all lesions have this classic target appearance with a lighter red–brown border that is likely caused by peripheral hemosiderin deposition. *A, Courtesy, Ronald P Rapini, MD. A, From Bolognia JL, Jorizzo JL, Schaffer JV. Dermatology, 3e. London: Saunders, 2012, with permission.*

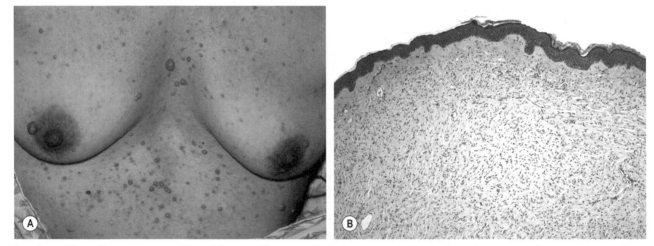

Fig. 18.11 Neurofibromas in a patient with neurofibromatosis. *A, Courtesy, Julie V Schaffer, MD. A, From Bolognia JL, Jorizzo JL, Schaffer JV. Dermatology, 3e. London: Saunders, 2012, with permission.*

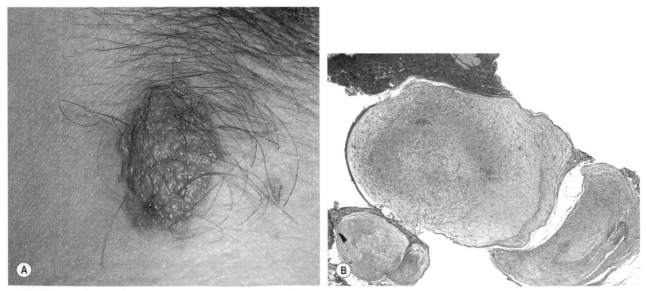

Fig. 18.12 Plexiform neurofibroma. The lesion can clinically resemble a melanocytic nevus; palpating the lesion may help. *A, Courtesy, Yale Dermatology Residents' Slide Collection.*

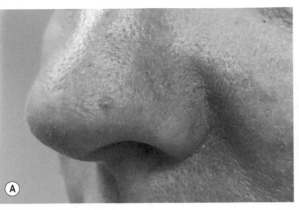 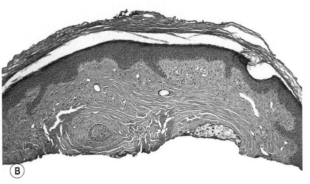

Fig. 18.13 Fibrous papule.

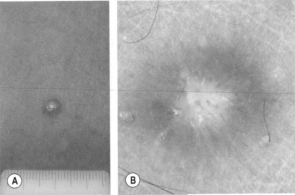 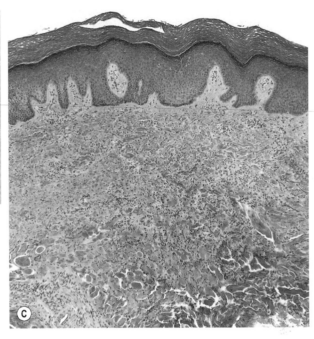

Fig. 18.14 Dermatofibroma. A clinical clue is dimpling around the lesion with lateral pressure; dermoscopy typically shows a central, whitish area. *A,B, Courtesy, Giuseppe Argenziano, MD, and Iris Zalaudek, MD. A, B, From Bolognia JL, Schaffer JV, Duncan KO, Ko CJ. Dermatology Essentials, 1e. Philadelphia: Saunders, 2014, with permission.*

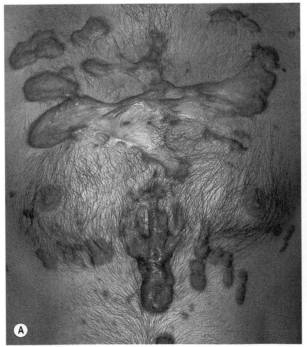 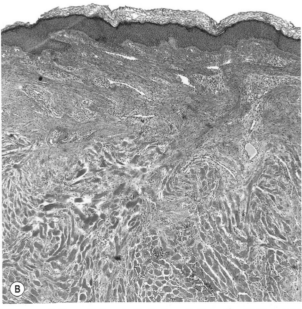

Fig. 18.15 Keloid. *A, Courtesy, Yale Dermatology Residents' Slide Collection. A, From Bolognia JL, Jorizzo JL, Schaffer JV. Dermatology, 3e. London: Saunders, 2012, with permission.*

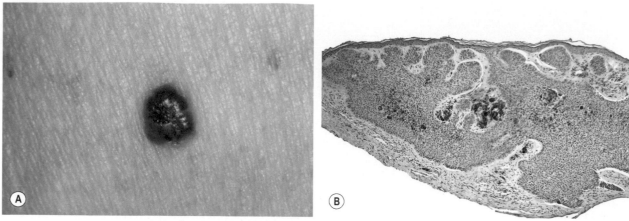

Fig. 18.16 Basal cell carcinoma, pigmented. *Courtesy, H. Peter Sawyer, MD. A, From Bolognia JL, Schaffer JV, Duncan KO, Ko CJ. Dermatology Essentials, 1e. Philadelphia: Saunders, 2014, with permission.*

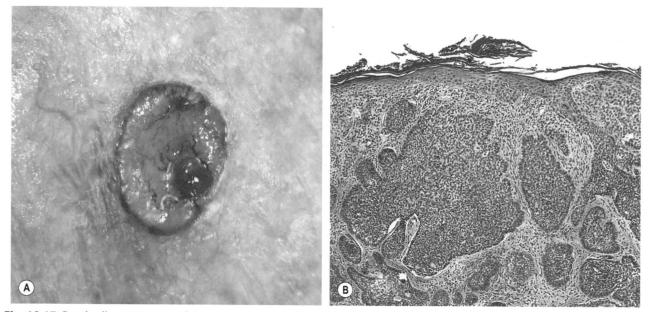

Fig. 18.17 Basal cell carcinoma, nodular. *A, Courtesy, Yale Dermatology Residents' Slide Collection.*

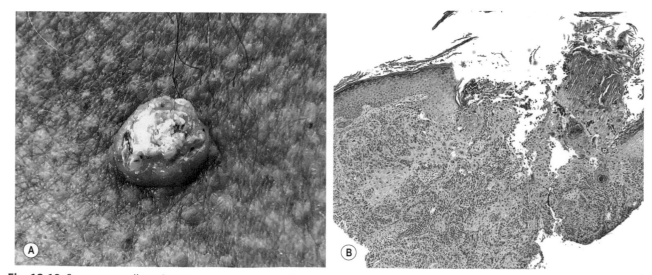

Fig. 18.18 Squamous cell carcinoma.

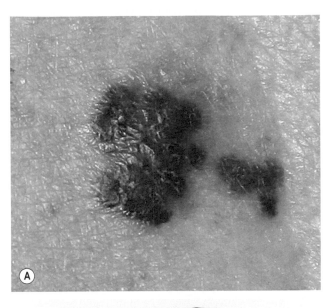

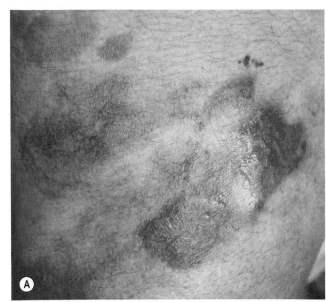

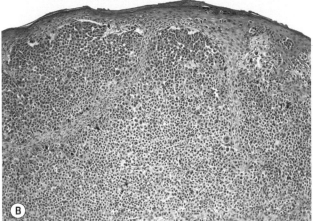

Fig. 18.19 Malignant melanoma. *A, Courtesy, Yale Dermatology Residents' Slide Collection.*

Fig. 18.20 Patch/plaque-stage mycosis fungoides. *A, Courtesy, Yale Dermatology Residents' Slide Collection.*

Dermal Cysts/Developmental Anomalies | 19

Although the most common cyst, the epidermoid cyst, may be located anywhere on the body, most cysts/tracts and developmental anomalies have characteristic locations (Fig. 19.1) and presentations (Fig. 19.2 – distinctive punctum; Figs. 19.3–19.8 – typical location). For midline lesions, the clinical presentation can be similar for different entities (i.e. dermoid cyst vs encephalocele), and imaging may be indicated. A combination of site and histopathologic findings are useful for cysts located on the neck (see Fig. 19.1B; Figs. 19.9–19.11); other anomalies have characteristic clinical presentations (Figs. 19.12–19.15). Over the lumbosacral spine, clues for an underlying spinal defect include segmental hemangiomas, a deep dimple, a pseudotail, and/or a deviated gluteal cleft (Figs. 19.16, 19.17).

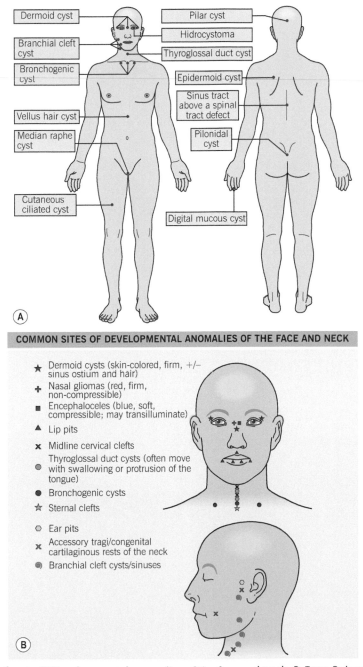

Fig. 19.1 A Common sites of cysts. **B** Developmental anomalies of the face and neck. *B, From Bolognia JL, Jorizzo JL, Schaffer JV. Dermatology, 3e. London: Saunders, 2012, with permission.*

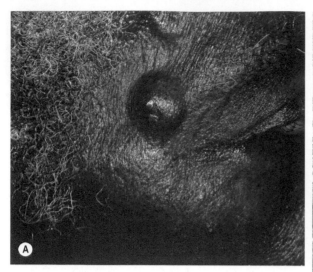

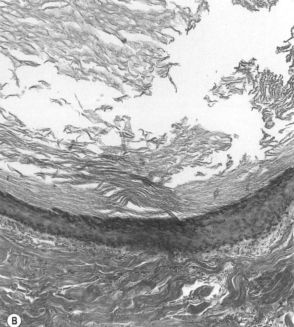

Fig. 19.2 Epidermoid cyst. A central punctum (pore) is often evident. Wall resembles normal epidermis with central flaky keratin.

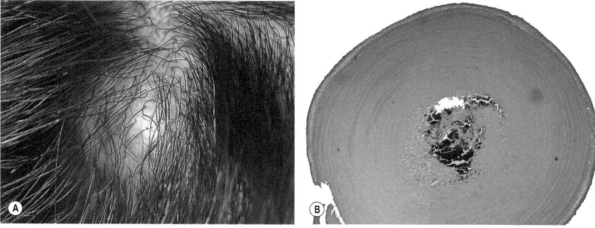

Fig. 19.3 Pilar cyst. This cyst is most common on the scalp. Wall lacks a prominent granular layer and surrounds dense keratin. *A, Courtesy, Mary Stone, MD. A, From Bolognia JL, Schaffer JV, Duncan KO, Ko CJ. Dermatology Essentials, 1e. Philadelphia: Saunders, 2014, with permission.*

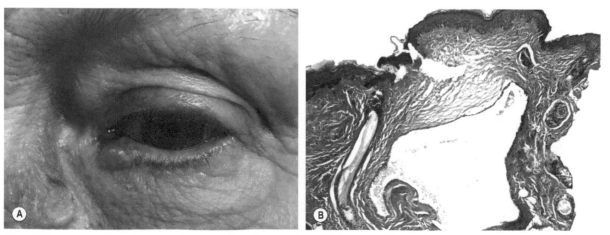

Fig. 19.4 Hidrocystoma. Translucent to blue papule, often on the eyelid margin. Biopsy findings include a space lined by epithelium with "snouts" on the cell surface.

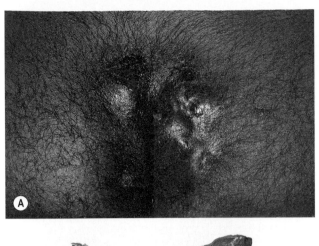

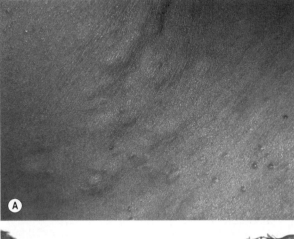

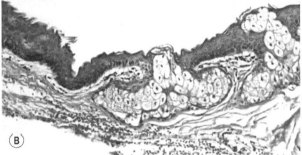

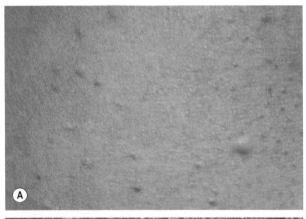

Fig. 19.6 Steatocystoma multiplex. This cyst can develop on any site; when multiple, lesions are typically larger than vellus hair cysts and present on the trunk. Wall with sebaceous glands and an inner rim that is bright pink and undulating. *A, Courtesy, Yale Dermatology Residents' Slide Collection.*

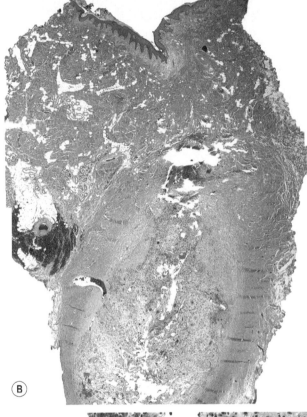

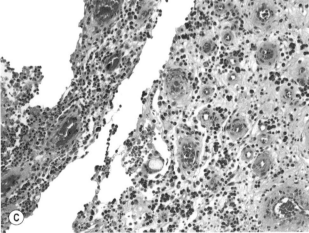

Fig. 19.5 Pilonidal sinus tracts. The most common location is the sacral area. Biopsy findings include epithelial lined tracts (not shown), acute and chronic inflammation, and free hair shafts. *A, Courtesy, Kalman Watsky, MD.*

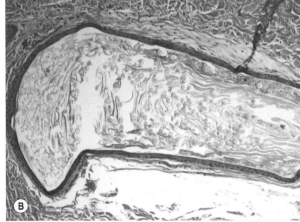

Fig. 19.7 Vellus hair cysts. Multiple lesions characteristically affect the trunk. Biopsy findings include epithelium that resembles the epidermis surrounding loose keratin and small round lightly pigmented vellus hairs. *A, Courtesy, Yale Dermatology Residents' Slide Collection.*

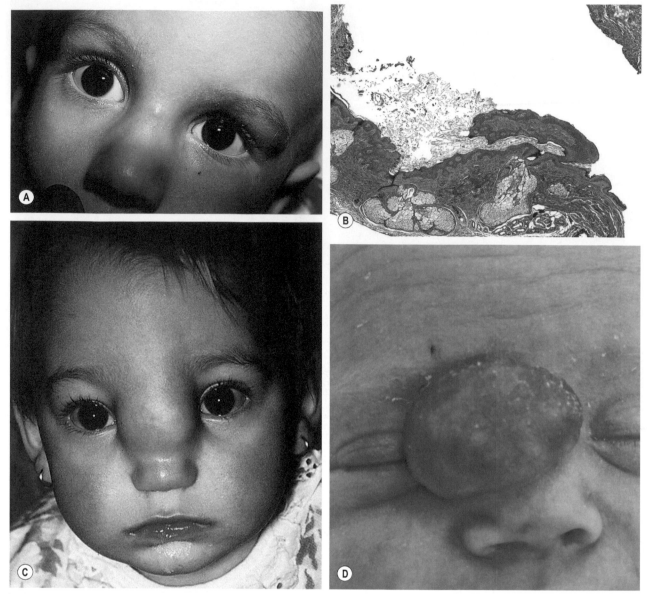

Fig. 19.8 Midline glabellar lesions. **A,B** Dermoid cyst. Wall contains adnexal structures. **C** Frontal encephalocele. **D** Nasal glioma. *C, Courtesy, Odile Enjolras, MD; D, Courtesy, Mary Chang, MD. A,C, From Schachner LA, Hansen RE. Pediatric Dermatology, 4e. London: Mosby, 2011, with permission. D, From Bolognia JL, Schaffer JV, Duncan KO, Ko CJ. Dermatology Essentials, 1e. Philadelphia: Saunders, 2014, with permission.*

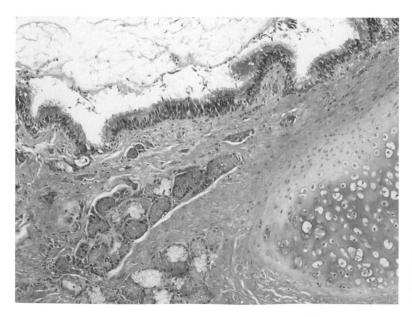

Fig. 19.9 Bronchogenic cyst. Wall is columnar; cartilage often present. *From Husain A. Thoracic Pathology. High Yield Pathology series. Philadelphia: Saunders, 2012.*

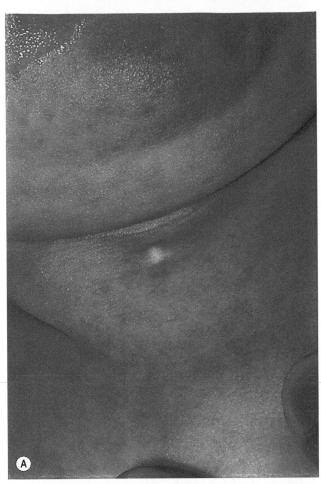

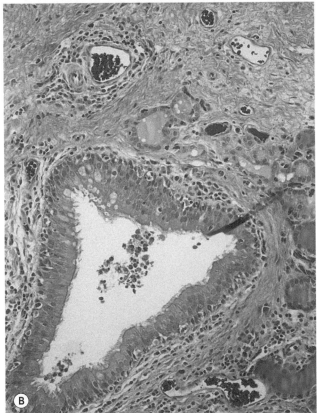

Fig. 19.10 Thyroglossal duct cyst. Wall with thyroid follicles. *B, Courtesy, Mary Stone, MD. A, From Schachner LA, Hansen RE. Pediatric Dermatology, 4e. London: Mosby, 2011. B, From Bolognia JL, Jorizzo JL, Schaffer JV. Dermatology, 3e. London: Saunders, 2012, with permission.*

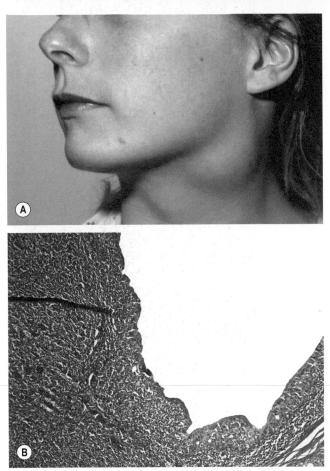

Fig. 19.11 Branchial cleft cyst. Columnar epithelium with dense inflammation. *A, From Myers EN. Operative Otolaryngology: Head and Neck Surgery, 2e. Philadelphia: Saunders, 2008.*

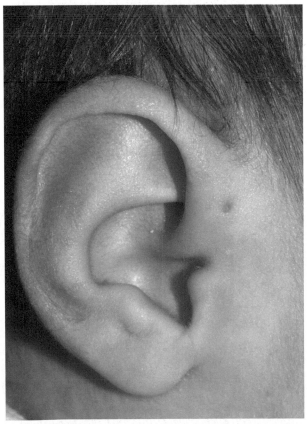

Fig. 19.12 Ear pit. *Courtesy, Julie V Schaffer, MD. From Bolognia JL, Jorizzo JL, Schaffer JV. Dermatology, 3e. London: Saunders, 2012, with permission.*

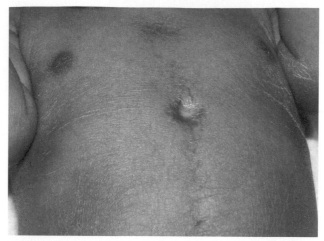

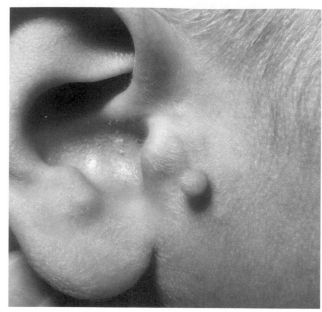

Fig. 19.13 Accessory tragus. *Courtesy, Antonio Torrelo, MD. From Schachner LA, Hansen RE. Pediatric Dermatology, 4e. London: Mosby, 2011.*

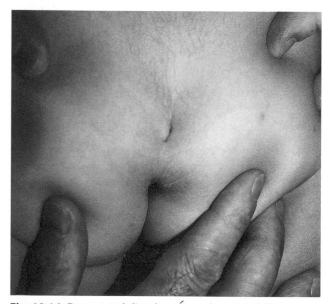

Fig. 19.15 Sternal cleft. *Courtesy, Julie V Schaffer, MD. From Bolognia JL, Jorizzo JL, Schaffer JV. Dermatology, 3e. London: Saunders, 2012, with permission.*

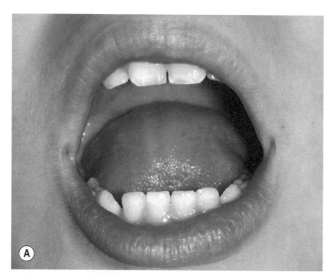

(A)

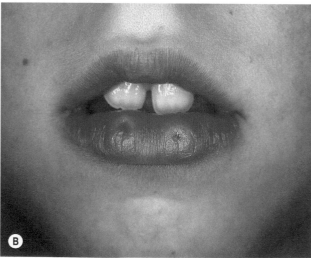

(B)

Fig. 19.14 Lip pit. *A, Courtesy NYU. B, Courtesy, Richard Antaya, MD and Julie V Schaffer, MD. A,B, From Bolognia JL, Jorizzo JL, Schaffer JV. Dermatology, 3e. London: Saunders, 2012, with permission.*

Fig. 19.16 Deep sacral dimple, a sign of an underlying myelomeningocele. *Courtesy, Seth J Orlow, MD, PhD. From Bolognia JL, Jorizzo JL, Schaffer JV. Dermatology, 3e. London: Saunders, 2012, with permission.*

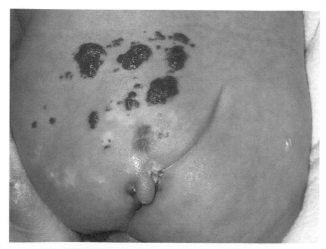

Fig. 19.17 Multiple cutaneous stigmata overlying a lipomeningomyelocele. *Courtesy, Richard Antaya, MD. From Bolognia JL, Jorizzo JL, Schaffer JV. Dermatology, 3e. London: Saunders, 2012, with permission.*

Small Papules Secondary to a Dermal Process | 20

The focus of this chapter is on dermal processes with minimal surface epidermal changes, in particular histiocytic/granulomatous disorders that produce multiple small papules on the skin. Entities in this chapter include lichen nitidus, histiocytoses, sarcoidosis, granuloma annulare, eruptive xanthoma, urticaria pigmentosa, and lichen myxedematosus. Dermal tumors/cysts (e.g. cherry angiomas, see Fig. 18.8A,B; neurofibroma, see Fig. 18.11A,B; steatocystomas, see Fig. 19.6A,B; vellus hair cysts, see Fig.19.7A,B), and epidermal tumors/ processes, which can also produce multiple papules (e.g. warts, see Fig. 7.16A,B; molluscum, see Fig. 7.17A,B; multiple facial papules, see Fig. 2.1), are not covered in this chapter. Papules with significant surface (epidermal) change are discussed in Chapter 6.

LICHEN NITIDUS

Clinical:
Shiny, tiny (≈1–2 mm) papules (Fig. 20.1)

Histopathologic:
Epidermal rete demarcating a lymphohistiocytic infiltrate in the superficial dermis

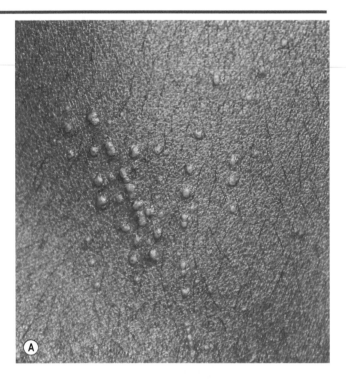

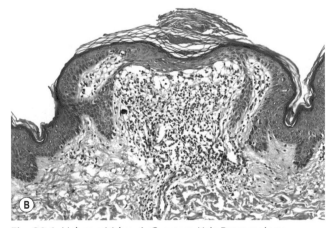

Fig. 20.1 Lichen nitidus. *A, Courtesy, Yale Dermatology Residents' Slide Collection.*

HISTIOCYTOSES

There are classic presentations of different histiocytoses (Fig. 20.2, Table 20.1), and the typical lesion is a dermal red–brown to pink papule for non–Langerhans cell histiocytoses. Such papules may also be seen in Langerhans cell histiocytosis (LCH), but the more common LCH lesion is an eroded and purpuric papule or plaque. In practice, there is significant overlap between various histiocytoses; the clinical distribution, other clinical lesions, and/or histopathologic features may be helpful in categorization.

Table 20.1 Classic features of selected histiocytoses		
Histiocytosis	**Classic clinical features**	**Classic histopathologic features**
Langerhans cell histiocytosis (Fig. 20.3A–C; see Figs. 2.14, 2.15, 6.22, 13.3)	• Eroded, purpuric papules/plaques in intertriginous zones • Ulcerations (see Chapter 10) • Pink to red–brown dermal-based papules without surface change	• Dermal Langerhans cells (Langerin+, CD1a+ [see Fig. 20.3C,D], S–100+) • Eosinophils may be present
Generalized eruptive histiocytoma (Fig. 20.3E,F)	• Favors the face and trunk • Red–brown papules	• Dermal histiocytic infiltrate (CD68+), often without obvious giant cells
Indeterminate cell histiocytosis	• Favors the trunk and proximal extremities • Red–brown papules	• Dermal histiocytic infiltrate (S–100+, CD68+, CD1a⁻, Langerin⁻)
Multicentric reticulohistiocytosis (Fig. 20.3G,H)	• Favors acral sites • Pink to red–brown papules	• Two-toned giant cells
Rosai–Dorfman disease (Fig. 20.3I–L)	• Red–brown papules or plaque(s)/nodule(s) • Massive, painless bilateral cervical lymphadenopathy is characteristic	• Emperipolesis • S100+ multinucleate cells (see Fig. 20.3J–L) • CD68+

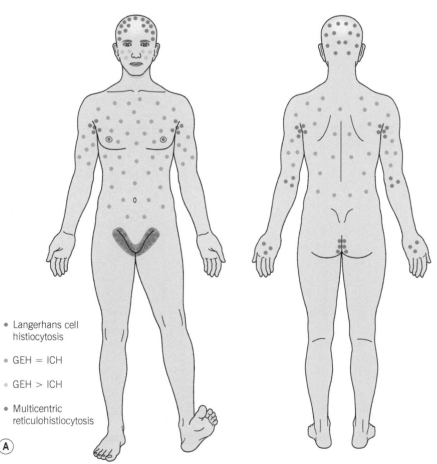

- Langerhans cell histiocytosis
- GEH = ICH
- GEH > ICH
- Multicentric reticulohistiocytosis

Ⓐ

Fig. 20.2 Histiocytoses. **A** Typical distribution of different histiocytoses. *GEH,* Generalized eruptive histiocytosis; *ICH,* indeterminate cell histiocytosis.

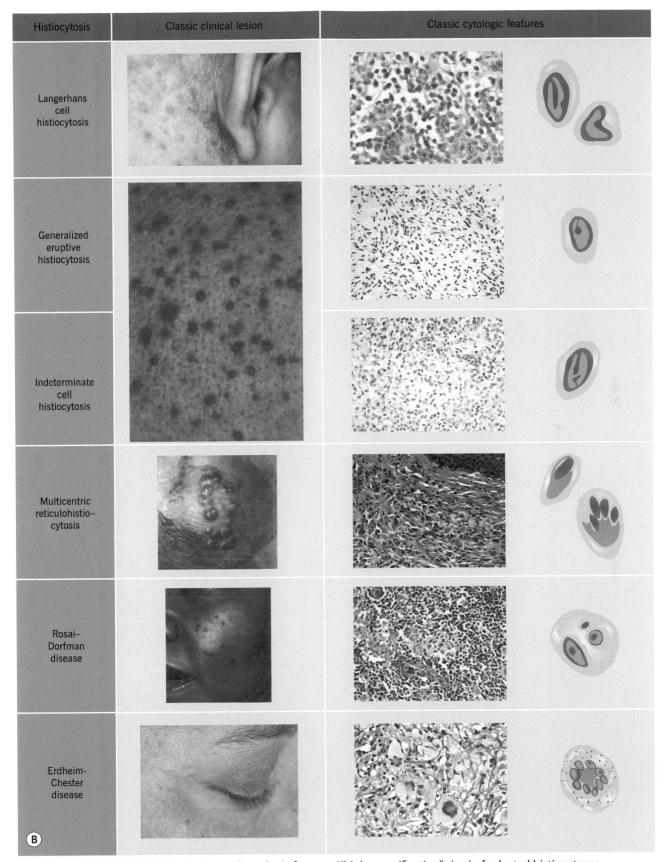

Fig. 20.2, cont'd **B** Classic clinical lesion and cytologic features ("high magnification" view) of selected histiocytoses. *Photographs courtesy, Irwin Braverman, MD; Julia Neckham, MD, and Michael Girardi, MD; Ingo Haase, MD, and Iliana Tantcheva-Poor, MD; Jean L Bolognia, MD, and Yale Dermatology Residents' Slide Collection. From Bolognia JL, Jorizzo JL, Schaffer JV. Dermatology, 3e. London: Saunders, 2012, with permission.*

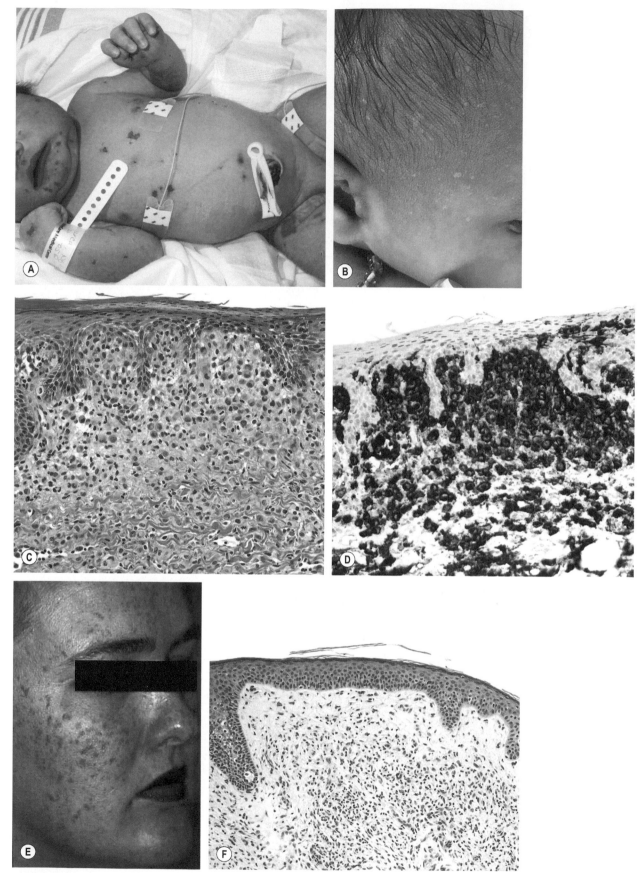

Fig. 20.3 Histiocytoses. **A–D** Langerhans cell histiocytosis. Lesions can appear hypopigmented in darker skin types. Langerhans cells are CD1a-positive (D). **E,F** Generalized eruptive histiocytoma.

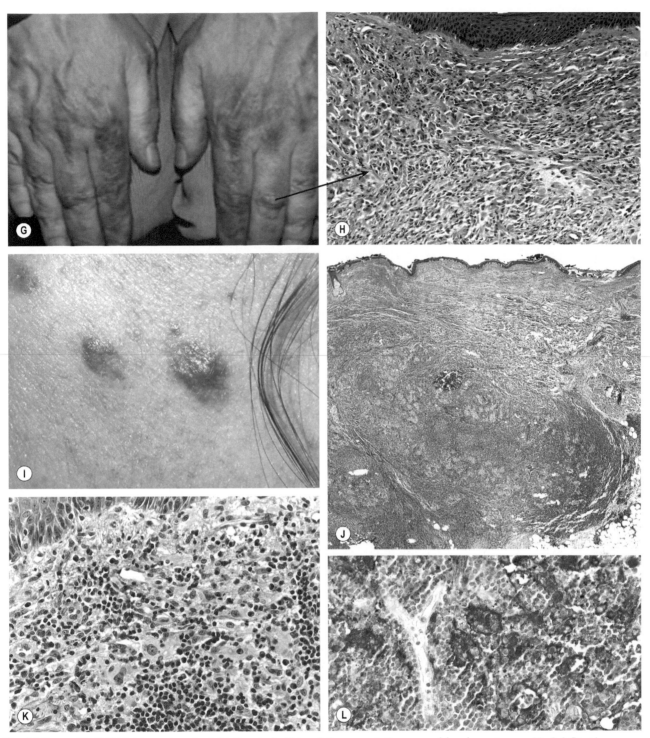

Fig. 20.3, cont'd G,H Multicentric reticulohistiocytosis. This subtle presentation resembles dermatomyositis. **I–L** Rosai–Dorfman disease. *A, Courtesy, Deborah S Goddard, MD, Amy E Gilliam, MD, and Ilona J Frieden, MD; B, Courtesy, Richard Antaya, MD; E,I Courtesy, Jennifer M McNiff, MD. G, Courtesy, Kalman Watsky, MD. A,G, From Bolognia JL, Schaffer JV, Duncan KO, Ko CJ. Dermatology Essentials, 1e. Philadelphia: Saunders, 2014, with permission.*

SARCOIDOSIS

Clinical:
May affect the skin only or be multisystemic (Fig. 20.4A)
Classically multiple red–brown to pink papules,
sometimes forming annular arrangements (Fig. 20.4H);
the nose is a typical site (see Fig. 2.7B)
Sarcoidosis can be a mimic of many other diseases
(Fig. 20.4D–F,I)

Any cutaneous site may be affected; there can be
associated alopecia or nail changes (Fig. 20.4G)
Sarcoidal lesions can develop during treatment with
checkpoint inhibitors

Histopathologic:
Classically, naked dermal granulomas (Fig. 20.4C)

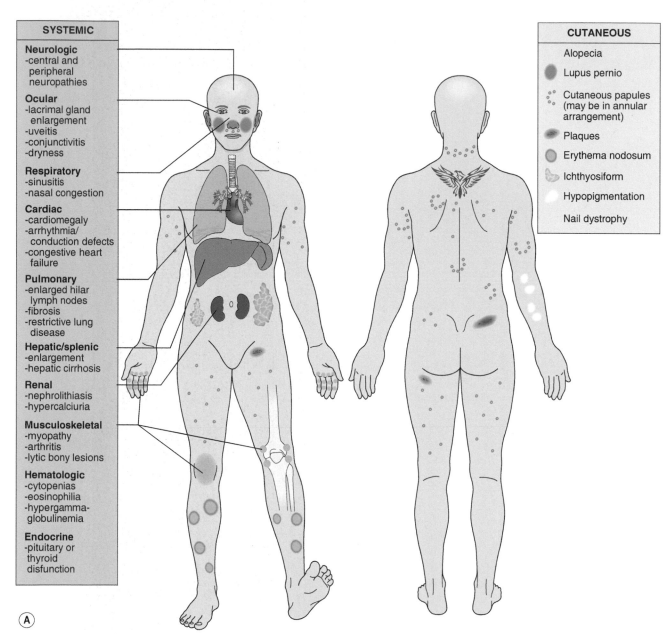

Fig. 20.4 Sarcoidosis. **A** Spectrum of systemic and cutaneous involvement in sarcoidosis.

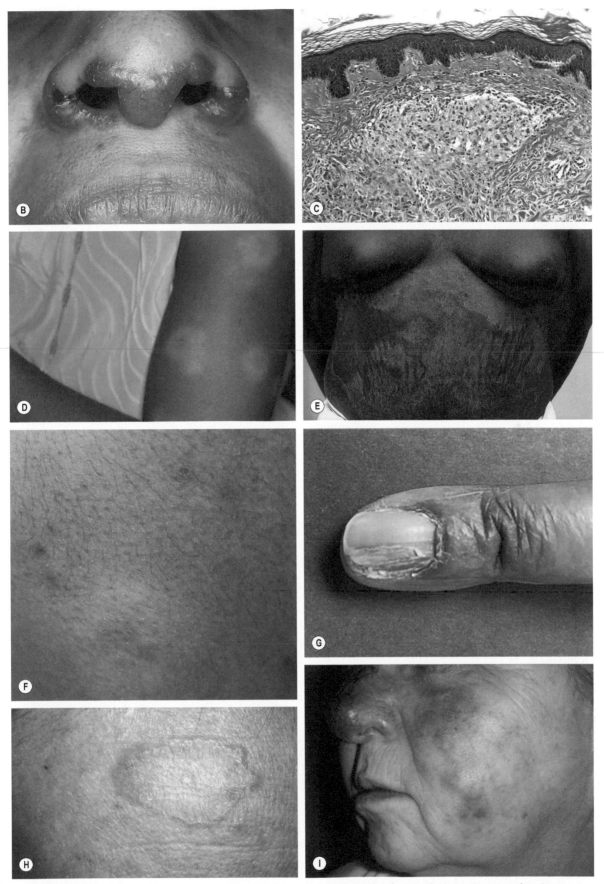

Fig. 20.4, cont'd **B,C** Sarcoidosis, classic papules with granuloma formation in the dermis. **D** Hypopigmented variant. **E** Ichthyosiform variant. **F** Thin, pink plaques surrounded by hypopigmentation. **G** Nail thinning caused by granulomas involving the nail matrix. **H** Pink papules in an annular arrangement. **I** Angiolupoid sarcoidosis. There is erythema and induration of the bilateral cheeks and the nose in this rare variant. *C,F, Courtesy, Yale Dermatology Residents' Slide Collection; D, Courtesy, Louis A Fragola, Jr, MD; E, Courtesy, Jean L Bolognia, MD; H,I, Courtesy, Irwin Braverman, MD. B,G, Courtesy, Jonathan Leventhal, MD and Jacob Siegel MD. D,E, From Bolognia JL, Schaffer JV, Duncan KO, Ko CJ. Dermatology Essentials, 1e. Philadelphia: Saunders, 2014, with permission.*

GRANULOMA ANNULARE

Clinical:
Often acral (see Fig. 1.51), but other sites can be involved
May be generalized (Fig. 20.5A)
Pink papules that can form annular arrangements
(Fig. 20.5B)

Histopathologic:
Dermal mucin surrounded by palisades of histiocytes
(Fig. 20.5C)

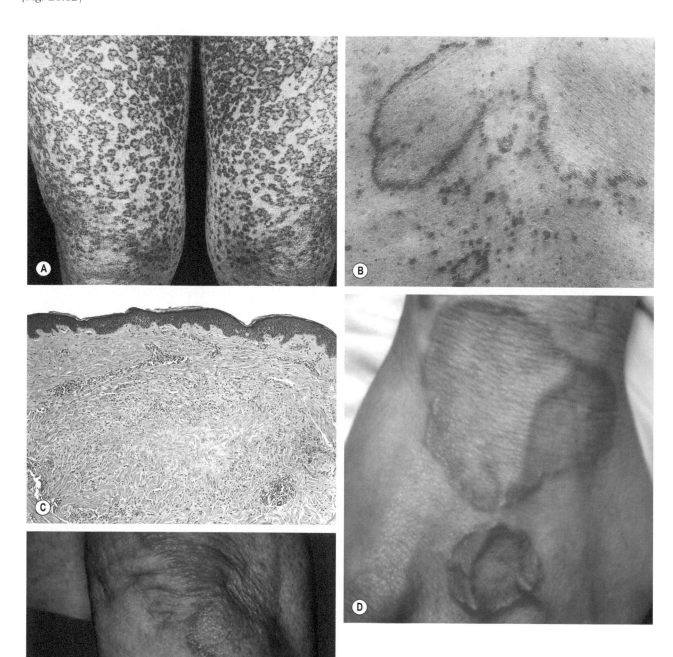

Fig. 20.5 A Granuloma annulare, generalized. **B** Granuloma annulare on the back. Some papules are in annular arrangements (**B,D,E**). **C** Palisading of histiocytes around dermal mucin. *A,B,D,E, Courtesy, Yale Dermatology Residents' Slide Collection. D,E, From Bolognia, Dermatology 3e, with permission. A, From Bolognia JL, Schaffer JV, Duncan KO, Ko CJ. Dermatology Essentials, 1e. Philadelphia: Saunders, 2014, with permission.*

ERUPTIVE XANTHOMA

Clinical:
Typically affects the buttocks/thighs (Fig. 20.6A)
In the setting of uncontrolled diabetes mellitus, and/or elevated lipids (i.e. hypertriglyceridemia)
Yellow–pink papules (Fig. 20.6B)

Histopathologic:
Intracellular and extracellular lipid (Fig. 20.6C)

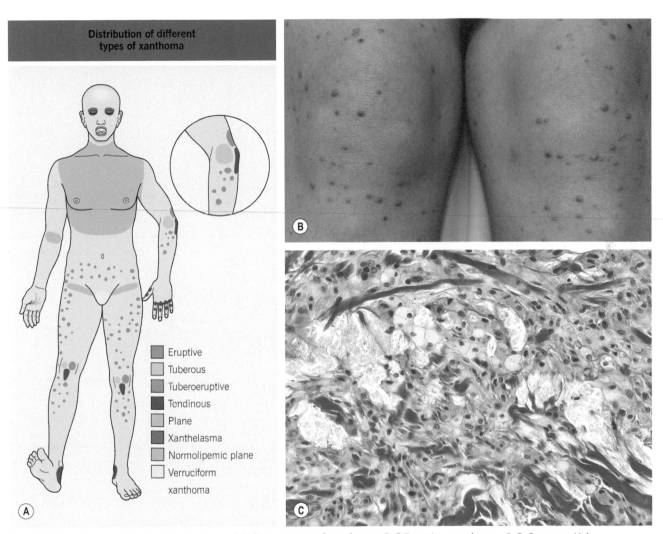

Distribution of different types of xanthoma

■ Eruptive
□ Tuberous
■ Tuberoeruptive
■ Tendinous
■ Plane
■ Xanthelasma
■ Normolipemic plane
□ Verruciform xanthoma

Fig. 20.6 Xanthoma. **A** Typical distribution of different types of xanthoma. **B,C** Eruptive xanthoma. *B,C, Courtesy, Yale Dermatology Residents' Slide Collection. A, From Bolognia JL, Schaffer JV, Duncan KO, Ko CJ. Dermatology Essentials, 1e. Philadelphia: Saunders, 2014, with permission.*

URTICARIA PIGMENTOSA

Clinical:
Favors the trunk (Fig. 20.7A,C; see Fig. 2.24A)
Red–brown papules that may urticate with stroking
(Darier's sign)

Histopathologic:
Dermal mast cells (Fig. 20.7B,D,E)

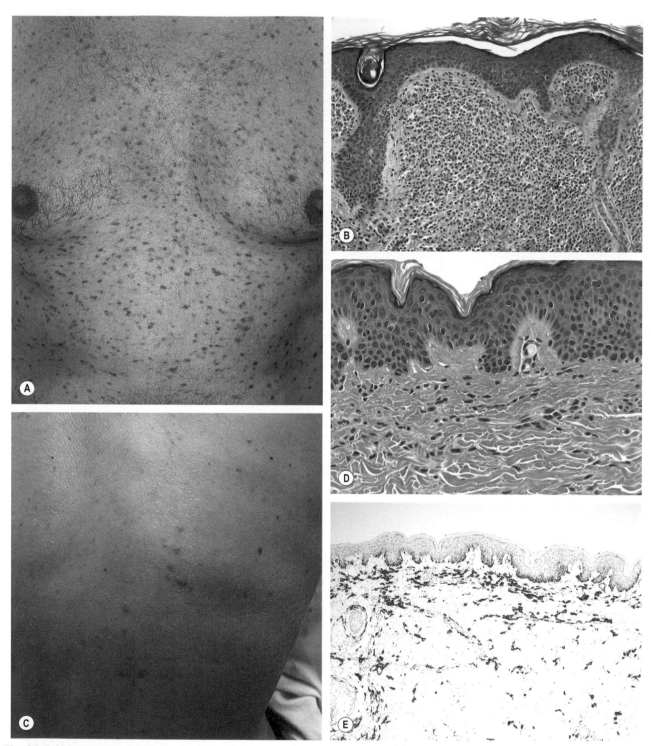

Fig. 20.7 Mastocytosis. **A,B** Urticaria pigmentosa presenting as numerous red–brown papules. **C,D** Mastocytosis that appears more urticarial clinically with a subtler infiltrate histopathologically. **E** CD117 staining is positive. *A, Courtesy, Michael Tharp, MD; C, Courtesy, Yale Dermatology Residents' Slide Collection; D,E, Courtesy, Nemanja Rodic, MD, PhD. A, From Bolognia JL, Schaffer JV, Duncan KO, Ko CJ. Dermatology Essentials, 1e. Philadelphia: Saunders, 2014, with permission.*

LICHEN MYXEDEMATOSUS (FIG. 20.8)

Clinical:
1- to 2-mm flesh-colored papules, sometimes in linear or clustered arrays
Scleromyxedema is the preferred term when there is an associated monoclonal gammopathy

Histopathologic:
Fibroblasts (spindle cells), often with increased stromal mucin

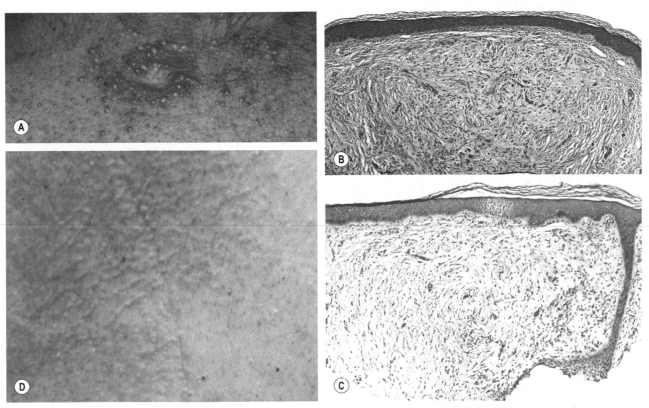

Fig. 20.8 A,B,C Lichen myxedematosus. **D** Scleromyxedema. Linear arrays of small papules. This patient had generalized involvement of the skin and an associated monoclonal gammopathy. *A, Courtesy, Kalman Watsky, MD. D, Courtesy, Jonathan Leventhal, MD.*

STEATOCYSTOMAS

Clinical:
Often on the trunk when multiple (see Fig. 19.6A)
May discharge an oily substance
Skin-colored papulonodules

Histopathologic:
Cyst wall lined by epithelium with a bright pink serrated surface (see Fig. 19.6B)

VELLUS HAIR CYSTS

Clinical:
Variably colored small papules (see Fig. 19.7A)

Histopathologic:
Cystic space containing keratin and vellus hairs (see Fig. 19.7B)

MILIA

Clinical:
White papules (see Fig. 2.1G)
If the surface is punctured, white material (keratin) can be extruded

Histopathologic:
Cystic space lined by epithelium resembling the normal epidermis

ACNE VULGARIS AND ACNE ROSACEA

(See Chapter 15)

Dermal Changes Caused by Deposition | 21

Certain materials, when deposited in the dermis, result in a characteristic clinical presentation, with particular histopathologic findings. Mucin deposition can be seen in a variety of disorders, with varying clinical presentations. Deposition may manifest as a broad, textural change or as papulonodules.

BROAD, TEXTURAL CHANGE

Macular/Lichen/Biphasic Amyloidosis

Clinical:

Predilection for the upper back (macular amyloidosis) and shins (lichen amyloidosis); biphasic forms have features of both macular (flatter lesions) and lichen amyloidosis (lesions are more raised)

Rippled, hyperpigmented plaques composed of linear arrays of monomorphous papules (Figs. 21.1, 21.2)

Histopathologic:

Light pink, smooth deposits in the papillary dermis, often with associated pigment incontinence; deposits are larger and associated with epidermal hyperplasia in lichen amyloidosis

Deposits stain with antibodies against cytokeratins

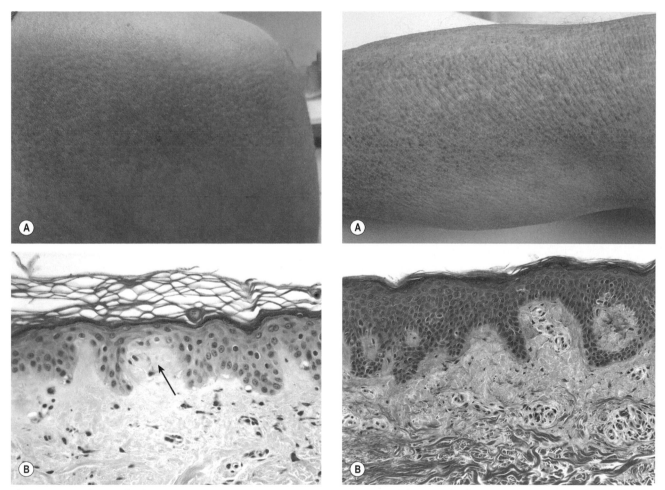

Fig. 21.1 Macular amyloidosis.

Fig. 21.2 Lichen amyloidosis. *A, Courtesy, Sean Christensen, MD PhD.*

Pretibial Myxedema (Fig. 21.3)

Clinical:
Pink plaque(s) that are nodular in later stages, especially on the lower extremity

Histopathologic:
Mucin throughout the reticular dermis

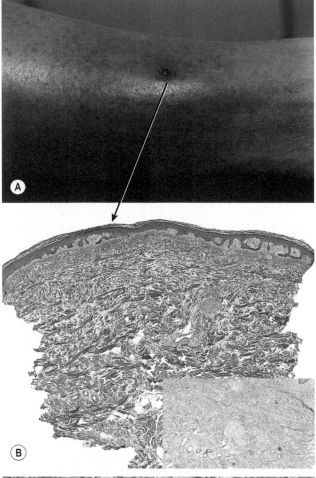

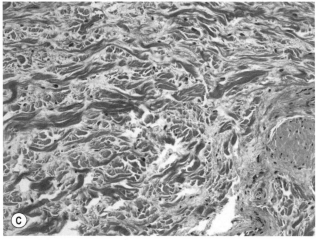

Fig. 21.3 Pretibial myxedema. **A** Early lesion of indurated erythema with a biopsy site. *A, Courtesy, Kalman Watsky, MD.*

Adult Colloid Milium (Fig. 21.4)

Clinical:
Brown to yellow translucent papules, especially on chronically sun-damaged skin of the face and/or hands but other sites may be affected

Histopathologic:
Nodules of pink, fissured material

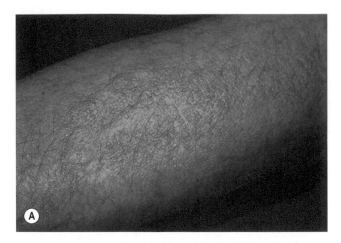

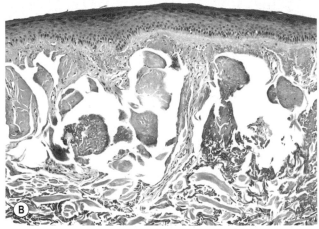

Fig. 21.4 Colloid milium. *A, From Lewis AT, Le EH, Quan LT, et al. Unilateral colloid milium of the arm. J Am Acad Dermatol. 2002;46:S5–7, © Elsevier.*

Scleromyxedema (Fig. 21.5, see Fig. 22.7)

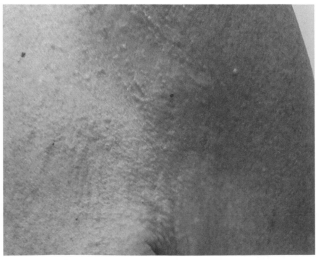

Fig. 21.5 Scleromyxedema. Thickening of skin with linear arrays of 1- to 2-mm papules. *Courtesy, Jonathan Leventhal, MD.*

Lipoid Proteinosis (Fig. 21.6)
Clinical:
Genodermatosis with mutations in *ECM1*
Characteristic hoarse voice and beaded papules along the eyelid margins
Waxy papules and plaques on extensor surfaces and face with scarring

Histopathologic:
Pink dermal material, sometimes with a vertical orientation in the upper dermis; material may be accentuated around adnexal structures

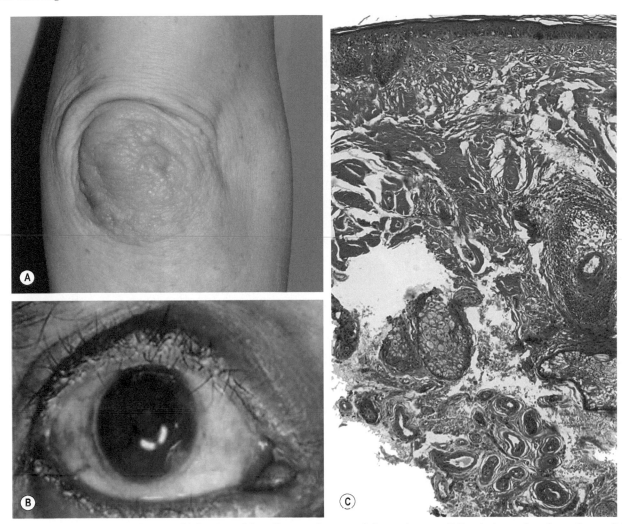

Fig. 21.6 Lipoid proteinosis. **A** Waxy thickening of the elbow and more subtly on the arm. **B** Beaded papules along the eyelid margin. **C** Thick, pink material in the dermis. *A, Courtesy, Julie V Schaffer, MD. A, From Bolognia JL, Jorizzo JL, Schaffer JV. Dermatology, 3e. London: Saunders, 2012, with permission. B, Yadava U et al. Pathology. 2006;38;600, with permission.*

Erythropoietic Protoporphyria (Fig. 21.7)
Clinical:
Genodermatosis, mutation in ferrochelatase
Sun-exposed skin is affected, especially the nose, cheeks, and dorsal hands
Erythema, erosions, waxy scarring

Histopathologic:
Pink dermal material around vessels (early lesions) and/or filling the upper dermis (later lesions)

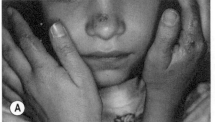
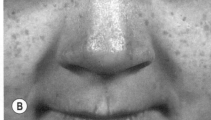
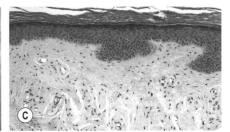

Fig. 21.7 Erythropoietic protoporphyria. *A, Courtesy, Yale Dermatology Residents' Slide Collection. B, Courtesy, Gillian Murphy, MD. From Bolognia JL, Jorizzo JL, Schaffer JV. Dermatology, 3e. London: Saunders, 2012, with permission.*

PAPULONODULES

Nodular Amyloidosis (Fig. 21.8)

Clinical:

Variably sized pink–orange, slightly translucent-appearing papulonodule(s)

Histopathologic:

Light pink material filling the dermis, interspersed plasma cells may be evident

Systemic Amyloidosis (Fig. 21.9)

Clinical:

Multiorgan disorder (e.g. kidneys, gastrointestinal tract, heart) with deposition of amyloid light-chain (AL) protein (immunoglobulin light-chain fragment)

Enlargement of the tongue
Waxy papules/plaques, commonly on the face
Periorbital purpura

Histopathologic:

Perivascular light pink, smooth deposits; apple-green birefringence with polarization

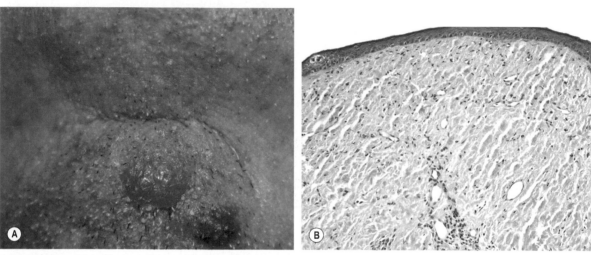

Fig. 21.8 Nodular amyloidosis. *A, Courtesy, Yale Dermatology Residents' Slide Collection.*

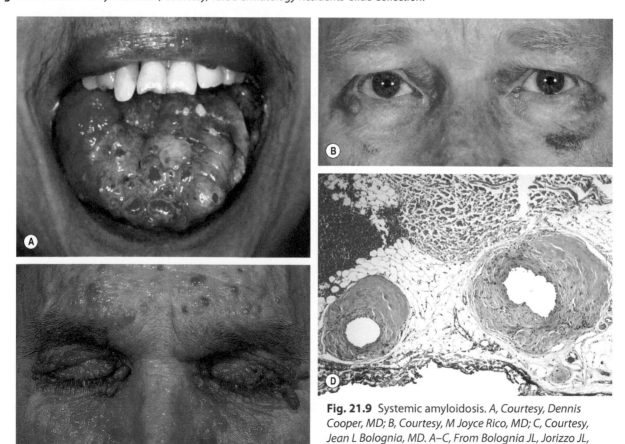

Fig. 21.9 Systemic amyloidosis. *A, Courtesy, Dennis Cooper, MD; B, Courtesy, M Joyce Rico, MD; C, Courtesy, Jean L Bolognia, MD. A–C, From Bolognia JL, Jorizzo JL, Schaffer JV. Dermatology, 3e. London: Saunders, 2012, with permission.*

Osteoma Cutis, Miliary Type

Clinical:
Multiple, small skin-colored to blue papules – often on the face (Fig. 21.10)

Histopathologic:
Dense pink material with small lacunae containing nuclei

Chronic Tophaceous Gout (Fig. 21.11)

Clinical:
Predilection for the ear or periarticular foci
Firm dermal/subcutaneous, pink–yellow papulonodules

Histopathologic:
Needle-like or feathery spaces within light blue–pink material surrounded by histiocytes

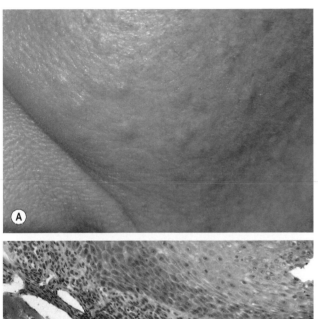

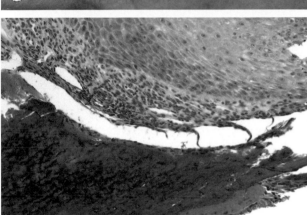

Fig. 21.10 Osteoma cutls. *A, Courtesy, Yale Dermatology Residents' Slide Collection. A, From Bolognia JL, Jorizzo JL, Schaffer JV. Dermatology, 3e. London: Saunders, 2012, with permission.*

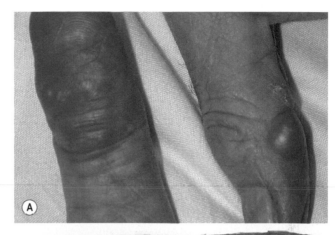

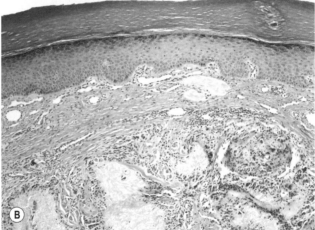

Fig. 21.11 Gout. Tophi on the digits. *A, Courtesy, Yale Dermatology Residents' Slide Collection.*

Calcinosis Cutis (Fig. 21.12)
Clinical:
Calcification can be the sequelae of a tissue injury
Calcium deposits in the skin are associated with limited systemic sclerosis and dermatomyositis
When superficial, white–yellow coloration is a clue; lesions tend to be rock hard

Histopathologic:
Bluish, chunky (sometimes granular) material

Eruptive Xanthoma (Fig. 21.13)
Clinical:
Associated with high lipid levels, uncontrolled diabetes mellitus, and thyroid disorders
Favors the extensor surfaces, especially the buttocks/thighs
Pink–red to yellow papules

Histopathologic:
Intracellular and extracellular lipids

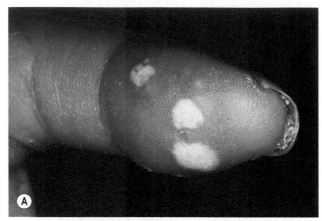

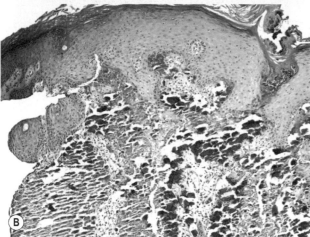

Fig. 21.12 Calcinosis cutis. *A, Courtesy, Yale Dermatology Residents' Slide Collection. A, Courtesy, Bolognia JL, Jorizzo JL, Schaffer JV. Dermatology, 3e. London: Saunders, 2012, with permission.*

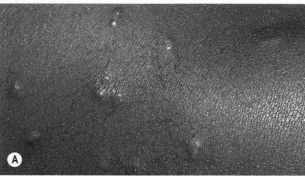

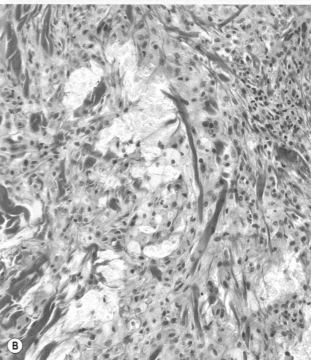

Fig. 21.13 Eruptive xanthomas. *A, Courtesy, Yale Dermatology Residents' Slide Collection.*

Xanthelasma (Fig. 21.14)
Clinical:
Yellowish papules and plaques on the eyelids, medial > lateral

Histopathologic:
Foamy cells in the dermis; typical features of eyelid with thin epidermis and vellus hairs

Digital Myxoid Cyst (Fig. 21.15)
Clinical:
Near a joint space of the finger
Bluish to skin-colored slightly translucent papulonodule

Histopathologic:
No epithelial lining (not a true cyst), increased dermal mucin, keratin typical of an acral site (stratum lucidum)

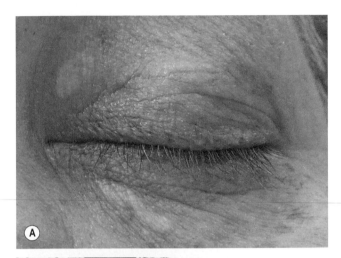

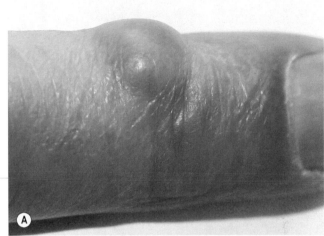

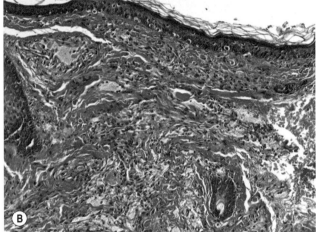

Fig. 21.14 Xanthelasma.

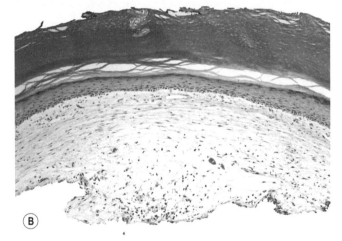

Fig. 21.15 Digital myxoid cyst with mucin in the dermis.
A, Courtesy, Yale Dermatology Residents' Slide Collection.

Focal Cutaneous Mucinosis (Fig. 21.16)
Clinical:
Localized, flesh-colored to pink papule

Histopathologic:
Mucin in the dermis

Follicular Mucinosis
(See Fig. 15.11)

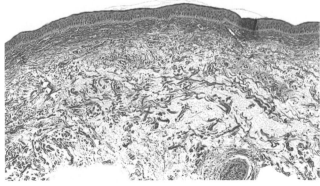

Fig. 21.16 Focal cutaneous mucinosis.

Erythema Elevatum Diutinum, Late Stage
(Fig. 21.17)

Clinical:

Symmetric, on extensor surfaces
Red–brown to purplish, soft to firm papulonodules
Associated with human immunodeficiency virus (HIV)
infection

Histopathologic:

Fibrosis with or without vasculitis, interspersed
neutrophils

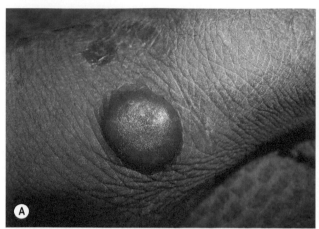

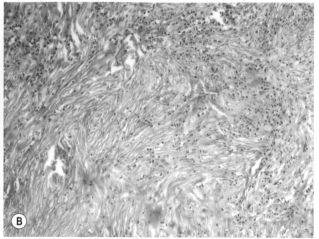

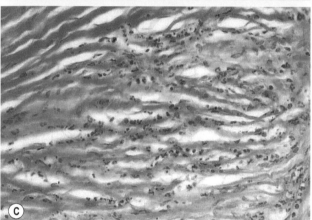

Fig. 21.17 Erythema elevatum diutinum, late stage. *A,
Courtesy, Rachel Moore, MD. A, From Bolognia JL, Jorizzo JL,
Schaffer JV. Dermatology, 3e. London: Saunders, 2012, with
permission.*

Sclerosing Disorders | 22

Induration, or hardening, of the skin can be a manifestation of systemic disease (e.g. systemic sclerosis); limited to the skin (e.g. morphea); or generalized or localized (e.g. graft-versus-host disease). Typically, these diseases favor certain sites (Fig. 22.1) with particular clinical clues; for example, sclerosis involving the subcutis often shows rippling of the skin (e.g. eosinophilic fasciitis; see Fig. 22.1). Induration of the skin can also be caused by exogenous substances (i.e. gadolinium – nephrogenic systemic fibrosis). This chapter covers graft-versus-host disease, systemic sclerosis, scleromyxedema, scleredema, eosinophilic fasciitis, linear melorheostotic scleroderma, morphea, and lichen sclerosus.

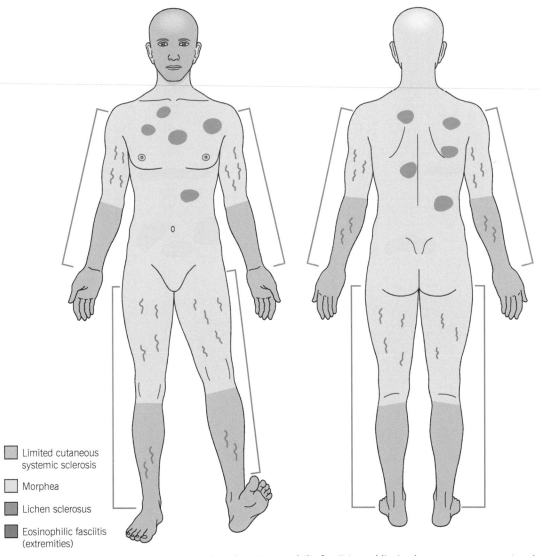

Limited cutaneous systemic sclerosis

Morphea

Lichen sclerosus

Eosinophilic fasciitis (extremities)

Fig. 22.1 Typical sites of involvement of sclerosing disorders. Eosinophilic fasciitis and limited cutaneous systemic sclerosis both involve the extremities, but the deeper involvement of the former is evidenced by rippling of the skin. Eosinophilic fasciitis can also involve the trunk. Morphea and extragenital lichen sclerosus tend to affect the trunk.

GRAFT-VERSUS-HOST DISEASE

Clinical:
Patients with chronic graft-versus-host disease can have skin findings that resemble many of the sclerosing disorders (Fig. 22.2, bolded text).

Histopathologic:
Depending on the type of clinical lesion, findings are variable. Acute, pink maculopapular rashes – interface change; lichenoid papules – denser, lichenoid inflammation below the epidermis; sclerotic lesions – morphea-like or lichen sclerosis–like

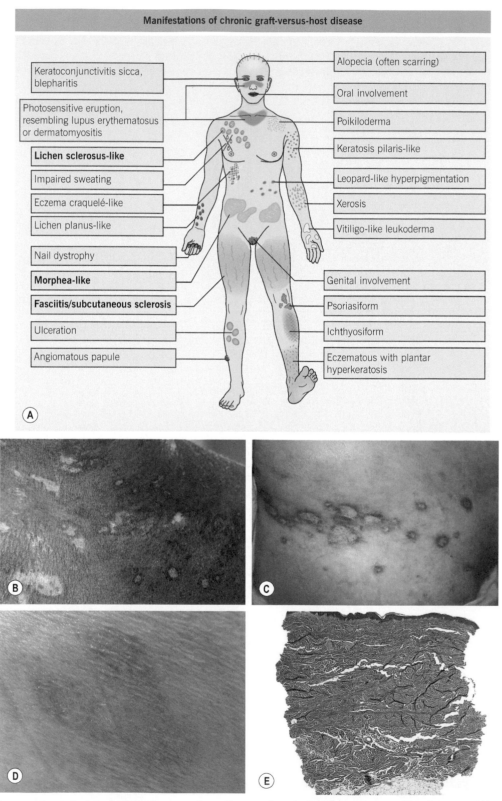

Manifestations of chronic graft-versus-host disease

Keratoconjunctivitis sicca, blepharitis

Photosensitive eruption, resembling lupus erythematosus or dermatomyositis

Lichen sclerosus-like

Impaired sweating

Eczema craquelé-like

Lichen planus-like

Nail dystrophy

Morphea-like

Fasciitis/subcutaneous sclerosis

Ulceration

Angiomatous papule

Alopecia (often scarring)

Oral involvement

Poikiloderma

Keratosis pilaris-like

Leopard-like hyperpigmentation

Xerosis

Vitiligo-like leukoderma

Genital involvement

Psoriasiform

Ichthyosiform

Eczematous with plantar hyperkeratosis

Fig. 22.2 Graft-versus-host disease. **A–C** Graft-versus-host disease, chronic. **B** Lichen sclerosus-like changes. **C** Morphea-like changes. Lesions can ulcerate. **D** Hyperpigmented lesion with superficial atrophy that was slightly indurated on palpation. **E** Biopsy findings can resemble those of morphea, or lichen sclerosus. *B,C, Courtesy, Yale Dermatology Residents' Slide Collection. A, From Bolognia JL, Schaffer JV, Duncan KO, Ko CJ. Dermatology Essentials, 1e. Philadelphia: Saunders, 2014, with permission.*

SYSTEMIC SCLEROSIS (SCLERODERMA)

Clinical:
Three main types of systemic sclerosis (Fig. 22.3)

Histopathologic:
Thickening of collagen in the dermis (identical to findings seen in morphea)

Systemic Sclerosis – Clues
Leukoderma – retention of perifollicular pigment, producing a "salt and pepper" appearance (Fig. 22.4; see Fig. 2.26)
Acral signs – in particular, the hands can show many features suggestive of systemic sclerosis (Fig. 22.5)
Telangiectasias – often on the face, borders are squared off (Fig. 22.6)

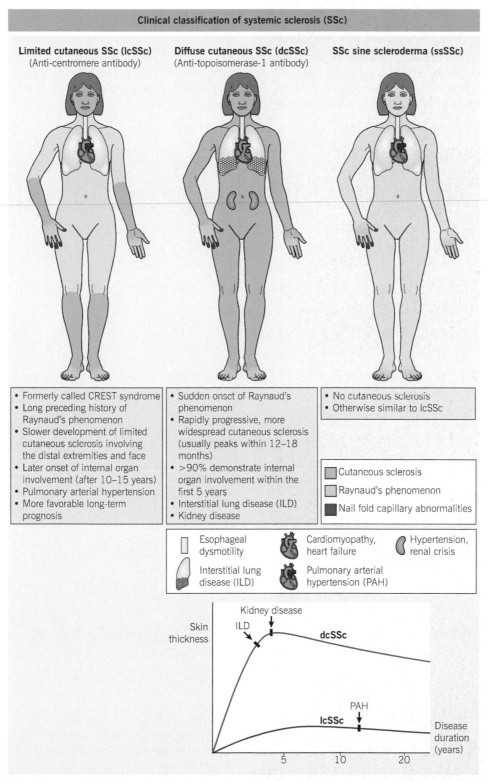

Fig. 22.3 Clinical classification of systemic sclerosis. *Courtesy, Karynne O Duncan, MD. From Bolognia JL, Schaffer JV, Duncan KO, Ko CJ. Dermatology Essentials, 1e. Philadelphia: Saunders, 2014, with permission.*

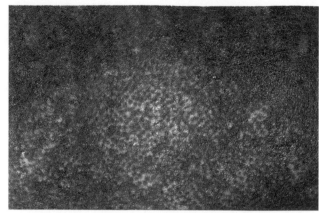

Fig. 22.4 Leukoderma of systemic sclerosis. *Courtesy, M Kari Connolly, MD. From Bolognia JL, Schaffer JV, Duncan KO, Ko CJ. Dermatology Essentials, 1e. Philadelphia: Saunders, 2014, with permission.*

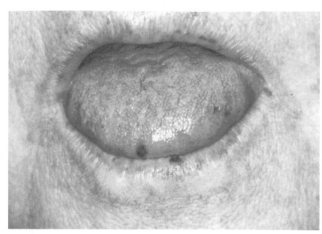

Fig. 22.6 Mat-like telangiectasias. *Courtesy, Irwin Braverman, MD.*

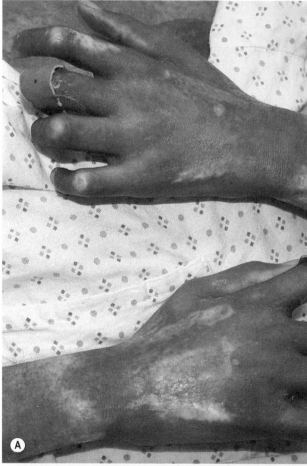

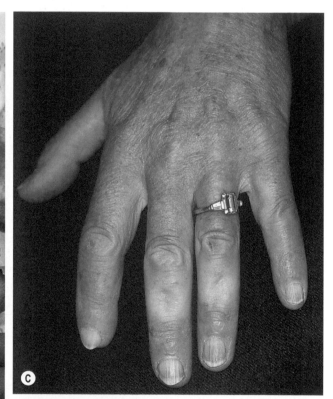

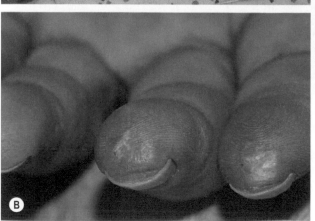

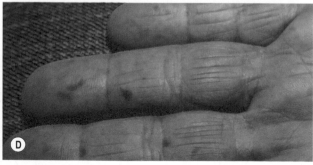

Fig. 22.5 Acral signs of systemic sclerosis. **A** Sclerodactyly. **B** Scarring secondary to digital pulp infarcts. **C** Edematous phase of systemic sclerosis. **D** Telangiectasias. *A, Courtesy, Yale Dermatology Residents' Slide Collection; B,D, Courtesy, Kalman Watsky, MD; C, Courtesy, Jean L Bolognia, MD. B,C,D, From Bolognia JL, Schaffer JV, Duncan KO, Ko CJ. Dermatology Essentials, 1e. Philadelphia: Saunders, 2014, with permission.*

SCLEROMYXEDEMA

Clinical:
Involves the hands and forearms, head (especially glabellar region), upper trunk, and thighs
Linear arrays of small papules may be evident overlying thickened or indurated skin (Fig. 22.7, see Figs. 20.8, 21.5)
Edema, especially of the hands, may be present

Histopathologic:
Increased fibroblasts and mucin

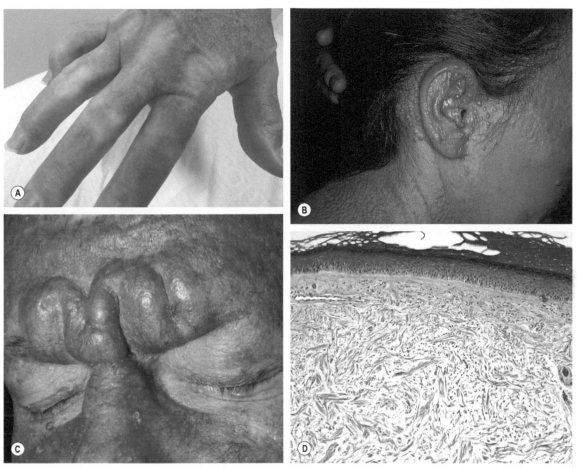

Fig. 22.7 Scleromyxedema. *A, Courtesy, Jonathan Leventhal, MD; B, Courtesy, Yale Dermatology Residents' Slide Collection; C, Courtesy, Joyce Rico, MD. B,C, From Bolognia JL, Schaffer JV, Duncan KO, Ko CJ. Dermatology Essentials, 1e. Philadelphia: Saunders, 2014, with permission.*

SCLEREDEMA

Clinical:
Typically involves the posterior neck and upper back
Less commonly involves the upper extremities and face
Induration +/− erythema (Fig. 22.8)

Histopathologic:
Increased space between collagen bundles +/− increased mucin

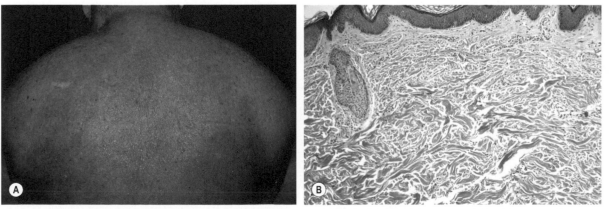

Fig. 22.8 Scleredema. *A, Courtesy, USC Residents' Collection. From Bolognia JL, Schaffer JV, Duncan KO, Ko CJ. Dermatology Essentials, 1e. Philadelphia: Saunders, 2014, with permission.*

EOSINOPHILIC FASCIITIS

Clinical:
Involves the extremities +/− the trunk
Induration often preceded by an edematous phase
Skin surface often rippled (Fig. 22.9)

Histopathologic:
Thickening and inflammation of the fascia +/− dermal involvement

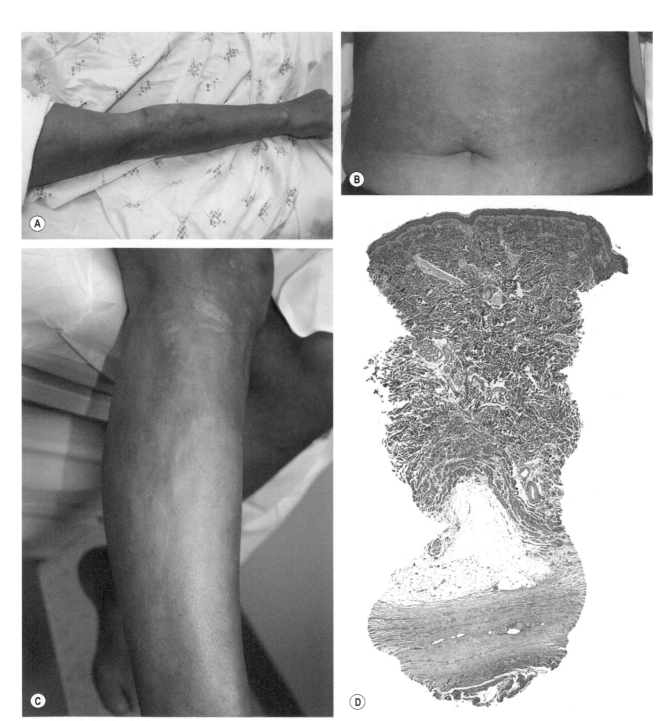

Fig. 22.9 Eosinophilic fasciitis. *A–C, Courtesy, Yale Dermatology Residents' Slide Collection.*

LINEAR MELORHEOSTOTIC SCLERODERMA

Clinical:
Often unilateral
Favors the extremities
Induration of the skin, rippling may be present (Fig. 22.10)
Involvement of bone (melorheostosis) may be associated

Histopathologic:
Adipocytes interspersed between thickened collagen
bundles

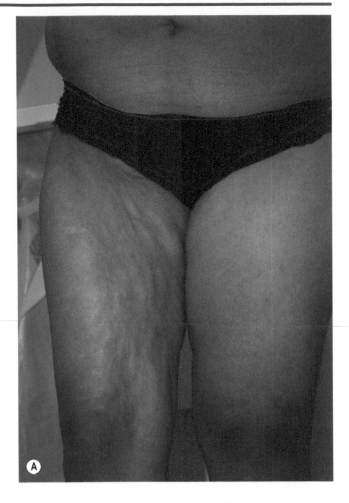

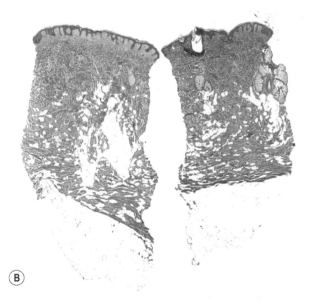

Fig. 22.10 Linear melorheostotic scleroderma. *A, Courtesy, Yale Dermatology Residents' Slide Collection.*

MORPHEA (CIRCUMSCRIBED, PLAQUE)

Clinical:
Favors pressure sites of the trunk (i.e. hips, waist, bra-line in women)

Discrete, indurated plaques, may be lilac-colored, hyperpigmented, or pink to reddish (Fig. 22.11)

Histopathologic:
Thickened collagen with decreased space (fenestrations) between collagen bundles, loss of fat around eccrine glands

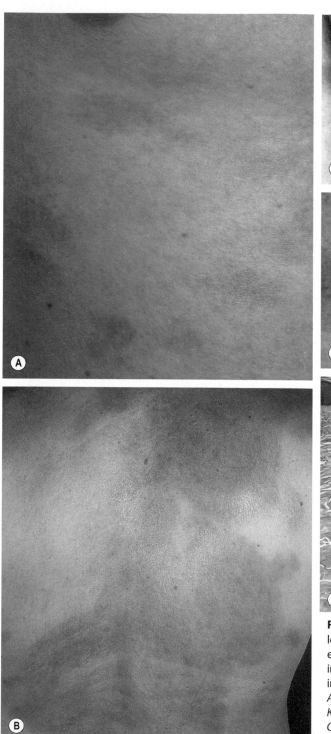

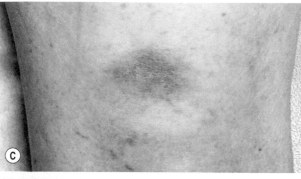

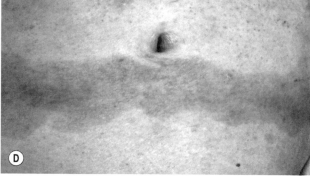

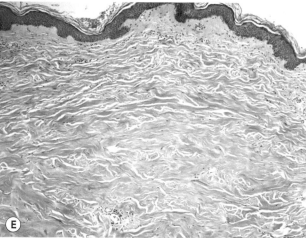

Fig. 22.11 Morphea, patch/plaque type. **A** Inflammatory stage; lesions have a characteristic lilac color. **B** Red–tan plaques with erythematous borders. **C** Oval pink–red plaque with subtle induration on palpation. **D** Late stage with hyperpigmentation in a characteristic configuration. **E** Thickened collagen bundles. *A, Courtesy, Yale Dermatology Residents' Slide Collection and Kamran Ghoreschi, MD. B, Courtesy, NYU Residents' Slide Collection. B, From Bolognia JL, Schaffer JV, Duncan KO, Ko CJ. Dermatology Essentials, 1e. Philadelphia: Saunders, 2014, with permission. C, Courtesy, Jonathan Leventhal, MD.*

MORPHEA, LINEAR

Clinical:

More commonly in children than in adults

Favors the head or extremities; on the extremities, a rippled appearance suggests deep involvement (Fig. 22.12)

Histopathologic features are the same as circumscribed morphea

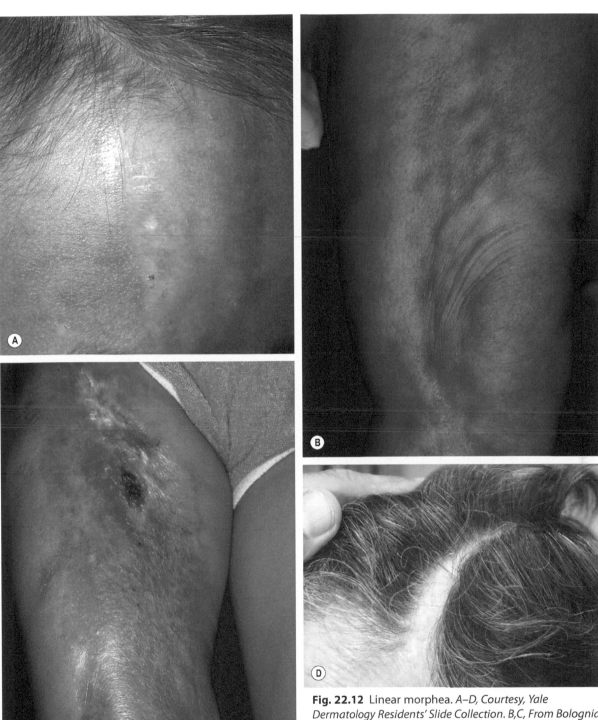

Fig. 22.12 Linear morphea. *A–D, Courtesy, Yale Dermatology Residents' Slide Collection. B,C, From Bolognia JL, Schaffer JV, Duncan KO, Ko CJ. Dermatology Essentials, 1e. Philadelphia: Saunders, 2014, with permission.*

LICHEN SCLEROSUS, EXTRAGENITAL

Clinical:
Predilection for the trunk (see Fig. 2.16A,B, for vulvar lichen sclerosus)

Atrophic, wrinkled, white macules and patches (Fig. 22.13)

Histopathologic:
Vacuolar change, dermal hyalinization, and underlying lymphocytes

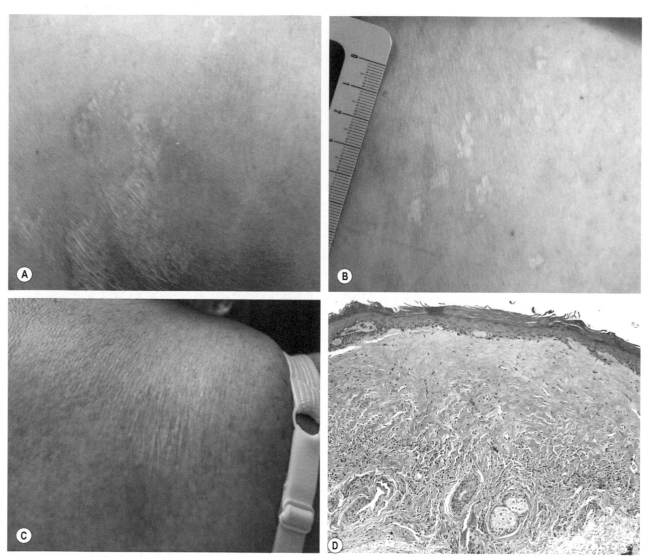

Fig. 22.13 Lichen sclerosus. *C, Courtesy, Yale Dermatology Residents' Slide Collection.*

Helminths/Arthropods 23

This chapter covers pediculosis, scabies, *Demodex* folliculitis, strongyloidiasis, tungiasis, cutaneous larva migrans, myiasis, tick bites, and filariasis.

PEDICULOSIS

Clinical:
Lice of different species primarily affect the head *(Pediculus humanus capitis)*, clothing *(Pediculus humanus corporis)*, and pubic hair/eyelashes *(Pthirus pubis)* (Figs. 23.1–23.4).

Histopathologic:
Lice and nits are generally not present in tissue sections as they do not burrow into or attach onto skin.

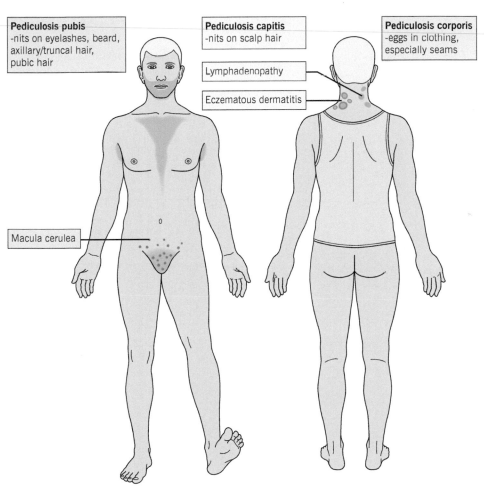

Pediculosis pubis
-nits on eyelashes, beard, axillary/truncal hair, pubic hair

Pediculosis capitis
-nits on scalp hair

Pediculosis corporis
-eggs in clothing, especially seams

Lymphadenopathy

Eczematous dermatitis

Macula cerulea

Fig. 23.1 Pediculosis, sites affected.

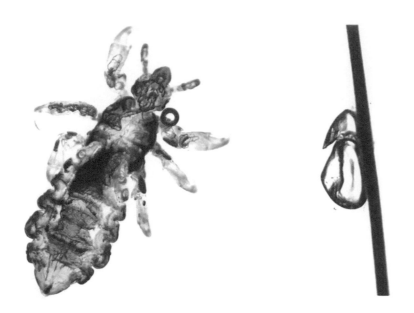

Fig. 23.2 Head louse (*Pediculus humanus capitis*) and an empty egg casing (the operculum is at the top) attached to a hair shaft.

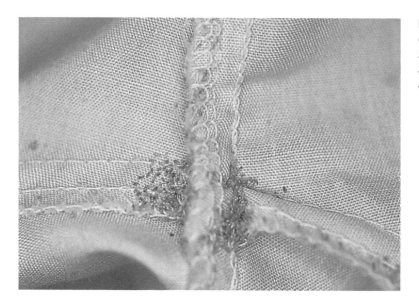

Fig. 23.3 Body lice eggs in the seams of clothing. *Courtesy, Yale Dermatology Residents' Slide Collection. From Bolognia JL, Jorizzo JL, Schaffer JV. Dermatology, 3e. London: Saunders, 2012, with permission.*

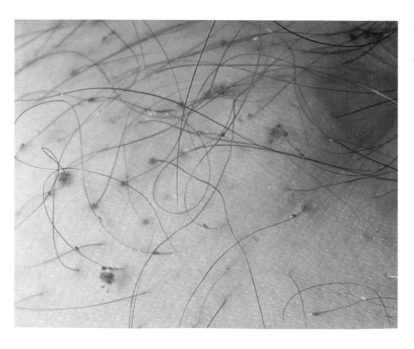

Fig. 23.4 Crab lice and eggs on pubic hair. *Courtesy, Louis A Fragola, MD. From Bolognia JL, Jorizzo JL, Schaffer JV. Dermatology, 3e. London: Saunders, 2012, with permission.*

SCABIES

Clinical:
Infestation with *Sarcoptes scabiei* var. *hominis*
Various skin manifestations (Figs. 23.5–23.8; see
Figs. 2.18G, 11.16, 13.5)

Histopathologic:
Within the stratum corneum, often with associated
neutrophils or parakeratosis, there are scybala (feces –
oval to round brown circles), egg casings (pink curlicues),
and/or mites

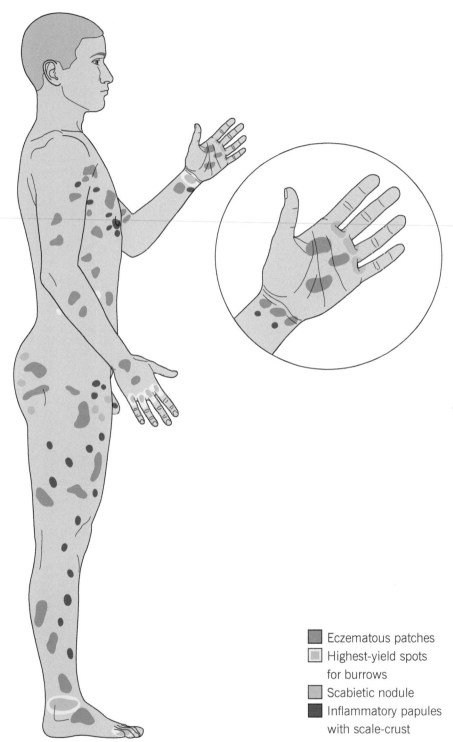

■ Eczematous patches
□ Highest-yield spots
  for burrows
■ Scabietic nodule
■ Inflammatory papules
  with scale-crust

Fig. 23.5 Range of cutaneous lesions in scabies. Crusted scabies may show prominent hyperkeratosis of acral sites.
From Bolognia JL, Schaffer JV, Duncan KO, Ko CJ. Dermatology Essentials, 1e. Philadelphia: Saunders, 2014, with permission.

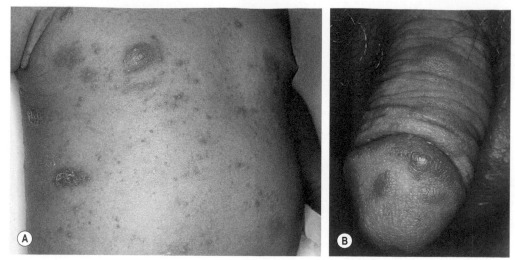

Fig. 23.6 Scabies infestation. **A** Eczematous patches and inflammatory papules. **B** Scabietic nodules. *A, Courtesy, Yale Dermatology Residents' Slide Collection. B, Courtesy, Robert Hartman, MD. A, From Bolognia JL, Jorizzo JL, Schaffer JV. Dermatology, 3e. London: Saunders, 2012, with permission. B, From Bolognia JL, Schaffer JV, Duncan KO, Ko CJ. Dermatology Essentials, 1e. Philadelphia: Saunders, 2014, with permission.*

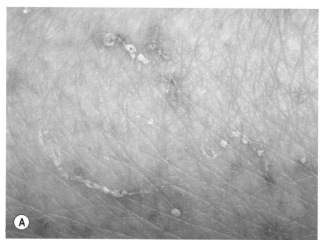

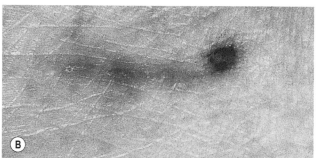

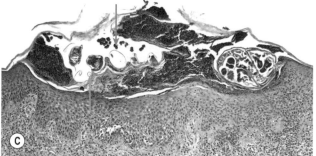

Fig. 23.7 Scabies. **A,B** Scabies linear burrow. **C** Microscopic mite (blue arrow), scybala (green arrow), and egg casings (orange arrow). *A, Courtesy, NYU Slide Collection. A, From Bolognia JL, Jorizzo JL, Schaffer JV. Dermatology, 3e. London: Saunders, 2012, with permission. B, Courtesy, Yale Dermatology Residents' Slide Collection.*

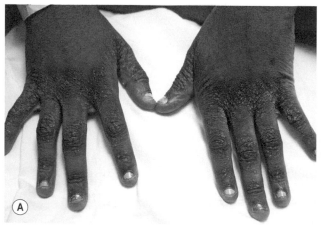

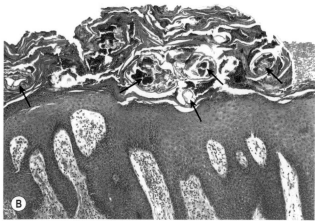

Fig. 23.8 Crusted scabies. The hyperkeratotic lesions, most typically on the hands, house numerous mites (arrows) and scybala (*). *Courtesy, Yale Dermatology Residents' Slide Collection.*

DEMODEX FOLLICULITIS

Clinical:
Caused by *Demodex* spp.
Erythematous papules and/or pustules on the face
(Figs. 23.9, 23.10)
Background of erythema and/or rosacea

Histopathologic:
Demodex are light purple tadpole shapes

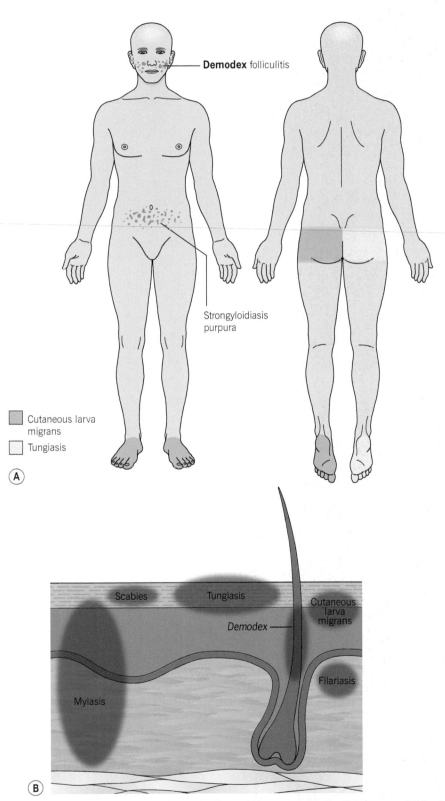

Fig. 23.9 Distribution of selected infestations. **A** Typical sites affected in *Demodex* folliculitis, strongyloidiasis, tungiasis, and cutaneous larva migrans. **B** Histopathologic location of selected arthropods/helminths. Microfilariae of filariasis are located in the dermis, but adult worms are in subcutaneous tissue or lymphatics.

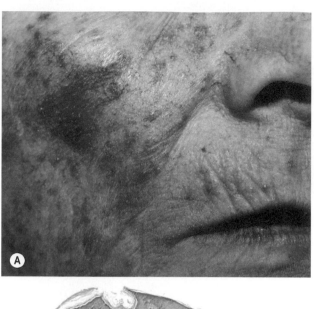

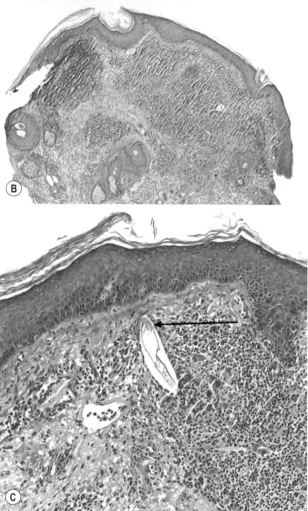

Fig. 23.10 *Demodex* folliculitis. *Demodex* mites are within follicles and in the dermis (arrow) surrounded by acute inflammation. *A, Courtesy, Kalman Watsky, MD.*

STRONGYLOIDIASIS

Clinical:

Caused by *Strongyloides stercoralis*
Thumbprint purpura, typically on the abdomen of immunocompromised hosts (see Fig. 23.9; Fig. 23.11)
Larva currens, serpiginous skin lesions, migrating up to 10 cm a day

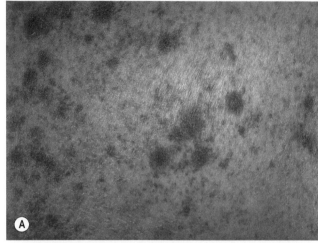

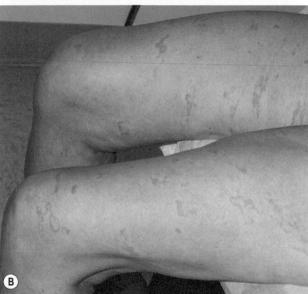

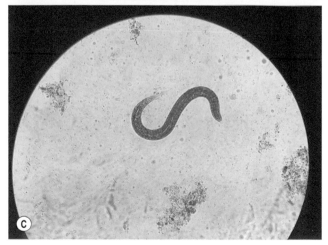

Fig. 23.11 Strongyloidiasis. **A** Strongyloidiasis hyperinfection. **B** Larva currens. **C** *Strongyloides* larva isolated from the stool. *A, Courtesy, Jean L Bolognia, MD. A, From Bolognia JL, Jorizzo JL, Schaffer JV. Dermatology, 3e. London: Saunders, 2012, with permission. B,C, From Pichard DC, Hensley JR, Williams E, et al. Rapid development of migratory, linear, and serpiginous lesions in association with immunosuppression. J Am Acad Dermatol. 2014;70:1130–4, © Elsevier.*

TUNGIASIS

Clinical:
Caused by infestation by a burrowing flea (e.g. *Tunga penetrans*)

Generally on the feet or the buttocks after contact with infested soil (see Fig. 23.9; Fig. 23.12)

Histopathologic:
Within the stratum corneum, a macroscopic organism with internal organs

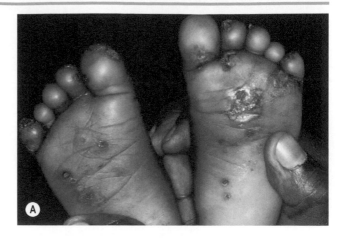

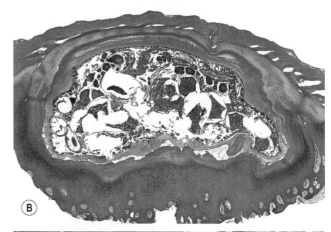

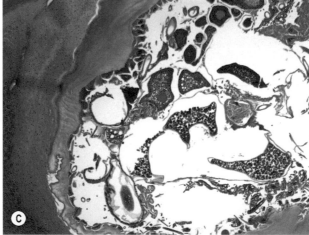

Fig. 23.12 Tungiasis. *A, Courtesy, Terri L Meinking, MD, Craig N Burkhart, MD, and Craig G Burkhart, MD. A, From Bolognia JL, Jorizzo JL, Schaffer JV. Dermatology, 3e. London: Saunders, 2012, with permission.*

CUTANEOUS LARVA MIGRANS (CREEPING ERUPTION)

Clinical:

Caused by animal hookworm larvae (e.g. *Ancylostoma caninum*, *A. braziliense*, and *Uncinaria stenocephala*) Commonly on feet or other body sites that have contacted contaminated soil or sand (e.g. buttocks; see Fig. 23.9) Serpiginous skin lesions (Fig. 23.13), migrating 1 to 2 cm day

Histopathologic:

Organisms may be evident in the stratum corneum or sometimes deeper

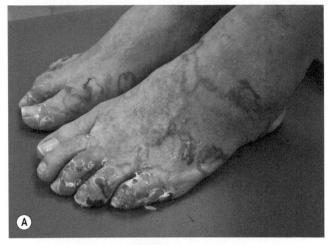

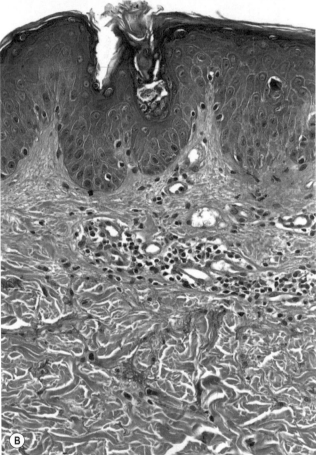

Fig. 23.13 Cutaneous larva migrans. *A, Courtesy, Peter Klein, MD. A, From Bolognia JL, Jorizzo JL, Schaffer JV. Dermatology, 3e. London: Saunders, 2012, with permission.*

MYIASIS

Clinical:
Infestation by fly larvae (e.g. *Dermatobia hominis*)
Presents as an erythematous nodule (Fig. 23.14) or as infestation of wounds

Histopathologic:
Larvae have an undulating outline, sometimes studded with yellowish spiny projections
Abundant skeletal muscle internally

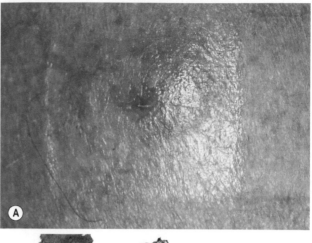

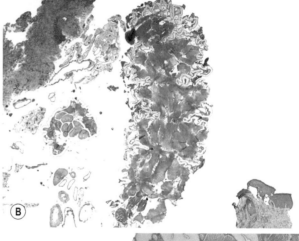

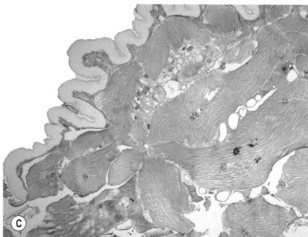

Fig. 23.14 Myiasis. *A, Courtesy, Yale Dermatology Residents' Slide Collection. A, From Bolognia JL, Schaffer JV, Duncan KO, Ko CJ. Dermatology Essentials, 1e. Philadelphia: Saunders, 2014, with permission.*

TICK BITES

Clinical:
Attached ticks (Fig. 23.15) have been mistaken for nodular melanoma
Careful examination will often reveal tick parts (e.g. legs)

Histopathologic:
Mouth parts often have a yellowish hue
Complex internal organs

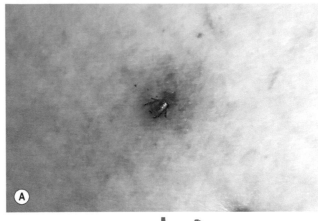

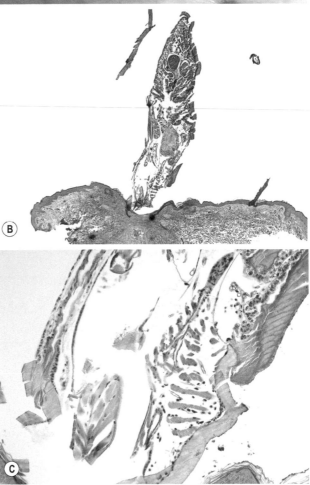

Fig. 23.15 Attached tick.

SUBCUTANEOUS FILARIASIS – ONCHOCERCIASIS (RIVER BLINDNESS)

Clinical:
Caused by *Onchocerca volvulus*, transmitted by black flies (*Simulium* spp.)
Various manifestations (Figs. 23.16–23.18)

Histopathologic:
Nodular lesions contain adult worms
Female worms have characteristic paired uteri internally

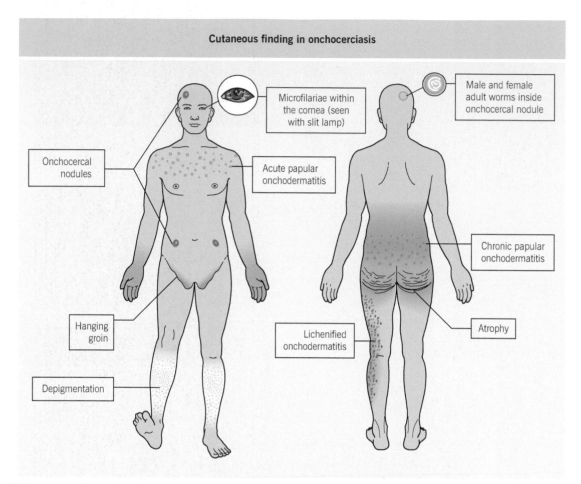

Fig. 23.16 Cutaneous findings in onchocerciasis. *From Bolognia JL, Jorizzo JL, Schaffer JV. Dermatology, 3e. London: Saunders, 2012, with permission.*

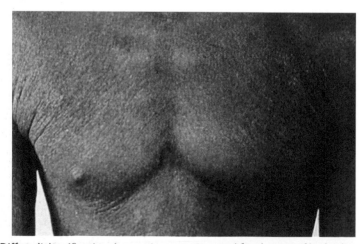

Fig. 23.17 Onchocerciasis. Diffuse lichenification, hyperpigmentation, and focal areas of leukoderma. *Courtesy, Omar P Sangüeza, MD. From Bolognia JL, Jorizzo JL, Schaffer JV. Dermatology, 3e. London: Saunders, 2012, with permission.*

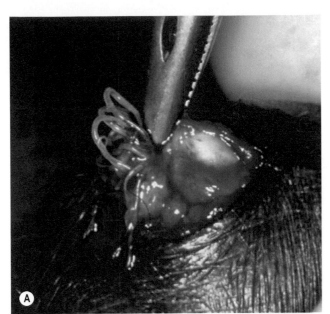

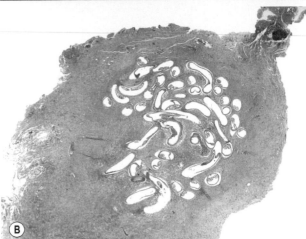

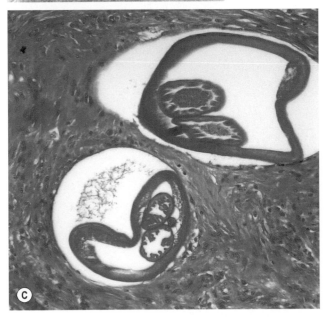

Fig. 23.18 Onchocercal nodule containing an adult worm.
*A, Courtesy, Steven A Nelson, MD and Karen E Warschaw, MD.
A, From Bolognia JL, Jorizzo JL, Schaffer JV. Dermatology, 3e.
London: Saunders, 2012, with permission.*

LYMPHATIC FILARIASIS

Clinical:
Caused by infection by tissue nematodes (e.g. *Wuchereria bancrofti*, *Brugia* spp.)
Lymphatics are occluded by adult worms, leading to chronic lymphedema, hanging groin, and elephantiasis (Fig. 23.19)

Histopathologic:
Organisms within lymphatics

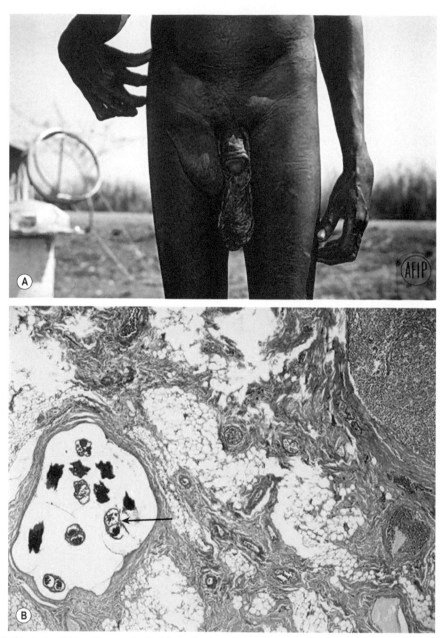

Fig. 23.19 Lymphatic filariasis. **A** Hanging groin. **B** A lymphatic vessel contains an adult worm (arrow). *A, Courtesy, Daniel Conner. A, From Tyring SK, Lupi O, Hengge UR. Tropical Dermatology. London: Churchill Livingstone, 2005. B, From Bolognia JL, Jorizzo JL, Schaffer JV. Dermatology, 3e. London: Saunders, 2012, with permission.*

Case Reviews

The focus of this chapter is to build on the major aims of this atlas – (1) visually analyzing something you may have never seen before, and (2) teaching the brain to "see" in a more educated manner, thus enhancing observational skills. The brief case reviews given are of presentations that may be classic, rare, or visually similar to another entity; these cases help demonstrate the nuances inherent to visual recognition of skin disease. Careful observation of clinical and histopathologic findings (which can be key to the diagnosis) and knowledge of the course of the disease lead to a working diagnosis, which can help determine management and treatment.

For a given patient, many of the principles and concepts in previous chapters come into consideration (Table 24.1), and this will happen seamlessly and automatically with greater experience. The process may be primarily epidermal or dermal, and the inflammatory cell type may be predictable from the clinical appearance. Importantly, although not emphasized in other chapters, in some situations, the clinical history and course are key elements. It helps to have seen something before, and particularly for unusual presentations, or something that seems novel, performing a biopsy can help confirm the clinical impression or point in a different direction.

Table 24.1 Clinical principles and concepts to consider when evaluating a case

History (i.e. age, comorbidities, medications, recent procedures, acute vs chronic)

Distribution (i.e. generalized, intertriginous)

Pattern (i.e. annular, linear) and morphology (i.e. primary lesion, color, topography)

Where is the action? (i.e. epidermal, dermal) Is there scale?

Is it inflamed? If so, on a clinical basis, what is predicted to be predominant cell type? (i.e. lymphocytic, neutrophilic, granulomatous)

Associated clues (i.e. nail changes, oral lesions)

Pertinent negatives

Histopathology

Course of disease

EPIDERMAL AND EPIDERMAL–DERMAL (INTERFACE) PROCESSES

Case 1

History: 63-year-old female with thyroid storm secondary to amiodarone, treated with thyroidectomy
Distribution: Trunk
Pattern and morphology: Scattered ichthyotic circular plaques*

*See Figs. 1.56, 5.26.

Epidermal process, appears noninflamed
Predicted histopathology: Hyperkeratosis
Course: Spontaneous resolution

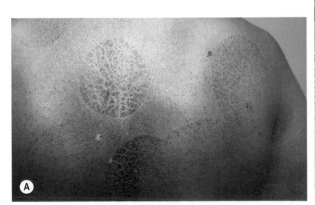
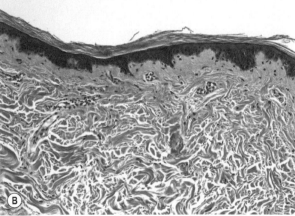

Fig. 24.1 Pityriasis rotunda. Biopsy findings include epidermal changes (slight hyperkeratosis and focal hypogranulosis) and minimal inflammation. This rare disease resembles an ichthyosis given the surface scale; the lesions are characteristically circular and involve the trunk. *A, Courtesy, Brittany Craiglow and Leon Luck.*

Case 2

History: Asymptomatic, new-onset
Distribution: Axillae
Pattern and morphology: Keratotic papules, centrally confluent

See Chapter 7

Epidermal process, appears noninflamed
Predicted histopathology: Hyperkeratosis

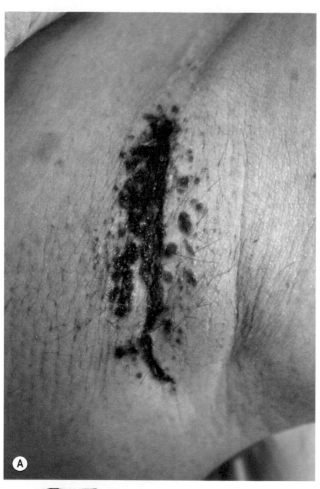

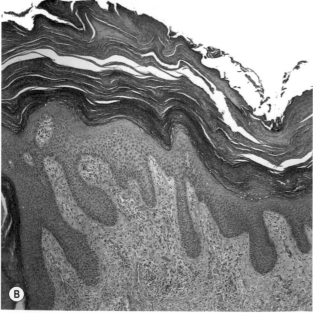

Fig. 24.2 Axillary granular parakeratosis. The stratum corneum contains retained keratohyaline granules; there is mild inflammation. Clinically, this appears to be an epidermal process, which is confirmed by the characteristic biopsy findings. *A,B, Courtesy, Yale Dermatology Residents' Slide Collection.*

Case 3

History: HIV-negative male, chronic lesions that appeared in adulthood
Distribution: Extremities
Pattern and morphology: Scattered hypopigmented, flat-topped papules

Epidermal process, appears noninflamed
Predicted histopathology: Epidermal change

See Chapter 7

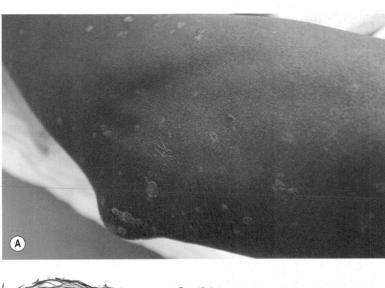

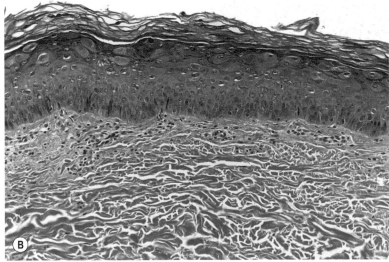

Fig. 24.3 Epidermodysplasia verruciformis. Biopsy findings include hyperkeratosis and altered cells with koilocytic change (keratinocytes have white space around nuclei with expanded light pink–purple cytoplasm) in the granular layer with minimal dermal inflammation. The characteristic biopsy findings of this epidermal process are key to the diagnosis. *A,B, Courtesy, Yale Dermatology Residents' Slide Collection.*

Case 4

History: 11-year-old male, new onset (Fig. 24.4A,B,D)
Distribution: Soles bilaterally
Pattern and morphology: Well-demarcated scaly plaques, pink-red, with fissures

Epidermal process, color suggests lymphocytic inflammation
Predicted histopathology: Spongiotic
Associated clues: No history of psoriasis

See Chapters 4 and 5.

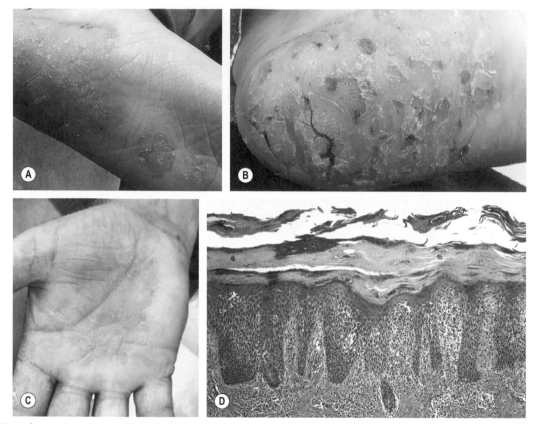

Fig. 24.4 Hyperkeratotic eczema. Clinically lesions resemble chronic eczematous dermatitis and/or psoriasis **(A,B)**; fissures are an important clue. In this patient, the soles were involved, although the central palm is characteristically affected, as shown in this photograph of another patient. The tips of digits may also be affected. Biopsy findings typically include acanthosis, spongiosis, and exocytosis of numerous lymphocytes (intraepidermal lymphocytes).

Case 5

History: 50-year-old male, long-standing rash with new-onset blisters

Distribution: Generalized on trunk and extremities

Pattern and morphology: Tense bullae* and well-demarcated psoriasiform plaques†

*See Chapter 12.
†See Chapter 5.

Bullous lesions and **epidermal thickening and scale**
Predicted histopathology: (of a plaque) Psoriasiform
(of a blister): Subepidermal split

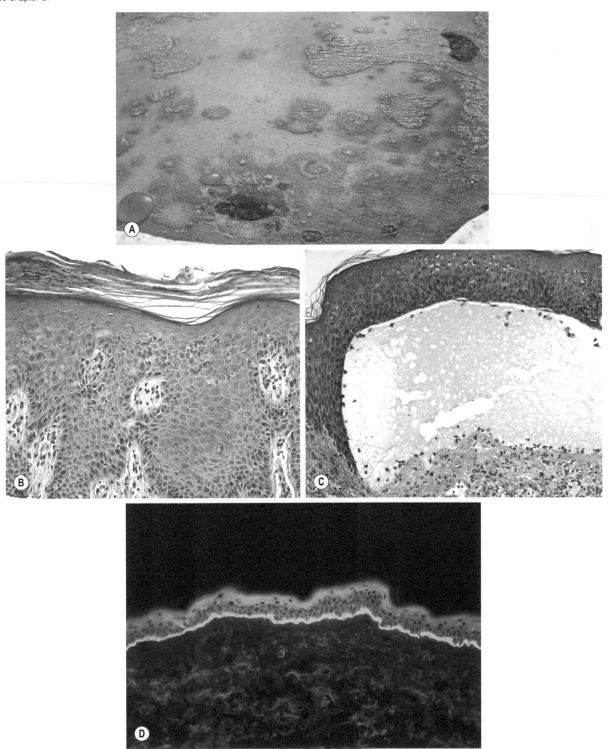

Fig. 24.5 Psoriasis and concomitant bullous pemphigoid. **B** Biopsy of a psoriasiform plaque had findings typical of psoriasis with parakeratosis, acanthosis, and hypogranulosis. **C** Biopsy of a tense blister had findings of a subepidermal split with eosinophils in the base, characteristic of bullous pemphigoid. Direct immunofluorescence testing was positive for linear deposition of IgG and C3 in a linear pattern at the dermal-epidermal junction. *A,B, Courtesy, Mary Tomayko, MD, PhD.*

Case 6

History: 26-year-old male, long-standing lesions, occasionally itchy
Distribution: Bilateral nipples/areolae

Pattern and morphology: Papillomatous plaques
Epidermal-based lesion*
Predicted histopathology: Epidermal hyperplasia

*See Chapter 7.

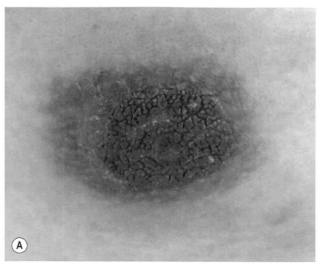

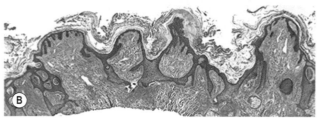

Fig. 24.6 Nevoid hyperkeratosis of the nipple and areola. There is hyperkeratosis and acanthosis of the epidermis that resembles changes of a seborrheic keratosis. *A, Courtesy, Mary Tomayko, MD, PhD.*

Case 7

History: 79-year-old Caucasian female
Distribution: Bilateral legs, especially shins
Pattern and morphology: Hyperkeratotic light pink-red papules, plaques, and nodules

Epidermal-based lesion*
Predicted histopathology: Epidermal hyperplasia
Associated clues: Multiple similar lesions on the legs

*See Chapter 7.

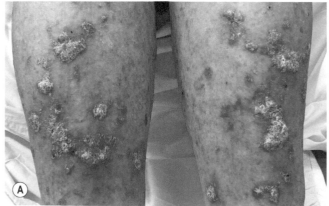

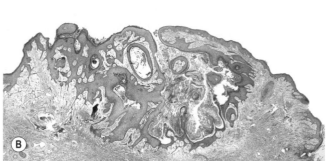

Fig. 24.7 Keratoacanthoma-like atypical squamous proliferations (eruptive squamous atypia). These lesions are often multiple, on the legs of severely sun-damaged skin. Biopsy findings can mimic squamous cell carcinoma or resemble keratoacanthoma, prurigo nodule, or hypertrophic lichen planus. A microscopic clue is the presence of thin, interconnecting basaloid strands flanking the lesion. These lesions generally respond well to conservative treatments.

Distribution: Eyelids and forehead/cheeks, hands over the joints, upper back and arms
Pattern and morphology: Pink to slightly purple patches,* minimal scale, focal erosions
Epidermal (Surface change) and **dermal process, appears inflamed**

Associated clues: Muscle weakness, nailfold telangiectasias, jagged cuticles
Predicted histopathology: Vacuolar change,* minimal inflammation, slightly dilated capillaries

*See Chapter 8; Fig. 2.6.

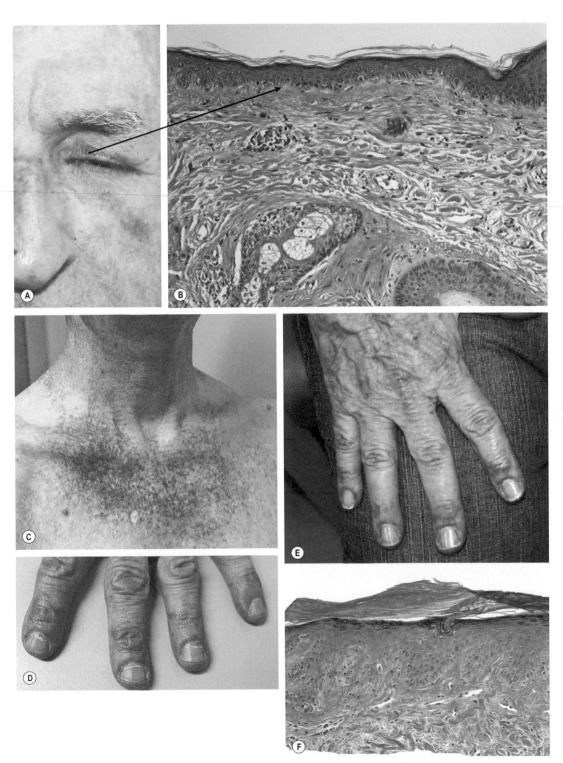

Fig. 24.8 A–E Dermatomyositis. The eyelids are involved by the so-called heliotrope rash (A). "Mechanic's hands" may be evident, with scaling along the adjacent sides of the index finger and thumb (D). Histologic findings include subtle interface vacuolar change, often with minimal inflammation (B,F). Despite the lack of inflammation, interface vacuolar processes often appear clinically inflamed (pink to violaceous). *A,C,E, Courtesy, Jeff Gehlhausen, MD, PhD; D, Courtesy, Yale Dermatology Residents' Slide Collection.*

Case 9

History: Stem cell transplant
Distribution: Trunk
Pattern and morphology: Erythematous macules and papules, becoming confluent*

Associated clues: Diarrhea and liver function abnormalities
Appears inflamed, suggesting a dermal process
Predicted histopathology: Mixed dermal infiltrate or subtle vacuolar interface

*See Chapter 8, Fig. 1.36.

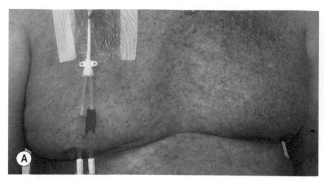
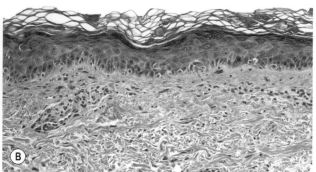

Fig. 24.9 Acute graft-versus-host disease. Classic histopathologic findings include interface vacuolar change with necrotic keratinocytes, sometimes extending into follicular epithelium. Interface vacuolar processes often appear clinically inflamed (pink to violaceous); inflammation is not always present. In this example, inflammation is mild. *A, Courtesy, Yale Dermatology Residents' Slide Collection.*

Case 10

History: Lesion waxes and wanes, new onset in adulthood
Distribution: Leg
Pattern and morphology: Linear,* eroded pink-red papules and slightly violaceous patches

Spongiotic (Weepy)† to **lichenoid** (violaceous)‡
appearance
Pink-purple color suggests lymphocytic inflammation
Predicted histopathology: Spongiotic to lichenoid

*See Fig. 1.28.
†See Chapter 4, Figs. 1.33, 1.41, 1.42.
‡See Fig. 1.35.

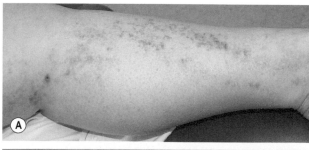
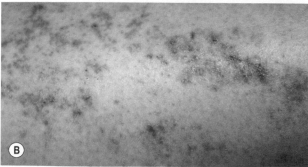
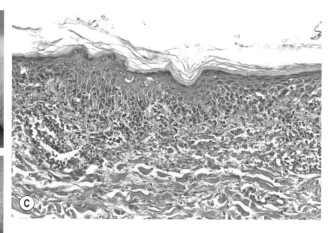

Fig. 24.10 Blaschkitis. Biopsy findings included lymphocytes at the junction of the epidermis and dermis, necrotic keratinocytes, and perivascular lymphocytes. Although histopathologic findings of Blaschkitis are typically spongiotic, interface patterns have been described. *A,B, Courtesy, Yale Dermatology Residents' Slide Collection; C, Courtesy Nemanja Rodic, MD.*

Distribution: Bilateral cheeks, symmetric
Pattern and morphology: Hyperpigmented patches
Color suggests pigment in the dermis, possibly caused by interface change

Predicted histopathology: Vacuolar change with pigment incontinence

See Figs. 1.53, 2.8, 8.12.

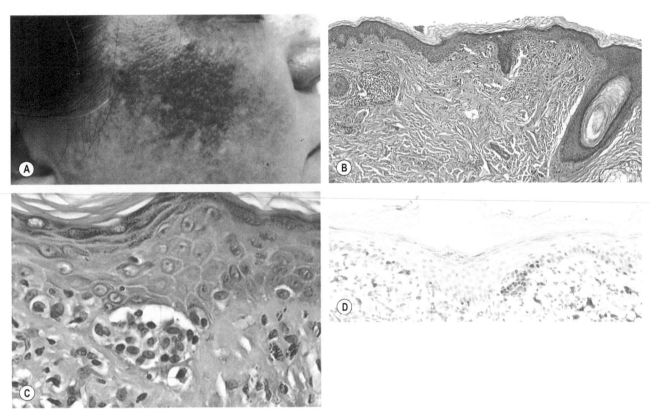

Fig. 24.11 Lichen planus pigmentosus. There is focal vacuolar change with pigment incontinence. Biopsy findings alone have some resemblance to melanoma *in situ* (**B**), with small cells clustered in nests and arranged singly at the dermal–epidermal junction (**C**). Some of these cells are positive with MITF (**D**), but correlation with the clinical findings avoids misdiagnosis as a melanocytic process. *A, Courtesy, Jeffrey Alter, MD.*

Case 12

History: 22-year-old female, slightly pruritic rash
Distribution: Trunk, inner arms, buttocks, hips
Pattern and morphology: Ashy gray to brown macules and patches on back and abdomen; inner arms (**C**), buttocks, and hips (**D**) with slightly scaly thin plaques with focal atrophy

See Figs. 1.46, 8.12, 18.20.

Atrophic patches and hyperpigmentation suggest an epidermal–dermal process
Predicted histopathology: Subtle epidermal changes, lymphocytic inflammation, pigment in dermis

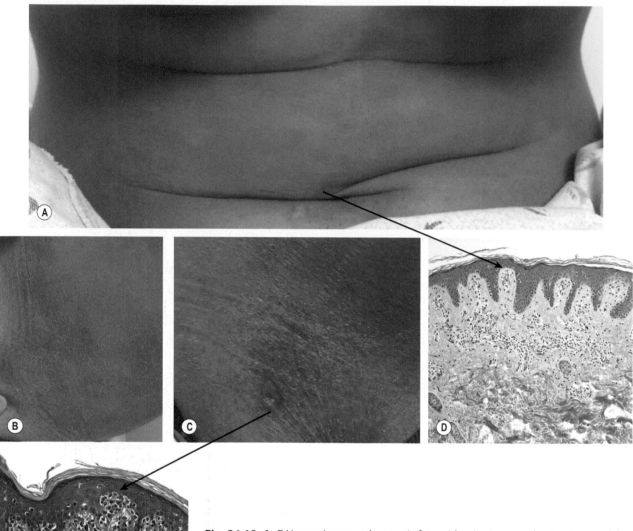

Fig. 24.12 A–E Hyperpigmented mycosis fungoides. Lesions on the trunk resemble erythema dyschromicum perstans (ashy dermatosis). Involvement of double-covered sites (see Fig. 1.16B) is typical of mycosis fungoides. The biopsy site in (C) is light pink. The patient had multiple biopsies from different sites, all showing an epidermotropic, atypical lymphocytic infiltrate, more subtle in (D) than (E). She had clonal rearrangement of the T-cell receptor gene, with an identical clone found in five different sites. She was treated with ultraviolet light B phototherapy. *E, Courtesy, Antonio Subtil, MD.*

Case 13

History: 70-year-old male, asymptomatic
Distribution: Flanks, inner arms
Pattern and morphology: Atrophic, reticulated, pink-red patches

Atrophy and color suggest an epidermal-dermal process
Pink-red color suggests lymphocytic inflammation
Predicted histopathology: Lymphocytic inflammation

See Figs. 1.46, 18.20.

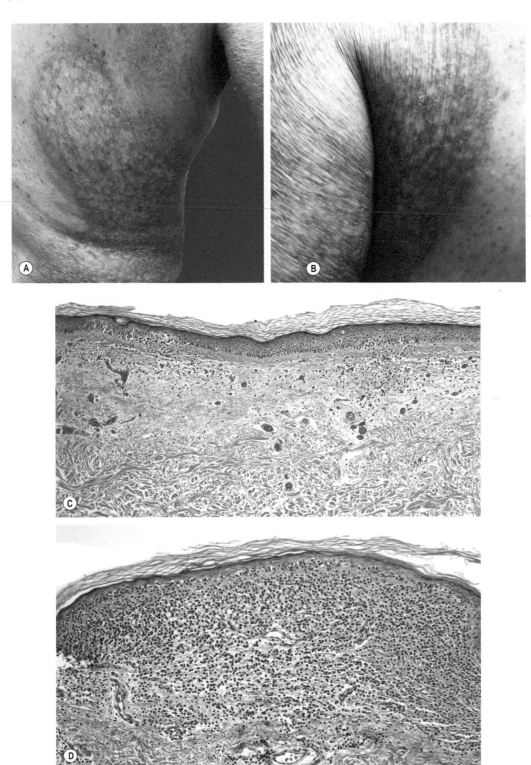

Fig. 24.13 Poikiloderma atrophicans vasculare (cutaneous T-cell lymphoma). An initial biopsy was suggestive, but not fully diagnostic, of the diagnosis, with epidermal atrophy, patchy lymphocytic inflammation, and dilated vessels (C). A second biopsy was taken because of high clinical suspicion and showed a dense lymphocytic infiltrate, with epidermotropic CD4+, CD5-, CD7- cells (D). *A,B, Courtesy, Jeffrey Alter, MD and Antonio Subtil, MD.*

Case 14

History: 3 weeks after starting ipilimumab
Distribution: Generalized
Pattern and morphology: Pink–red macules and papules, slightly scaly

Mostly dermal process, some surface change
Pink-red color suggests lymphocytic inflammation
Predicted histopathology: Epidermal changes with dermal inflammation*

*See Figs. 1.35, 2.25.

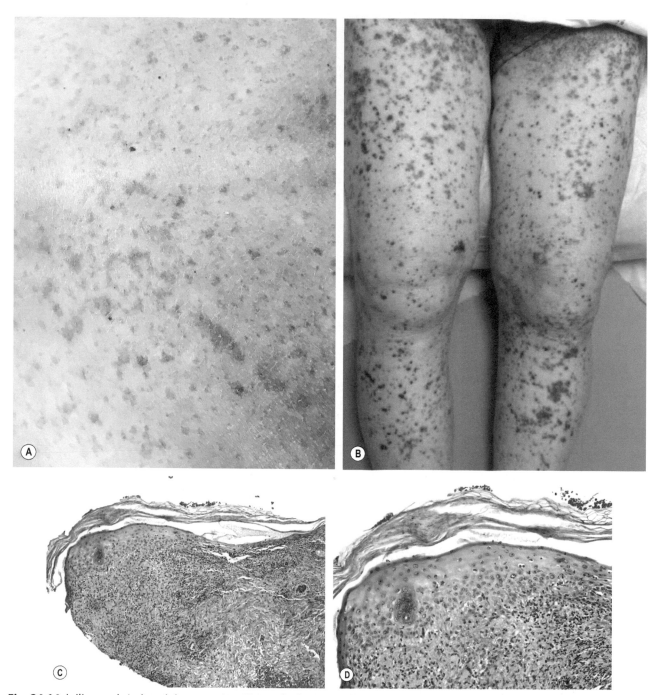

Fig. 24.14 Ipilimumab-induced drug reaction. Biopsy findings include parakeratosis, interface change, and dermal lymphocytic inflammation (C,D). *A,B, Courtesy, Jennifer N Choi, MD.*

History: Pruritic
Distribution: Generalized
Pattern and morphology: Hyperpigmented flat-topped papules,* coalescing into plaques in some areas

Color suggests dermal inflammation, lymphocytic
Associated clue: Lacy, focally eroded plaques on the buccal mucosa
Predicted histopathology: Lichenoid*

*See Figs. 2.13, 6.7–6.13.

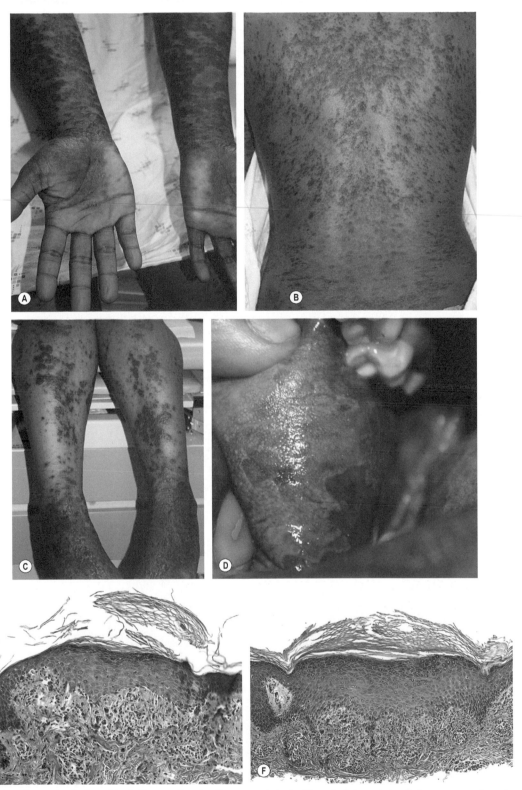

Fig. 24.15 Lichen planus. In darker skin, inflammation is often associated with a dark brown to dark gray–purple color. Biopsy findings from the shoulder (E) and wrist (F) showed similar features, with hyperkeratosis, hypergranulosis, lichenoid inflammation, and pigment incontinence. *A–F, Courtesy, Yale Dermatology Residents' Slide Collection.*

History: Lichen planus elsewhere
Distribution: Anterior shins
Pattern and morphology: Flat-topped plaques with linear scale*

*See Chapter 7, Figs. 6.7–6.13.

Epidermal change (scale), **pink-purple color suggests dermal inflammation**
Associated clues: Multiplicity, Wickham's striae
Predicted histopathology: Lichenoid*

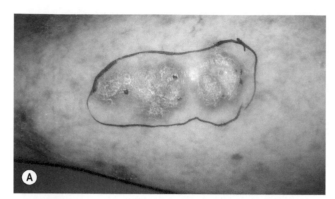

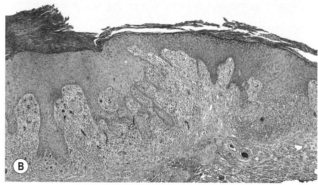

Fig. 24.16 Hypertrophic lichen planus. Individual lesions of hypertrophic lichen planus can mimic squamous cell carcinoma clinically and histopathologically. Biopsy clues include hypergranulosis and lichenoid inflammation accentuated at the tips of elongated rete (B). *A, Courtesy, Yale Dermatology Residents' Slide Collection.*

Case 17

History: 7-year-old male
Distribution: Extremities
Pattern and morphology: Pink–red eroded papules, some in linear arrays
Epidermal change (scale), **color suggests dermal lymphocytic inflammation**

Associated clues: Spontaneous blistering, nail dystrophy
Predicted histopathology: Hyperkeratosis and acanthosis; with history of spontaneous blistering and nail changes, a subepidermal split might be predicted

See Chapters 6 and 7.

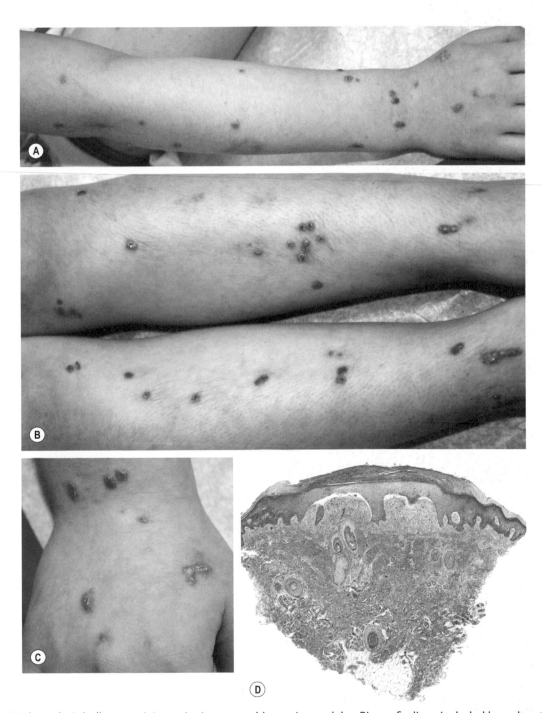

Fig. 24.17 Epidermolysis bullosa pruriginosa. Lesions resemble prurigo nodules. Biopsy findings included hyperkeratosis and acanthosis, but also a subepidermal split. The subepidermal clefting below the epidermal changes is key to the diagnosis, but it may be overlooked histopathologically as well. In such cases, the patient may be misdiagnosed as having prurigo nodules. Some of the redness clinically is likely caused by slightly increased vessels and by lymphocytic inflammation. *A–C, Courtesy, Richard Antaya, MD.*

PURPURA

History: 55-year-old female, history of metastatic endometrial carcinoma
Distribution: Legs

*See Chapter 9.

Pattern and morphology: Retiform purpura*
Epidermal (scale) and **dermal** (purpura)
Predicted histopathology: Vascular occlusion

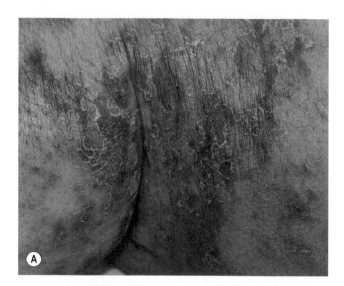

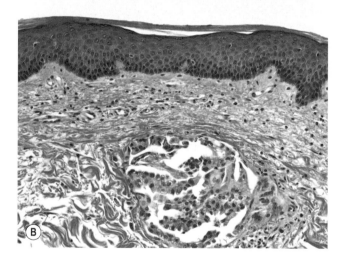

Fig. 24.18 Retiform purpura on the leg secondary to vascular occlusion by metastatic endometrial carcinoma. Hyperkeratosis corresponds to the surface scale. *A, Courtesy, Swapna Reddy, MD.*

DERMAL PROCESSES – GRANULOMATOUS

History: 58-year-old male
Distribution: Scalp, face
Pattern and morphology: Annular papules* with hyperpigmentation

*See Figs. 1.25, 20.4; Chapter 20.
^See Fig. 15.9.

Dermal process, pink-gray color
Pertinent negative: Conchal bowl^ spared
Predicted histopathology: Dermal inflammation and/or alteration (e.g. scarring, atrophy, pigment incontinence)

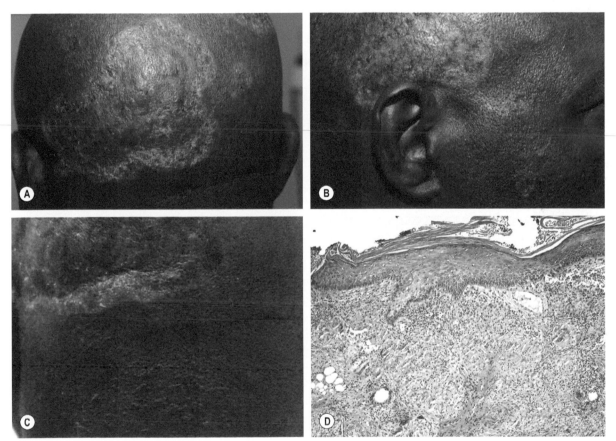

Fig. 24.19 Sarcoidosis. In darker skin, granulomatous inflammation can be skin-colored to pink to hypo- or hyperpigmented. Biopsy findings: granulomatous inflammation, and the type of inflammation helps in suggesting against discoid lupus erythematosus, as does the sparing of the conchal bowls. *A,C, Courtesy, Yale Dermatology Residents' Slide Collection; B, Courtesy, Kalman Watsky, MD.*

History: 84-year-old female with acute myelogenous leukemia
Distribution: Legs
Pattern and morphology: Red–brown plaques

Dermal process, pink-brown color suggests granulomatous inflammation*
Predicted histopathology: Granulomatous

*See Fig. 1.48.

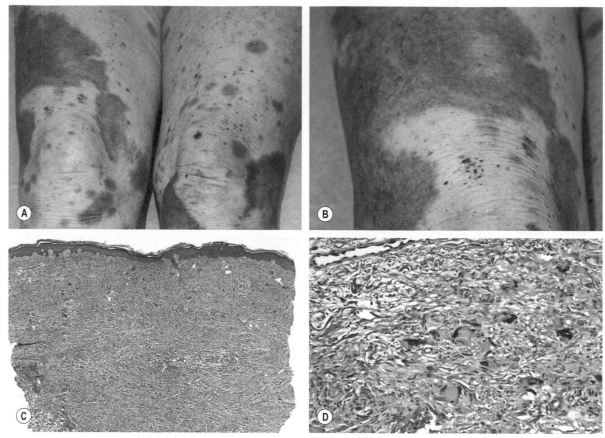

Fig. 24.20 Necrobiotic xanthogranuloma (NXG). Although NXG is classically periorbital, it can affect other sites. Biopsy findings were centered in the dermis and included foci of altered collagen surrounded by numerous bizarre giant cells, histiocytes, and lymphocytes.

Case 21

History: 49-year-old female
Distribution: Forehead*
Pattern and morphology: Annular plaques

Dermal process, pink color suggests lymphocytic inflammation, but pattern on forehead suggests a granulomatous disorder
Predicted histopathology: Granulomatous†

*See Fig. 2.9.
†See Fig. 1.48.

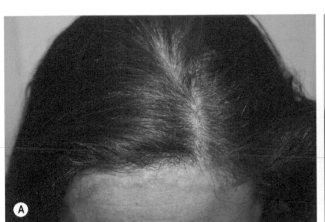

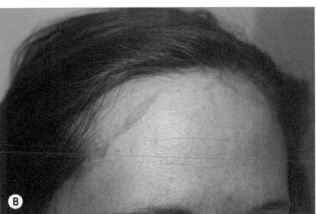

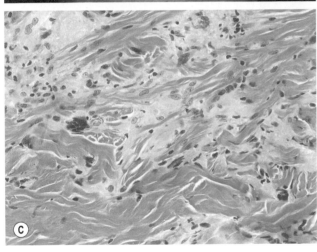

Fig. 24.21 Annular elastolytic giant cell granuloma. Although some consider this a variant of granuloma annulare, the clinical presentation is classically annular plaques on the forehead/scalp and/or other sun-exposed sites. There is minimal epidermal change clinically. Histologic findings are based in the dermis and include giant cells with elastophagocytosis. Granulomatous disorders may be pink in color in lighter skin types and are not always red-brown. *A–C, Courtesy, Yale Dermatology Residents' Slide Collection.*

DERMAL PROCESSES – NEUTROPHILIC

Case 22

History: 62-year-old male several days status post multiple procedures using IV contrast
Distribution: Scattered over face and body
Pattern and morphology: Raised, translucent papules, some crusted

*See Chapter 16; Fig. 2.7.

Epidermal change (crusting, pseudovesiculation), **translucency suggests neutrophilic inflammation***
Predicted histopathology: Neutrophilic
Course: Spontaneous resolution

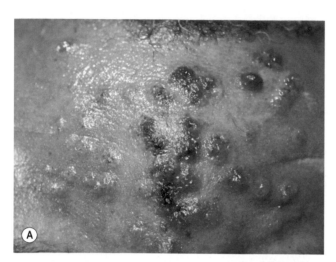

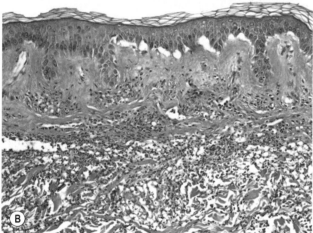

Fig. 24.22 Iododerma. Neutrophilic infiltrates that are more superficial can produce yellow coloration (pustular); deeper neutrophilic infiltrates are classically hot-red but can have this translucent, blistered appearance. *A, Courtesy, Yale Dermatology Residents' Collection.*

History: 80-year-old female seen several months after excision of a right leg squamous cell carcinoma; she had been putting her leg in a hot water bath daily
Distribution: Right leg

Pattern and morphology: Scattered purpuric* papules
Hot-red color suggests neutrophilic inflammation or a purpuric component
Predicted histopathology: Neutrophilic*

*See Chapters 9 and 16.

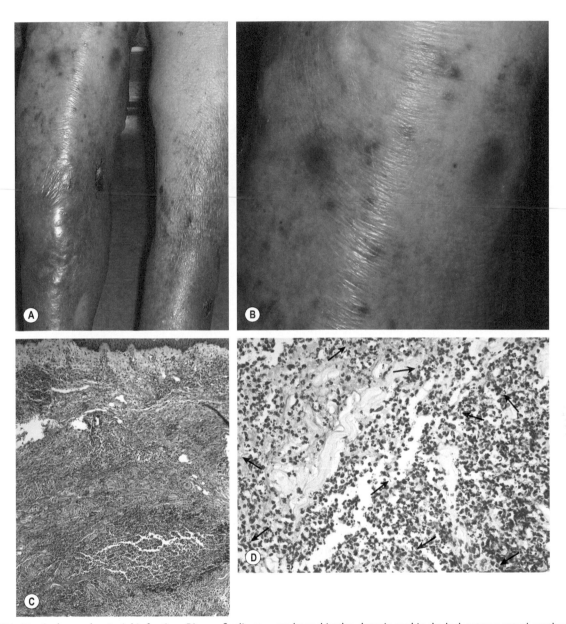

Fig. 24.23 Atypical mycobacterial infection. Biopsy findings were based in the dermis and included extravasated erythrocytes as well as neutrophilic abscesses (C) with rare acid-fast bacteria (arrows) (D).

DERMAL PROCESSES – TUMOR, DEPOSITION, THICKENING

Case 24

History: 74-year-old female (Fig. 24.24A,C,D)
Distribution: Anterior shins
Pattern and morphology: Indurated plaques studded with firm, pseudovesicular papules
Firmness on palpation suggests dermal deposition* of material

*See Chapter 21.

Predicted histopathology: Dermal edema or other material
Pertinent negative: No thyroid abnormality
Course: Improvement with compression

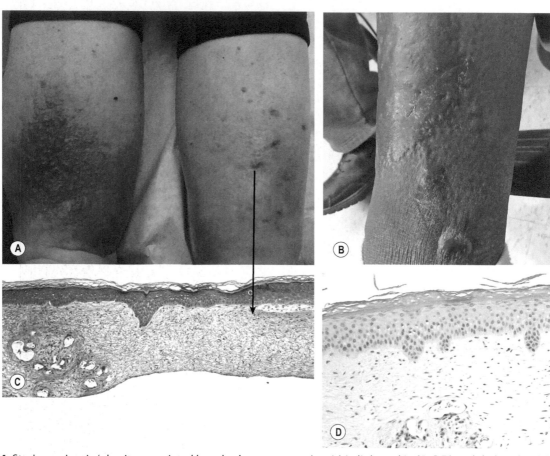

Fig. 24.24 Stasis mucinosis (obesity-associated lymphedematous mucinosis) in lighter skin **(A,C,D)** and darker skin **(B)**. Biopsy of a raised papule with dermal edema, clustered vessels, and slightly increased dermal mucin (C,D). *A, Courtesy, Ronnie Klein, MD.*

History: 44-year-old female, history of mixed connective tissue disorder, on hydroxychloroquine
Distribution: Back and extremities

Pattern and morphology: Gray patches
Color suggests dermal deposition of pigment
Predicted histopathology: Deposition of dermal pigment

See Fig. 1.53

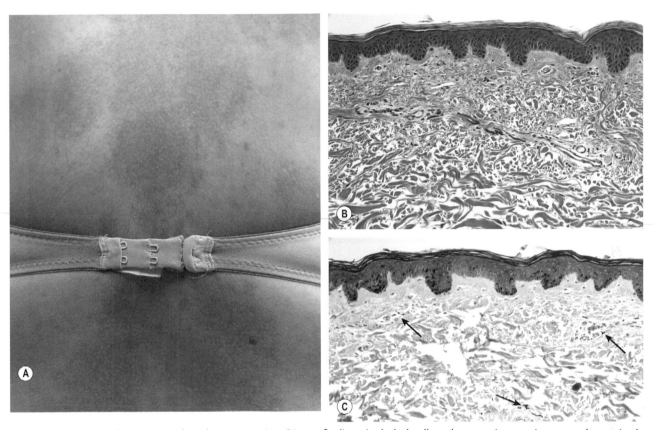

Fig. 24.25 Hydroxychloroquine-induced pigmentation. Biopsy findings included yellow–brown pigment in macrophages in the dermis, particularly around vessels. The dermal pigment stained with Fontana Masson (arrows) and did not stain with Perls' stain for iron. Hydroxychloroquine-related pigmentary change has a predilection for the shins; the pigment may stain with Fontana Masson alone or also stain with Perls' stain for iron. *A, Courtesy Jennifer M McNiff, MD.*

History: 61-year-old male kidney transplant recipient on tacrolimus, mycophenolate mofetil, and prednisone; recent onset, asymptomatic lesion
Distribution: Solitary on left sole
Pattern and morphology: Firm 1-cm discrete nodule with surface hyperpigmentation

*See Chapter 18.

Dermal lesion*
Predicted histopathology: Melanocytic lesion vs. other dermal tumor

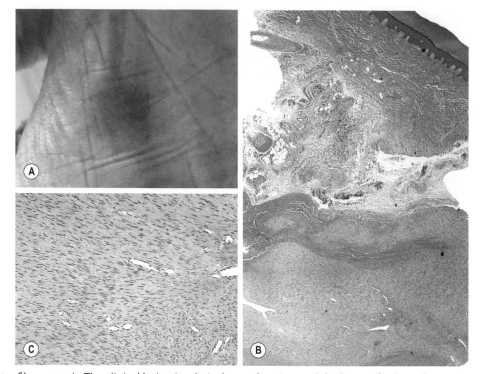

Fig. 24.26 Plantar fibromatosis. The clinical lesion is relatively nondescript, and the biopsy finding of sweeping fascicles of spindle cells was key to making the diagnosis.

Case 27

History: 58-year-old male liver transplant recipient on tacrolimus and azathioprine
Distribution: Left nose
Pattern and morphology: Somewhat translucent light pink papule

*See Chapter 18.

Dermal-based lesion*
Predicted histopathology: Dermal-based, tumor-like basal cell carcinoma

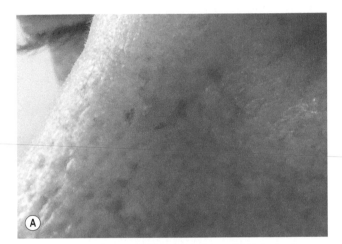

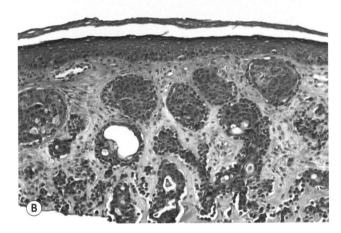

Fig. 24.27 Adnexal tumor with some features of syringoma. The clinical appearance is not specific. Biopsy findings included epithelial islands with ductal differentiation that involved the base of the specimen. The features were difficult to pigeon-hole, and the base was excised to ensure complete removal given the patient's immunosuppressed status and higher risk of developing skin cancer.

History: 57-year-old male, new onset
Distribution: Generalized on trunk and extremities
Pattern and morphology: 1–3 mm red papules
Color suggests a dermal mixed or lymphocytic infiltrate

Predicted histopathology: Mixed or lymphocytic dermal infiltrate
Associated clues: Fevers

See Chapters 18, 20

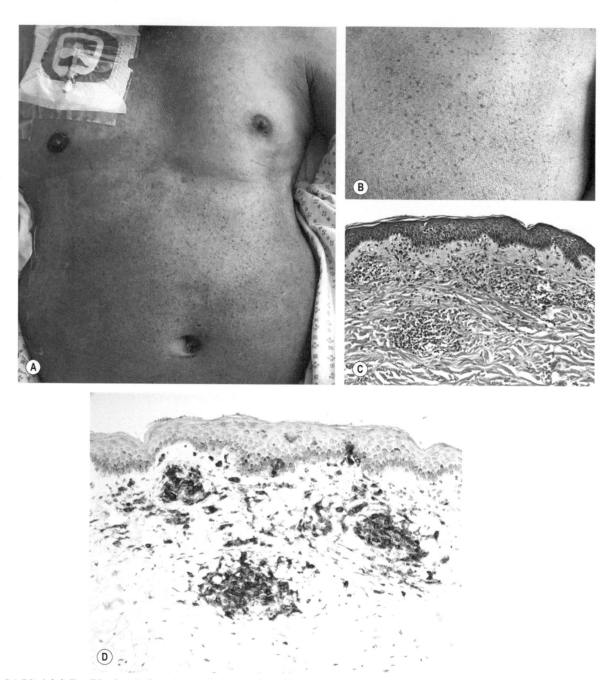

Fig. 24.28 Adult T-cell leukemia/lymphoma in the setting of human T-cell leukemia virus type 1 (HTLV-1). The 1- to 3-mm papules clinically **(A,B)** correspond to small collections of atypical lymphocytes in the dermis **(C)** that characteristically express CD25 **(D)**. Biopsy findings were essential to diagnosing the skin lesions. *A,B, Courtesy, Jacob Siegel, MD.*

History: 55-year-old female, sudden onset
Distribution: Extremities then trunk
Pattern and morphology: Swelling with induration and puckering

Puckering suggests deep dermal change
Predicted histopathology: Sclerosis*

*See Chapter 22.

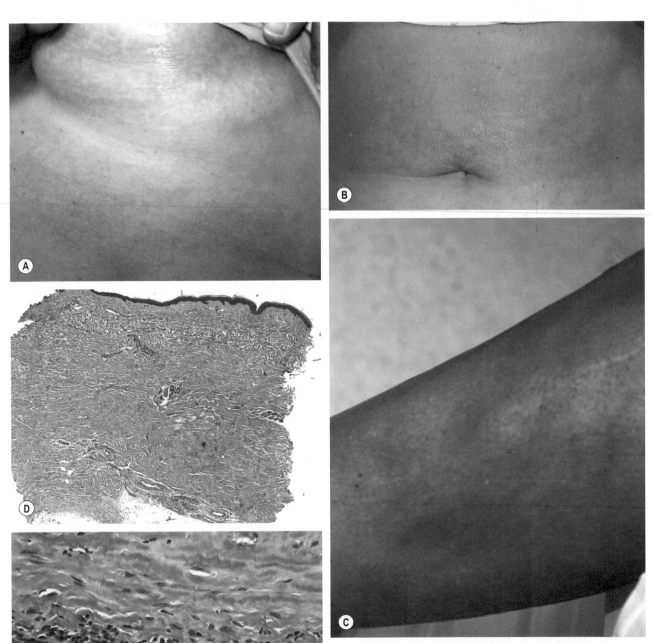

Fig. 24.29 Eosinophilic fasciitis. Biopsy findings included fascial thickening and inflammation (E), but the dermal changes alone (sclerotic collagen) resembled morphea (D). *A–C, Courtesy, Yale Dermatology Residents' Slide Collection.*

Index

Page numbers followed by "*f*" indicate figures, "*t*" indicate tables, and "*b*" indicate boxes.